Substance Use and Addiction in Adolescents

Editors

SIVABALAJI KALIAMURTHY
JOSÉ FLORES

CHILD AND ADOLESCENT PSYCHIATRIC CLINICS OF NORTH AMERICA

www.childpsych.theclinics.com

Consulting Editor
JUSTINE LARSON

October 2026 • Volume 35 • Number 4

ELSEVIER

1818 Market Street • Suite 3323 • Philadelphia, Pennsylvania, 19103-2899

http://www.theclinics.com

CHILD AND ADOLESCENT PSYCHIATRIC CLINICS OF NORTH AMERICA Volume 35, Number 4
October 2026 ISSN 1056–4993, ISBN-13: 978-0-443-43282-8

Editor: Joanna Gascoine
Developmental Editor: Sukirti Singh

Publishing Office: *Child and Adolescent Psychiatric Clinics of North America* (ISSN 1056-4993) is published quarterly by Elsevier Inc.,1818 Market Street, Philadelphia, PA 19103, United States. Periodicals postage paid at New York, NY and additional mailing offices. USA POSTMASTER: Send address changes to *Child and Adolescent Psychiatric Clinics of North America*, Elsevier Customer Service Department , 3251 Riverport Lane, Maryland Heights, MO 63043, USA. Months of issue are January, April, July, and October. Subscription prices are $392 per year (US individuals), $100.00 per year (US & Canadian students), $436.00 per year (Canadian individuals), $502.00 per year (international individuals), and $200.00 per year (international students). For institutional access pricing please contact Customer Service via the contact information below. International air speed delivery is included in all *Clinics* subscription prices. All prices are subject to change without notice. Orders, claims, and journal inquiries: Please visit our Support Hub page https://service.elsevier.com for assistance.

Reprints. For copies of 100 or more of articles in this publication, please contact the Commercial Reprints Department, Elsevier Inc., 360 Park Avenue South, New York, New York 10010-1710 Tel.: 212-633-3874; Fax: 212-633-3820, E-mail: reprints@elsevier.com.

Child and Adolescent Psychiatric Clinics of North America is covered in *MEDLINE/PubMed (Index Medicus), ISI, SSCI, Research Alert, Social Search, Current Contents,* and *EMBASE/Excerpta Medica.*

Contributors

CONSULTING EDITOR

JUSTINE LARSON, MD, MPH, DFAACAP
Associate Division Chief for Psychiatry, Children's National Hospital, Washington, DC

EDITORS

SIVABALAJI KALIAMURTHY, MD, FASAM
Assistant Professor, Department of Psychiatry and Pediatrics, The George Washington University School of Medicine and Health Sciences, Attending Physician, Division of Psychiatry, Children's National Hospital, Assistant Professor, Department of Psychiatry, Howard University, Washington, DC; Instructor (Voluntary), Yale University, New Haven, Connecticut

JOSÉ FLORES, MD, PhD, MPH
Board Certified Psychiatrist, Psych Bright Health, Office of Diversion and Reentry, Los Angeles County, CA, USA

AUTHORS

OMAR ABBAS, MD
Resident Physician, Department of Psychiatry and Neuroscience, School of Medicine, University of California Riverside, Riverside, California

SABIHUL ALAM, MD, JD
Attending Physician, Division of Behavioral Health, Riverside University Health System, Riverside, California

KAMMARAUCHE ANENI, MBBS, MHS
Assistant Professor, Child Study Center, Biomedical Informatics and Data Science, Yale School of Medicine, New Haven, Connecticut

DEEPA CAMENGA, MD, MHS, FAAP
Associate Professor, Department of Emergency Medicine, Department of Pediatrics, Yale School of Medicine, Yale, New Haven, Connecticut

JENNIFER C. CREEDON, MD
Associate Professor, Department of Clinical Psychiatry, Louisiana State University Health New Orleans School of Medicine, New Orleans, Louisiana

JORDAN DAVIS, PhD
Assistant Clinical Professor, Department of Child and Adolescent Psychiatry, NYU Grossman School of Medicine, New York, New York

EDDER DUARTE, MD, PhD
Child and Adolescent Psychiatry Fellow, Department of Psychiatry and Neuroscience, School of Medicine, University of California Riverside, Riverside, California

PANTEA FARAHMAND, MD
Assistant Clinical Professor, Department of Child and Adolescent Psychiatry, NYU Grossman School of Medicine, New York, New York

LISA R. FORTUNA, MD, MPH
Professor and Chair, Department of Psychiatry and Neuroscience, School of Medicine, University of California, Riverside, Riverside, California

FALISHA GILMAN, MD
Assistant Clinical Professor, Department of Psychiatry, Yale University School of Medicine, New Haven, Connecticut

BRADY J. HEWARD, MD
Associate Professor, Department of Psychiatry, University of Vermont Larner College of Medicine, Burlington, Vermont

PETER R. JACKSON, MD
Associate Professor, Department of Psychiatry, University of Vermont Larner College of Medicine, Burlington, Vermont

SKYLAR A. JONES, BA
Study Coordinator, The Jane and Terry Semel Institute for Neuroscience and Biobehavioral Sciences, University of California, Los Angeles, Los Angeles, California

SIVABALAJI KALIAMURTHY, MD, FASAM
Assistant Professor, Department of Psychiatry and Pediatrics, The George Washington University School of Medicine and Health Sciences, Attending Physician, Division of Psychiatry, Children's National Hospital, Assistant Professor, Department of Psychiatry, Howard University, Washington, DC; Instructor (Voluntary), Yale University, New Haven, Connecticut

DEBRA E. KOSS, MD, DFAACAP, DFAPA
Clinical Assistant Professor, Department of Psychiatry, Rutgers Robert Wood Johnson Medical School, Piscataway, New Jersey

MARGARET R. KUKLINSKI, PhD
Endowed Professor in Prevention in Social Work, Director, Social Development Research Group, School of Social Work, University of Washington, Seattle, Washington

PRIANKA KUMAR, MD, MPH
Resident Physician, Department of Psychiatry, University of California San Diego, San Diego, California

SUREN NAJARYAN, MD
Resident Physician, Department of Psychiatry and Neuroscience, School of Medicine, University of California Riverside, Riverside, California

ELIZABETH NGARACHU, MBChB, MMed, Psych
Student, Division of Health and Behavioral Science, Seattle Pacific University, Seattle, Washington

JENNIFER J. PARK, PhD
Postdoctoral Associate, Department of Psychiatry, Yale University School of Medicine, New Haven, Connecticut

MICHELLE V. PORCHE, EdD
Professor In-Residence, Department of Internal Medicine, University of California, Riverside, School of Medicine, Riverside, California

MARC N. POTENZA, MD, PhD
Professor, Child Study Center, Department of Neuroscience, Yale University School of Medicine, New Haven, Connecticut, Connecticut Council on Problem Gambling, Wethersfield, Connecticut, Connecticut Mental Health Center, New Haven, Connecticut

MIKAELA PULSE, PhD
Postdoctoral Scholar, Department of Psychiatry and Neurosciences, University of California, Riverside, School of Medicine, Riverside, California

NATALIA RAMOS, MD, MPH
Assistant Clinical Professor, Department of Psychiatry and Biobehavioral Sciences, University of California, Los Angeles David Geffen School of Medicine, Los Angeles, California

ROSS SHEGOG, PhD
Professor, Department of Health Promotion and Behavioral Sciences, UTHealth School of Public Health, Houston, Texas

JENNY SHEN, PhD
Postdoctoral Fellow, Department of Psychiatry and Biobehavioral Sciences, University of California, Los Angeles David Geffen School of Medicine, Los Angeles, California

JORGE C. SRABSTEIN, MD
Clinical Professor, Department of Psychiatry and Behavioral Sciences, George Washington University, School of Medicine and Health Sciences, Rockville, Maryland; Medical Director, Department of Psychiatry and Behavioral Sciences, Children's National Hospital, Washington, DC

LEILA M. VAEZAZIZI, MD
Assistant Clinical Professor, Department of Psychiatry, NYU Grossman School of Medicine, New York, New York

Contents

CHILD AND ADOLESCENT PSYCHIATRIC CLINICS

FORTHCOMING ISSUES

January 2027
Antipsychotics in Children and Adolescents
Adelaide S. Robb, Khushbu Gandhi, and Faith R. Kelley, *Editors*

April 2027
Family-Based Interventions in Child and Adolescent Psychiatry
Khalid I. Afzal, Karam Radwan, *Editors*

July 2027
College Mental Health
Brian Skehan and Vivien Chan, *Editors*

RECENT ISSUES

July 2026
The Behavioral Health Crisis Care Continuum for Youth
Jonathon W. Wanta, Rebecca Marshall, Vera Feuer, *Editors*

April 2026
Assessing and Treating Children and Adolescents Exposed to Trauma
Lisa M. Amaya-Jackson, Ruth S. Gerson and Sarah Vinson, *Editors*

January 2026
Transforming Systems of Care for Girls
Consuelo C. Cagande, Lisa R. Fortuna, and Elizabeth McGuire, *Editors*

SERIES OF RELATED INTEREST
Psychiatric Clinics
https://www.psych.theclinics.com/
Pediatric Clinics
https://www.pediatric.theclinics.com/

AACAP Members: Please go to www.jaacap.org for information on access to the Child and Adolescent Psychiatric Clinics. *Resident* Members of AACAP: Special access information is available at www.childpsych.theclinics.com.

THE CLINICS ARE AVAILABLE ONLINE!
Access your subscription at:
www.theclinics.com

Preface

Substance Use and Addiction in Adolescents

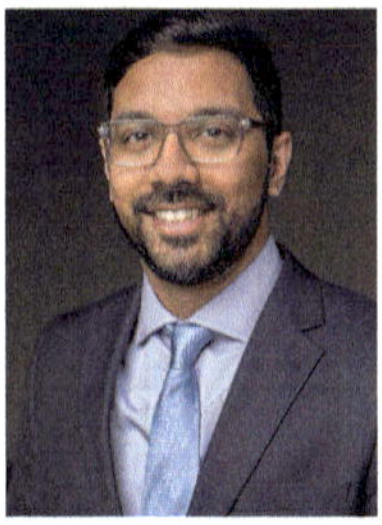

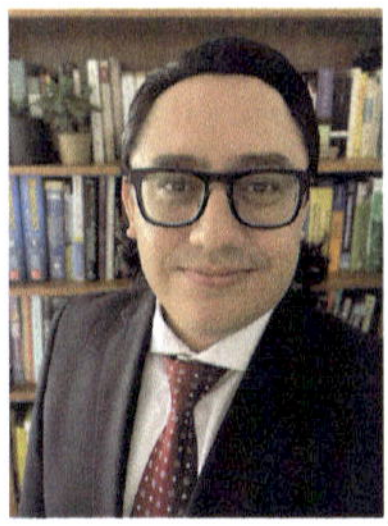

Sivabalaji Kaliamurthy, MD José Flores, MD, PhD, MPH
Editors

Adolescent substance use and addiction sit among the most pressing and rapidly evolving challenges in child and adolescent psychiatry today. Alcohol, nicotine, and cannabis remain the most commonly used psychoactive substances among adolescents. Monitoring the Future data from 2025 continue to highlight substantial exposure across developmental stages, with past-year alcohol use reported by 11% of eighth graders, 24% of tenth graders, and 41% of twelfth graders; cannabis use by 8%, 16%, and 26%, respectively; and nicotine vaping by 9%, 14%, and 20% of students across the same grade levels.[1] Over the past decade, the landscape has shifted dramatically, marked by the rising potency of substances, an increasing normalization of use among youth, the widening disparities in access to prevention and treatment, and the growing intersection of substance use with complex psychiatric comorbidities. Cannabis products now contain significantly higher concentrations of tetrahydrocannabinol (THC) than in prior generations, with average THC potency in confiscated cannabis products increasing several-fold over the past two decades,[2] while fentanyl has transformed the lethality of opioid exposure, with synthetic opioid–involved overdose deaths among US youth aged 15 to 24 years increasing from 4652 deaths in 2018 to 6723 deaths in 2022.[3] Nicotine use has also re-emerged through vaping and novel nicotine delivery systems that have fundamentally altered both the pharmacology and the social ritual of nicotine consumption among adolescents, while behavioral addictions increasingly compete for clinical attention alongside more traditional substance use disorders. At the same time, adolescents face these risks during a uniquely vulnerable developmental period, where neurodevelopment, identity formation, peer influence, and family systems all shape both risk and recovery. These are the factors that determine whether a clinical encounter can redirect a catastrophic trajectory toward recovery, resilience, and health, and the tools for working with them are what this issue reviews.

Child Adolesc Psychiatric Clin N Am 35 (2026) xiii–xvii
https://doi.org/10.1016/j.chc.2026.07.001 childpsych.theclinics.com
1056-4993/26/© 2026 Published by Elsevier Inc.

These changes demand more than just updated clinical knowledge; they demand new frameworks developmentally calibrated for prevention, identification, and treatment, and built around the systems where adolescents actually live, in other words, frameworks that are family-centered and systemically integrated. Traditional models of addiction care, often developed for adults, are insufficient when applied to adolescents without adaptation: for instance, buprenorphine-induction protocols that ignore adolescent dosing and consent challenges or harm-reduction models designed for adults that may inadequately account for school environments, parental oversight, and the neurodevelopmental vulnerability that shape adolescent decision making and risk perception. Similarly, digital interventions and screening approaches that rely on independent health care engagement may overlook adolescents' dependence on caregivers, concerns regarding privacy, and limited access to confidential treatment spaces. Even diagnostic frameworks themselves may be insufficiently developmentally calibrated; behavioral addictions involving gaming, social media, or artificial intelligence (AI) chatbots challenge traditional substance-centered conceptions of addiction, while culturally and structurally mediated experiences among LGBTQ+ youth and racially and ethnically minoritized adolescents demonstrate how discrimination, trauma, family rejection, and sociopolitical context fundamentally shape both risk and engagement in care. Youth require approaches that account for developmental stage, school systems, confidentiality challenges, family involvement, and the reality that many present with substance use in the context of depression, anxiety, trauma, psychosis, or other cooccurring psychiatric illness rather than in isolation.

This issue of *Child and Adolescent Psychiatric Clinics of North America* brings together a diverse group of clinicians, researchers, and educators who are deeply engaged in advancing care for adolescents with substance use disorders. Previous issues of *Child and Adolescent Psychiatric Clinics of North America*[4–6] have provided a strong foundational framework for understanding adolescent substance use disorders. These works have emphasized core domains, including epidemiology and trends in youth substance use, the neurobiological underpinnings of adolescent vulnerability, and the role of developmental, genetic, and psychosocial risk factors. Prior issues have also detailed evidence-based approaches to screening, assessment, and treatment, including screening, brief intervention, and referral to treatment (SBIRT) models, prevention strategies, and disorder-specific management across substances such as alcohol, cannabis, opioids, stimulants, and tobacco. More recent focused issues, centered on cannabis, have highlighted emerging concerns related to increasing potency, neurocognitive effects, and psychiatric comorbidities.

Collectively, these contributions have established a critical knowledge base that has shaped how clinicians conceptualize and approach substance use in adolescents. This issue seeks not to repeat that foundation, but to build upon it by expanding the discussion toward newer clinical realities, underexplored populations, implementation challenges, and systems-level interventions that increasingly define modern adolescent addiction care.

One way to conceptualize the breadth of this special issue is to imagine adolescent substance use care across three intersecting axes: x, y, and z. The x-axis might reflect the continuum of substance use, from no use to early use to substance use disorder and overdose risk. Adolescents move across this continuum in dynamic and often nonlinear ways, requiring clinicians to intervene at multiple stages rather than waiting for severe pathologic condition to emerge. The y-axis might then reflect the level of evaluation or intervention, from individual screening or clinical care to institutional, community, and advocacy-based responses. Effective adolescent addiction treatment rarely exists solely within the walls of a clinic. The z-axis would reflect the modifiers that shape presentation and treatment, including substance type, whether adolescents have cooccurring conditions, and the developmental, cultural, and identity-related context. No two adolescents with substance use disorder present in the same way.

Several of the articles we received map clearly onto the x-axis, reflecting the continuum from early prevention and identification to severe substance use disorders and overdose risk. Aneni and colleagues examine how digital interventions can expand SBIRT models across adolescent-serving systems, addressing barriers related to confidentiality, access, workforce limitations, and implementation fidelity. Heward and colleagues explore harm-reduction approaches for adolescents, emphasizing naloxone distribution, safer-use counseling, and risk-reduction strategies for youth who may not yet engage in traditional abstinence-based treatment models. Farahmand and colleagues review the evolving landscape of adolescent nicotine use disorders, including high-potency vaping products, shifting nicotine delivery systems, neurodevelopmental vulnerability to nicotine exposure, and emerging behavioral and pharmacologic treatment approaches. Kaliamurthy and Kumar focus on adolescent opioid use disorder in the fentanyl era, highlighting counterfeit pill exposure, overdose prevention, medications for opioid use disorder, and emerging adolescent-centered models of addiction treatment.

The y-axis is reflected in articles that expand where and how intervention occurs. Koss and Gilman position advocacy as a core competency for child and adolescent psychiatrists, arguing that effective substance use care increasingly requires engagement with policy, workforce development, financing, and systems-level reform. Alam and Kaliamurthy examine the legal and ethical complexities surrounding adolescent consent and confidentiality, demonstrating how confidentiality itself can function as a therapeutic and preventive intervention that shapes disclosure, engagement, overdose prevention, and access to care. Collectively, these articles emphasize that adolescent addiction care extends well beyond the clinic and is increasingly shaped by schools, legislation, digital infrastructure, electronic medical records, public health systems, and broader sociopolitical forces.

Finally, the z-axis is reflected in articles that emphasize heterogeneity and complexity. Srabstein examines bullying as an important but often overlooked psychosocial determinant of adolescent substance use, reviewing evidence that victimization, perpetration, and trauma-related sequelae are associated with increased risk of substance use and may influence both clinical presentation and treatment needs. Fortuna and colleagues examine how structural racism, trauma exposure, immigration stress, cultural identity, and inequities in screening and treatment shape substance use trajectories among racially and ethnically minoritized youth. Shen and colleagues explore substance use among LGBTQ+ youth through frameworks of minority stress and intersectionality, highlighting the roles of family rejection, discrimination, trauma exposure, and sociopolitical stressors in shaping risk and resilience. A separate contribution from Fortuna and colleagues addresses adolescents with cooccurring bipolar disorder and substance use disorders, emphasizing developmental neurobiology, diagnostic complexity, suicidality, and the need for integrated family-centered treatment approaches. Potenza and Park broaden the conceptualization of addiction itself by examining behavioral addictions involving gaming, gambling, social media, pornography, and AI chatbots within digitally mediated developmental environments. Collectively, these contributions underscore that adolescent substance use disorders do not emerge in isolation, but rather within intersecting developmental, psychiatric, sociocultural, and structural contexts that profoundly shape risk, treatment engagement, and recovery.

Across all three axes, one theme remains consistent: the strength of our clinical urgency often exceeds the strength of our evidence base. Many of the interventions used in adolescents are extrapolated from adult literature, supported by limited pediatric-specific trials, or implemented in systems that were never designed for youth with cooccurring psychiatric and substance use disorders. Questions remain regarding the optimal use of medications for opioid use disorder in adolescents, the psychiatric consequences of high-potency cannabis exposure, effective family-based interventions for youth with severe substance use, and how best to integrate peers, schools, and digital platforms into sustained recovery models. In some areas, such as vaping, behavioral addictions, and contingency management in adolescents, the field is still defining basic standards of care.

This issue therefore serves not only as a clinical guide but also as a roadmap for future inquiry. By identifying where evidence is strong, where it is emerging, and where major gaps remain, these articles help define priorities for research, implementation science, policy development, and workforce training. The goal is not simply to improve treatment of substance use disorders once they are fully established, but to create systems capable of identifying risk earlier, intervening more effectively, and supporting recovery in ways that are realistic for adolescents and families.

Adolescent addiction psychiatry is no longer a niche area of practice. It sits at the center of pediatric mental health, emergency care, school health, and public policy. As clinicians, we are increasingly called upon to respond not only to substance use itself but also to the broader developmental and psychiatric context in which it occurs. We are deeply grateful to the authors who contributed their expertise to this issue and to the editorial team for the opportunity to assemble this collection. We hope this issue provides readers with practical guidance, new perspectives, and renewed urgency in addressing one of the most consequential areas in child and adolescent mental health. Most importantly, we hope it helps move the field closer to a future in which evidence-based, developmentally appropriate addiction care is not the exception for adolescents, but the standard.

Sivabalaji Kaliamurthy, MD
Division of Psychiatry and
Behavioral Medicine
Children's National Hospital
The George Washington University School
of Medicine and Health Sciences

Department of Psychiatry
Howard University

Department of Psychiatry
Yale University
New Haven, CT 06511, USA

José Flores, MD, PhD, MPH
PsychBright Health &
Office of Diversion and Reentry
Los Angeles County, CA, USA

E-mail addresses:
Skaliamurt@childrensnational.org (S. Kaliamurthy)
jose.flores.mdphd@gmail.com (J. Flores)

REFERENCES

1. Miech RA, Patrick ME, O'Malley PM, et al. Monitoring the Future national survey results on drug use, 1975–2025: Overview and detailed results for secondary school students. In: Monitoring the Future Monograph Series. Ann Arbor (MI): Institute for Social Research, University of Michigan; 2026.
2. Chandra S, Radwan MM, Majumdar CG, et al. New trends in cannabis potency in USA and Europe during the last decade (2008–2017). Eur Arch Psychiatry Clin Neurosci 2019;269(1):5–15. https://doi.org/10.1007/s00406-019-00983-5.
3. Miller M, Wheeler-Martin K, Bunting AM, et al. Changes in synthetic opioid–involved youth overdose deaths in the United States: 2018–2022. Pediatrics 2025;155(6):e2024069488. https://doi.org/10.1542/peds.2024-069488.
4. Hsiao R, Ryan SA. Substance use disorders, part 1. Child Adolesc Psychiatric Clin N Am 2016;25(3).
5. Hsiao R, Ryan SA. Substance use disorders, part 2. Child Adolesc Psychiatric Clin N Am 2016;25(4).
6. Riggs P, Hinckley JD, Ross JM. Adolescent cannabis use. Child Adolesc Psychiatric Clin N Am 2023;32(1).

Digital Interventions to Facilitate Screening, Brief Interventions, and Referral to Treatment for Substance Use Among Adolescents

Kammarauche Aneni, MBBS, MHS[a,b,*],
Elizabeth Ngarachu, MBChB, MMed Psych[c],
Margaret R. Kuklinski, PhD[d], Ross Shegog, PhD[e],
Deepa Camenga, MD, MHS[f,g]

KEYWORDS

• Adolescent • Substance use • Digital interventions • Barriers to access • SBIRT

KEY POINTS

- Substance use in adolescence is linked to short-term and long-term morbidity and mortality.
- Adolescent-focused substance use prevention and treatment services remain limited and difficult to access, highlighting the need for scalable and accessible approaches.
- Digital interventions can improve access to substance use services through enhanced *screening* processes and *brief intervention* delivery; but evidence supporting *referral to treatment* is needed.
- Brief digital interventions have shown efficacy for improving antecedents to drug use (eg, knowledge and self-efficacy) and reducing substance use among adolescents.

BACKGROUND

Introduction

Although rates of adolescent substance use have steadily decreased since 2020,[1] substance use remains one of the most common causes of preventable morbidity

[a] Child Study Center, Yale School of Medicine, New Haven, CT, USA; [b] Biomedical Informatics and Data Science, Yale School of Medicine, New Haven, CT, USA; [c] Student, Division of Health and Behavioral Science, Seattle Pacific University, Seattle, WA, USA; [d] Social Development Research Group, School of Social Work, University of Washington, Seattle, WA, USA; [e] Department of Health Promotion and Behavioral Sciences, UTHealth School of Public Health, Houston, TX, USA; [f] Department of Emergency Medicine, Yale School of Medicine, New Haven, CT, USA; [g] Department of Pediatrics, Yale School of Medicine, New Haven, CT, USA
* Corresponding author. Child Study Center, 230 S Frontage Road, New Haven, CT 06519.
E-mail address: uche.aneni@yale.edu

Child Adolesc Psychiatric Clin N Am 35 (2026) 617–636
https://doi.org/10.1016/j.chc.2026.05.001 childpsych.theclinics.com
1056-4993/26/

Abbreviations	
AI	artificial intelligence
AR	augmented reality
BSTAD	Brief Screener for Tobacco, Alcohol or Other Drugs
CDS	clinical decision support tool
CHADIS	Child Health and Development Interactive System
CRAFFT	Car, Relax, Alone, Forget, Family or Friends, Trouble
cSBI	computerized Screening and provider Brief Intervention system
EHR	electronic health record
MR	mixed reality
S2BI	Screening to Brief Intervention
SBIRT	Screening, Brief Intervention and Referral to Treatment
SODAS	Stop Options Decide Act Self-Praise
SUD	substance use disorder
VR	virtual reality
XR	extended reality

and mortality in adolescents. By the end of high school, nearly half of all adolescents in the United States have tried alcohol, cannabis, or nicotine-containing products.[2] Since 2020, the rates of drug-related hospitalizations, deaths, and health-related spending have concurrently increased for this population,[3–6] underscoring the increasing severity of consequences related to the highly potent drug supply that adolescents can easily access.[7] These factors underscore the importance of early identification of adolescents at risk of substance use problems and early intervention to prevent these short-term and long-term consequences.

The SBIRT model (Screening, Brief Intervention and Referral to Treatment) is a public health approach to identify people at risk for substance use problems early, provide immediate counseling (brief intervention) for those with risky patterns, and connect those with severe issues to specialized treatment, aiming to reduce alcohol/drug-related harm across various settings.[8,9] The American Academy of Pediatrics recommends SBIRT across settings where adolescents receive health care services.[10] Although the US Preventive Services Task Force highlights that evidence for SBIRT for adolescents is inconclusive (largely due to insufficient studies),[11,12] it remains a widely used public health approach for addressing substance use among adolescents. Traditionally, SBIRT is delivered via a face-to-face encounter between a clinician and an adolescent. However, data indicate that not all adolescents receive face-to-face SBIRT services during routine health care visits.[13,14] For example, a recent study showed that approximately 57% of primary care clinicians provide screening at every well-child visit, less than 40% use a validated substance use screening tool, and only 1 in 3 complete all aspects of the SBIRT.[15]

Multiple studies have documented barriers to widespread adoption and implementation of clinician-delivered SBIRT that span all socioecological domains (individual, relational, organizational, community, and systemic). Systems-level factors include the lack of payment models that support the implementation of SBIRT.[8] In health care settings, multiple organizational-level barriers also disrupt the implementation of SBIRT, including lack of private spaces to facilitate adolescent openness in completing the screener[13,16] and lack of readily available behavioral health clinicians within the practice where the child is seen.[17] Community level factors include the lack of community-based substance use prevention and treatment programs where adolescents reside.[18]

Within the health care setting, limited clinician time,[19] lack of training,[19] lack of knowledge about intervention/treatment resources,[16,19,20] and limited provider incentive and reimbursement for delivering these services are commonly cited clinician-level barriers to SBIRT.[16,20,21] On the patient level, adolescents report concerns with confidentiality[19] and stigma[22,23] as barriers to discussing substance use with their clinician. Parent denial[21,22] and challenges with transportation and childcare services[24,25] can also negatively impact parent motivation to participate in clinician-recommended interventions.

The use of digital technology may mitigate barriers across these socialecological domains, given that over 90% of US adolescents have access to smartphones,[26] and nearly 75% of people 10 years and older own mobile phones globally.[27] *Screening*: For example, several studies show that digital screening takes less time than clinician-administered screens[28] and therefore could improve provider efficiency. Studies have shown that digital screeners, especially those that are self-administered by the adolescent, result in a higher likelihood of reporting substance use,[28] thus mitigating concerns related to confidentiality and stigma. Unlike paper-based screeners, which require interpretation, digital screeners can automatically calculate risk scores to inform the provider's clinical decision-making. *Brief Interventions*: Digital interventions that reach adolescents and parents directly can obviate the need for transportation or clinician time to deliver an intervention. Since these interventions are readily accessible to adolescents via their devices, they can also mitigate challenges posed by provider lack of time and training, a lack of available behavioral health providers and/or extended treatment waitlists. Other benefits of digital interventions include the ability to design tailored interventions for specific adolescent populations, the option to use gamification to foster engagement, and the capacity to deliver interventions with fidelity. *Referral to Treatment*: Accessible digital or online databases may also facilitate referral or linkage to treatment services.

Yet, digital interventions are not widely implemented across adolescent-serving settings. The purpose of this paper is to provide a broad overview of digital interventions that address different aspects of the SBIRT continuum (**Fig. 1**). First, we review the history of the use of digital technologies across the various components of SBIRT. We then summarize the evidence for a variety of digital interventions that focus on screening, brief intervention, or treatment referral. Finally, we discuss the current limitations and challenges with implementing digital SBIRT interventions in health care settings, and review areas for future research.

Evolution of Digital Interventions for Substance Use Prevention and Treatment

The use of digital technology to facilitate substance use prevention and treatment initially involved screening applications that began in the late 1980s and early 1990s

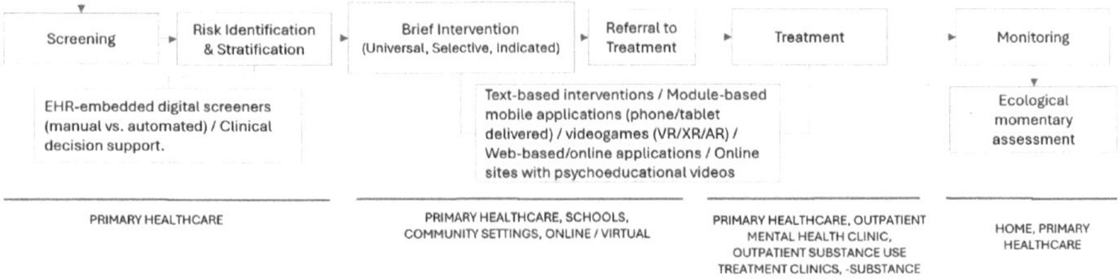

Fig. 1. An SBIRT Framework for applying digital behavioral change interventions for preventing and treating substance use among adolescents.

with the translation of validated screeners into computerized formats,[29] the use of computers for screening for high risk behaviors like substance use among adolescents in clinical settings,[30] and the use of computers to deliver substance use prevention content to improve adolescent decision-making.[31] Subsequent applications in the 2000's adapted evidence-based strategies for prevention and treatment into more interactive computer programs.[32] With the advent of newer technologies such as smartphones and tablets, text-based interventions,[33–35] games[36,37] and extended reality (XR)[38,39] including virtual reality (VR), augmented reality (AR), and mixed reality (MR) interventions rose. Similarly, the rise in wearable smart technology, such as the Apple Watch and Fitbit for passive sensing, allowed for studies exploring the utility of wearable technology for ongoing monitoring of substance use, although nearly all studies have been conducted among adults.[40–42] The rise in the application of artificial intelligence (AI) has allowed the investigation of its use in substance use risk prediction,[43] using a wide variety of data sources including national survey data, electronic health record data, social media data, game-based data, and neuroimaging data.[43–49]

Although these newer technologies are continually developing, most existing interventions use computer-based, text-based, game-based, or app-based platforms. In this section, we describe how digital technologies have been used to facilitate substance screening, brief prevention/treatment interventions, and referral to treatment (see **Fig. 1**).

Screening

Digital screeners for adolescent substance use and risk stratification are designed to improve substance use screening rates and foster early identification and timely intervention. They may be self-administered by the adolescent or clinician-administered using a mobile device such as a smartphone, tablet, or computer. They may also exist on a web-based platform outside of the electronic health record (EHR) or be integrated into the EHR. Tablet-administered digital screeners can be used with privacy shields, which provide privacy in a busy waiting room. Digital screeners include validated screeners such as the CRAFFT (Car, Relax, Alone, Forget, Family or Friends, Trouble),[50] BSTAD (Brief Screener for Tobacco, Alcohol or Other Drugs),[51] or S2BI (Screening to Brief Intervention)[52] in a mobile or web-based application.

One of the first studies to examine the utility of digital technologies for adolescent substance use screening found that tablet-based screening was a valid alternative to clinician-administered screening, using the CRAFFT screener. [28] They also found that the digital screener took significantly less time to complete compared to clinician-administered screens and had relatively high sensitivity and specificity across three common substances (alcohol, cannabis, tobacco).[28] Another study, evaluating the psychometric properties of a digitally delivered widely validated screener for adolescent substance use (S2BI) found that the digitally administered screener sufficiently stratified adolescents into 4 risk categories (no past-year use, use without a substance use disorder [SUD], mild or moderate SUD, and severe substance use disorder) with high sensitivity and specificity (75%–98%) across 3 substances (alcohol, cannabis, tobacco/nicotine).[52] A more recent study comparing the self-administered CRAFFT to clinician-administered CRAFFT used a web-based online platform, Child Health and Development Interactive System (CHADIS), designed to support the *detection, prevention and treatment of a wide range of behavioral and developmental problems among children and adults*.[53] The study comprised a national sample of adolescents (N = 130,688) aged 12 to 20 years from multiple regions across the US (Northeast, Midwest, South, and West). They found that self-administered screening was associated with a significantly higher likelihood of reporting substance use, suggesting that adolescents are more forthcoming when using digital screens, which may be perceived as less stigmatizing.[54] Other studies have also found that standardizing screening procedures using tablets can reduce bias in screening and foster earlier detection of substance use by up to 6 months.[55]

Despite the advantages and evidence of digital technology for substance use screening, a major challenge remains barriers with integrating these approaches within existing workflows,[56] which impact adoption across health care settings.

Brief interventions for substance use prevention and treatment

Many existing digital interventions support only the delivery of brief interventions to address substance use, although there are very few digital platforms, like CHADIS referenced earlier, which is currently developing a computerized Screening and provider Brief Intervention system (cSBI) called CHADIS-cSBI that combines screening and brief interventions for implementation in pediatric primary settings.[57] In this section, we describe digital interventions that support delivery of brief interventions to address substance use.

Unlike face-to-face interventions, digital brief interventions can be completed at any time with high fidelity and may not require the involvement of a clinician. Brief digital interventions typically consist of 1 to 5 sessions[58,59] and include universal (interventions targeting all adolescents regardless of risk),[60,61] selective (interventions targeting high risk youth),[60,61] or indicated (interventions targeting adolescents with early substance use) interventions (**Table 1**).[37,60,61] Similar to digital screening tools, brief digital interventions may be self-administered or clinician-administered using a variety of software program modalities (eg, App-based, web-based, and text-based) and hardware delivery channels (desktop, computer, smart-phone, tablet) (see **Table 1**). Digital interventions employ a variety of learning methods to foster skill acquisition for behavioral change (gamification, tutorials, simulation, drills, and quizzes)[62–65] (see **Table 1**).

Evidence-based digital interventions have been tested across a variety of settings (eg, school, primary care, emergency department, juvenile justice settings, online settings) for a variety of substances, including alcohol, tobacco, nicotine, and illicit drugs.[60,61,66] Most interventions are designed for adolescents (eg, eCHECKUP TO GO, LifeSkills Training Program, SafERteens, PlaySmart, Invite Only VR),[38,67–71] although some focus on parents (eg, Family Check-Up Online)[72] or on both parents and adolescents (eg, Pathways for African American Success, PNC-txt & PP-txt).[73–75] Most of the indicated interventions are designed for health care and juvenile justice settings as adjuncts to ongoing care or as part of a clinician-delivered interventions (eg, ProjectChill, U-Connect, PNC-txt, e-TOKE).[76–79] Conversely, many universal interventions are designed for school or community settings (eg, Climate Schools program).[75,80]

Many of the published digital brief interventions are grounded in established health behavior theories. For example, several universal and selective digital interventions are grounded in the social cognitive/learning theory,[38,60,67] while indicated and treatment-oriented digital interventions are often grounded in social norms theory, motivational interviewing, or transtheoretical models.[77,79] Interventions involving parents also use relational theories,[32,73] such as family systems theory, which describes how interactions within members of a family can influence behaviors and health outcomes. These interventions use a variety of methods to encourage theory-informed behavior change (see **Table 1**), including games or gamification (eg, PlaySmart, Invite only VR),[37–39,67,81,82] tutorials (eg, Stop Options Decide Act Self-Praise (SODAS)),[83,84] quizzes (eg, POP4Teens),[85,86] drill and practice (eg, MobileCoach),[87] and simulated

Table 1
Nomenclature for types of digital interventions targeting adolescent substance use

Categories	Sub-category	Intervention Type	Definition
Risk priority population	Prevention	Universal	Applicable to all adolescents regardless of substance use risk.
		Selective	Tailored to adolescents at higher risk for substance use (eg, adolescents who have experienced trauma) but have not used substances.
		Indicated	Tailored for adolescents who have initiated substance use but do not have a substance use disorder.
	Treatment	Treatment	Target adolescents with diagnosed substance use disorders.
Administration		Self	Accessed and used directly by the end-user without any clinician input.
		Facilitated	Administered by a trained clinician or facilitator using a mobile device.
Delivery channel	Nonmobile	Desktop	Accessed using a desktop computer.
	Mobile	Computer-based	Accessed using a mobile computer.
		Phone or Smartphone	Accessed using a phone or smartphone.
		Tablet	Accessed using a tablet.
Program modality		App-based	Accessed using an application, which may be stored on a mobile or nonmobile device.
		Web-based	Accessed using an internet browser, which may be accessed using a mobile or nonmobile device with internet connection.
		Text-based	Interventions that are delivered using text messages
Methods	Game-based	Game or gamification	Digital interventions that employ games or gamification in design and delivery. Games are *a system where players are engaged in an artificial conflict under a set of rules with a quantifiable outcome (eg, win, lose).*[62] *Gamification involves the use of game elements (eg, win/lose, time pressure, narrative storylines) in nongame contexts.*[63] Games includes VR, AR and MR games and can be accessed using mobile and nonmobile devices.
	Nongame based	Tutorials	Interventions that employ tutorials. Tutorials are structured methods of instruction that involve the use of interactive stepwise modules that can include evaluative prompts/ questions and feedback.[64]

(*continued on next page*)

Table 1
(*continued*)

Categories	Sub-category	Intervention Type	Definition
		Simulation	An experiential method for learning and practice where users mimic real-world experiences in a safe controlled environment.[65] Simulations may be used in a game or outside of a game.
		Drill-and-practice	Interventions that involve drill-and-practice. Drill-and-practice involves presenting a user with a question, requiring a response and providing an evaluation of the question and feedback.[64] It is repetitive in the sense that multiple questions on a specific concept are presented to the learner to enhance understanding.
		Tests/Quizzes	Involve the use of questions to assess and instill knowledge and skill. Can be used in game or nongame interventions.

experiences (eg, Alcohol Alert).[88] These methods are not mutually exclusive and may be used together in a digital intervention.

Several systematic reviews have evaluated the effectiveness of digital brief interventions on reducing or preventing substance use in adolescents.[35,60,61,89,90] For example, a systematic review of 39 digital interventions found that they were effective in increasing knowledge, reducing favorable attitudes toward drugs, and reducing the intention to use drugs, all of which are known predictors of abstinence from substances.[61] One systematic review and meta-analyses of digital interventions for cannabis use found that effects for prevention interventions were sustained up to 12 months.[66] However, another systematic review and meta-analysis evaluating digital interventions for adolescents with problematic drug use found a small but significant effect size for alcohol, but null findings for smoking cigarettes or cannabis.[91] Other systematic reviews have shown short-term efficacy in reducing drug use for primary care-based, game-based, and text-based digital brief interventions.[35,37,92] A meta-analysis of text-based interventions to reduce alcohol and tobacco among adolescents and young adults revealed a moderate effect size of 0.25.[35] A systematic review on game-based interventions addressing adolescent substance use found that at least two-thirds of the included 26 games had some effect in improving attitudes related to substance use and in reducing substance use.[37] A systematic review and meta-analysis by the author found significant reductions for alcohol, cannabis and tobacco with effect sizes ranging from 0.2 to 0.4.[60] Our findings also suggested that interventions that include booster sessions were more likely to be effective, and that interventions that involve parents tend to have larger effect sizes.[60] Although evidence for mediators and moderators of digital intervention effectiveness is still emerging, preliminary evidence suggests that digital interventions that involve multiple sessions and digital interventions that foster skill practice tend to be more effective in reducing substance use compared to those that simply provide information, regardless of digital modality.[60,61] Furthermore, digital interventions that are universal or selective tend to be more effective in improving antecedents to drug use and preventing drug use than digital interventions that are treatment focused, regardless of intervention modality or setting.[66,93] Given the mixed findings with efficacy of brief digital interventions, future work that identifies specific mediators and moderators of digital intervention efficacy would directly inform clinical application and integration of effective digital interventions across health care settings.

Clinical Vignettes Illustrating Screening and Brief Intervention Clinical Workflows that Integrate Digital Technology

Kiisha, Age 16: Low-Risk for Substance Use Disorder

The evening before Kiisha's annual physical, she receives a previsit questionnaire via her patient portal. Kiisha completes the questionnaire, which includes the CRAFFT screen, on her tablet, and the results are linked to Kiisha's electronic health record (screening). Because Kiisha's CRAFFT results indicate low-risk, she is automatically provided with positive reinforcement and invited to participate in a brief, evidence-based, universal digital substance use prevention intervention to empower and strengthen her skills. The intervention is an interactive program where she learns about the risks of drug use through quizzes, learns and practices coping skills to manage stress, and learns strategies to refuse drugs if offered. During Kiisha's annual physical, an embedded clinical decision support tool (CDS) tool alerts the primary care provider (PCP) to the CRAFFT results and the completion of the universal digital intervention. The PCP praises Kiisha for completing the intervention and encourages her to continue avoiding drug use (positive reinforcement).

Abel, Age 14: Moderate-Risk for Substance Use Disorder

Abel presents for his annual physical examination at his PCP's office. After checking in at the front desk, he receives a link on his phone to complete a previsit questionnaire, including the CRAFFT, which he fills out in the waiting room (screening). Before seeing Abel, a built-in EHR-embedded CDS informs the PCP that Abel is medium-risk and that a brief intervention is recommended. During the visit, the CDS tool guides the PCP through a brief intervention (clinician-facilitated) and provides a list of digital, selective interventions the PCP can offer Abel (brief intervention). The PCP also provides a QR code for Abel to scan, granting him access to an evidence-based digital substance-use prevention video game. Abel is encouraged to begin the intervention at the clinic and is informed that he can also complete it outside the clinic. The PCP also schedules a follow-up visit in 1 month to check in on Abel's progress with the video game intervention.

Referral to treatment

Digital technologies can also facilitate clinicians' referral of eligible adolescents for addiction treatment. Although online treatment program locators such as the Substance Abuse and Mental Health Services Administration (SAMHSA's) findtreatment.gov or https://www.211ct.org/exist, to date, few studies have investigated the effectiveness of technology-supported referral to treatment; however, evidence indicates that such referrals are feasible. For example, a quality improvement study at a large pediatric primary care network found that an embedded EHR algorithm that risk-stratified the adolescent and prompted a recommendation for referral increased the overall number of referrals to addiction treatment services.[94] However, evidence for improved treatment engagement or substance use outcomes is lacking.

Jada age 16, High risk—primary care clinic

Jada, a 16-year-old girl, completes a digital CRAFFT screener on a tablet after checking in for her physical examination appointment (screening). An EHR-embedded CDS tool alerts her

PCP that Jada is *high-risk* and prompts the PCP to provide recommendations for treatment (brief intervention). The CDS tool also includes a referral order for local substance use treatment programs, with descriptions of programs that the PCP can give to the patient (referral to treatment). Additionally, the CDS provides a list of digital, selective or indicated interventions the PCP can send to Jada's phone. The PCP encourages Jada to complete the digital intervention while waiting for an intake and as an adjunct to local treatment options.

Luis, age 16, High-risk—outpatient mental health clinic

Luis shares with his outpatient therapist that he has been using alcohol to cope with his anxiety. His therapist completes a substance use history assessment and diagnoses him with a moderate alcohol use disorder. Together with Luis, she uses the SAMHSA online treatment locator to find treatment locations amenable to Luis. She also reviews the c4tbh.org/program-review to find a digital program that Luis can access while waiting for substance use treatment services. The therapist's clinic has partnered with Alcohol eCHECKUP TO GO (https://echeckuptogo.com/programs/alcohol) and can provide Luis with access to this online intervention.

DISCUSSION

Overall, existing research demonstrates that digital *screening tools* are feasible and effective in detecting substance use. Digital *brief interventions* are feasible and acceptable, with promising early efficacy, particularly for interventions that support skill practice and for universal or selective interventions; however, digital technologies are generally underdeveloped for *referral to treatment* and the evidence of how digital technology can support referral to treatment and treatment engagement is lacking. Existing literature also highlights substantial opportunities for further study and refinement of these interventions. Additionally, numerous practical barriers limit the real-world implementation and sustainability of even the most effective digital interventions for SBIRT in health care settings.

Workflow challenges and lack of evidence to support referral to treatment practice: A foremost challenge in implementing digital SBIRT is the need to use platforms outside the electronic health record.[56,95] Although several studies have evaluated the implementation of digital interventions for adolescent substance use across health care settings, including primary care,[28,54,96] school-based,[97] and ED settings,[98,99] few are embedded within the electronic health record. As such, this may limit uptake among clinicians who would need to work outside of their usual workflow to review screening results.

Although digital technology can support referral to treatment, there remains a general lack of evidence to inform clinical practice. Our review found only one study that has examined the feasibility of digital technology for referrals, while evidence of whether digital approaches for referral to treatment impact treatment engagement or substance use outcomes are nonexistent to the best of our knowledge. Current practice relies on clinicians to be aware of treatment resources while clinicians cite lack of knowledge of treatment programs as a barrier to implementing SBIRT. Existing online treatment locators exist outside of the electronic health record and as such outside of many clinical workflows making the use of these locators challenging to adopt. Implementation approaches to embedding these locators within clinical practice workflows across health care settings are needed.

Accessibility: Clinicians are often unaware of available and effective digital interventions to recommend to adolescents and their parents. Although several websites have compiled lists of evidence-based digital interventions (eg, c4tbh.org/program-reviews, blueprintsprograms.org), the practicality of accessing these resources in busy clinical settings is limited. Furthermore, most digital programs, which are available online are not accessible without an institutional subscription, making it challenging for a youth or family to directly access, or for a clinician to adopt without organizational buy-in. Overall, there are no systematic approaches for clinicians to access these resources at the point of care. In addition, even if screening is completed electronically and available to clinicians within the electronic health record, a lack of embedded linkage infrastructure that supports referral to treatment when indicated can impact clinician uptake of these clinical decision-support tools.

Privacy: Privacy concerns also limit the reach of digital SBIRT interventions. Both clinicians and patients report concerns about privacy around substance use information shared on digital platforms.[100] Many mobile applications do not disclose security features on the platform, such as how the data will be used or who will have access to the data.[101] Clinicians may also make recommendations to patients for certain apps without necessarily knowing whether there are any privacy concerns.[100] The MIND platform rates digital interventions based on access, cost, privacy, clinical evidence, usability, and the application's ability to integrate with existing workflows and includes a privacy quality rating based on the app's privacy policy, the location where collected data is stored, and how the data is used and shared, which can assist clinicians in making an assessment of whether to recommend a particular application. The American Psychiatric Association's App Evaluation Model,[102,103] on which the MIND platform is based or the FASTER (Framework to Assist Stakeholders in Technology Evaluation for Recovery)[104] can help guide clinicians in recommending a digital intervention or health care administrators in curating digital interventions for their health care settings.

Digital divide and culturally tailored interventions: Although owning a mobile device can improve access to evidence-based interventions, challenges with accessing digital interventions may inadvertently exacerbate inequities.[105] Adolescents who live in communities impacted by digital redlining may be unable to access these interventions due to poor internet access even if clinicians make recommendations about these interventions, resulting in inequitable reach of these interventions among vulnerable populations.[105] Available digital interventions are predominantly in English language limiting access to adolescents who do not speak English. Furthermore, digital interventions that are culturally tailored for adolescents of racial ethnic minority groups are generally lacking.[90,106,107] Our recent systematic review found only 6 interventions that included some cultural tailoring for Black adolescents,[90] while other systematic reviews have also documented a lack of tailored interventions for American Indian/Alaska Native and Hispanic youth[106] as well as a lack of inclusion of adolescents who identify as American Indian/Alaska Native in studies that have tested digital interventions regardless of cultural tailoring.[60]

Engagement: Engagement in digital interventions, particularly self-administered interventions, is increasingly noted as a challenge.[61,108] Studies have found that digital interventions can have high drop-out rates or low adherence.[61] Factors that contribute to poor engagement include a lack of interest or motivation, privacy concerns, complexity of tasks, and a lack of engaging content. Considering these factors in intervention design is crucial to ensuring digital interventions that adolescents enjoy and want to use.[109]

Costs: Out-of-pocket costs also restrict the reach and sustainability of digital interventions for substance use prevention. Few digital interventions are covered by health insurance, and even fewer have the U.S. Food and Drug Administration (FDA) approval, which is typically a prerequisite for coverage. Currently, only 2 digital interventions for substance use (reset and reset-O) have FDA approval, but these are interventions for adults. In 2024, the Centers for Medicare and Medicaid approved three new reimbursement codes for using digital interventions,[110] but the impact of these codes is yet unknown. Outside of the research setting, many digital SBIRT interventions require a subscription or fee, which can be paid by the individual or organization (eg, workplace or school). These fees help cover maintenance and updates necessary to keep the system functional and relevant. Without a way of continued coverage to maintain these digital interventions, their sustainability would be impacted.

Challenges with AI: Clinicians also report concern with AI-powered interventions, particularly generative AI.[111] Recent adolescent deaths related to the use of unmonitored generative AI interventions underscores this challenge.[112] Although many self-administered digital interventions are unmonitored, these interventions usually have limited avenues for participants to disclose concerning information. As generative AI begins to be integrated into digital interventions, there will be a need to be an acceptable process for monitoring performance activities in these interventions.

FUTURE DIRECTIONS

Given the current limitations in clinical reach, there are vast opportunities for future research and development. In this section, we describe two areas that require future work to harness the full potential of digital technology for adolescent substance use prevention and treatment.

Research

Screening: Although evidence indicated feasibility of digital screeners, adoption of the practice varies across health care settings. Implementation studies that inform effective strategies for embedding and adopting the use of digital screeners into the clinical workflow across various health care settings can improve uptake. *Brief interventions*: As mentioned earlier, evidence on the effectiveness of digital interventions for adolescent substance use is mixed, and few assess long-term efficacy. We found only 1 study that demonstrated sustained effects up to 7 years postintervention of the digital intervention (SODAS).[113] This study offered booster sessions after completion of digital intervention, which may indicate that additional exposure to digital content may contribute to sustained effects over time. Future research is needed to continue to rigorously develop and test novel digital interventions for substance use SBIRT to inform the adoption, implementation and sustainability of these approaches. Specific areas that warrant further research include understanding the mediators (eg, theory-driven constructs of change such as self-efficacy) and moderators (eg, type of intervention, number of sessions, intervention modality, health care setting, risk level targeted) of digital intervention efficacy, developing and testing culturally tailored interventions for adolescents who identify as Black, Hispanic, or American Indian/Alaska Native, and conducting cost-effectiveness studies that evaluate the cost-benefit ratio of digital interventions relative to in-person interventions. *Referral to Treatment:* Effectiveness-Implementation studies to inform best practices for using digital technology to support referral to treatment and treatment engagement across adolescent-serving settings are sorely needed.

Emerging Technologies (Extended Reality-Interventions, Artificial Intelligence, and Wearable Technologies)

Novel applications of digital technology for screening, risk identification, and stratification include the use of AI or machine learning for substance use risk prediction.[43–49] A recently funded study testing an AI model, the Duke Predictive Model of Adolescent Mental Health (Duke-PMA), had an AUROC of 75 to 84 in predicting adolescents who will develop mental illness.[114] An ongoing study will be testing the Duke-PMA AI model in real-world settings across clinics in North Carolina. Similar studies that focus on real-time substance use risk identification and connection with intervention services are needed to close the gap in access to prevention and treatment interventions among adolescents. Games can collect performance data (eg, time to complete a task, accuracy on quizzes) during gameplay, which can be used to assess risk for substance use.[49] Furthermore, games including XR games can be designed to capture biometric data (heart rate, skin conductance) during game play that can be used to assess risk and tailor intervention activity during game play based on this data in real time. Novel studies are exploring the utility of in-game biometric data to assess substance use risk using AI/ML algorithms among adolescents and young adults, with implications for improving risk assessment, monitoring and tailoring game play.[49,115] Ecological momentary assessments using self-report data collected from smartphones and/or objective data using wearable technology that include sensors from wrist/arm/chest bands or transdermal patches are promising modalities for collecting real-time data on substance use risk.[42,116,117] Although the use of wearable technology has been investigated among adults,[41,42] it's use among adolescents is in its infancy.[42,116,117] Novel technologies such as XR-games have focused on targeting vaping and alcohol use. The application of these newer technologies to develop interventions that target other substances, such as cannabis, which is rising among youth, is an area for future work. Finally, digital interventions that use novel technologies and are culturally tailored to specific populations, or that involve parents, are promising areas for future work.

SUMMARY

Digital interventions for screening, brief intervention, and referral to treatment of adolescent substance use are feasible across adolescent-serving settings. Digital screening tools can improve early detection of adolescent substance use and overcome barriers related to clinician time, workflow inefficiencies, privacy, and confidentiality. Digital brief interventions have shown some efficacy for preventing and reducing adolescent substance use, but little research has focused on digital interventions to facilitate referral to treatment. Future studies that clarify factors that contribute to digital intervention efficacy, effective implementation strategies, and cost-effectiveness of digital SBIRT approaches will further enhance evidence-informed integration of these approaches to support routine health care practice.

CLINICS CARE POINTS

- Evidence demonstrates the effectiveness of digital technologies for adolescent substance use screening and brief intervention; however little research has focused on referral to treatment.
- Multiple challenges limit the wide-scale implementation of digital interventions into real-world clinical practice. Adapting existing interventions into site-specific workflows may facilitate clinician uptake.
- Clinicians can access online lists of evidence-based digital interventions (eg, c4tbh.org/program-reviews, blueprintsprograms.org) to support clinical decision-making around digital substance use interventions.

GENERATIVE AI STATEMENT

Generative AI was used to find references. Each reference was cross-checked and reviewed for accuracy.

FUNDING

This work was supported by the National Institutes on Drug Abuse under award number K23DA059638 (PI: Aneni). The content is solely the responsibility of the authors and does not necessarily represent the official views of the National Institutes of Health.

DISCLOSURE

The authors have nothing to disclose.

REFERENCES

1. Miech R.A., Johnston L.D., Patrick M.E., et al., Monitoring the Future national survey results on drug use, 1975-2024: Overview and key findings for secondary school students. Monitoring the Future Monograph Series, Institute for Social Research, University of Michigan; Ann Arbor (MI), Available at https://monitoringthefuture.org/mtf2025vol1/ (Accessed 17 April 2025).
2. Farokhnia M, Harris JC, Speed SN, et al. Lifetime use of alcohol and cannabis among U.S. adolescents across age: exploring differential patterns by sex and race/ethnicity using the 2019 NSDUH data. Drug Alcohol Depend Rep 2023;10:100214. https://doi.org/10.1016/j.dadr.2023.100214.
3. Friedman J, Hadland SE. The overdose crisis among U.S. adolescents. N Engl J Med 2024;390(2):97–100.
4. EBSCO. Economic impact of addiction | Research Starters | EBSCO Research. EBSCO, Available at: https://www.ebsco.com/research-starters/economics/economic-impact-addiction (Accessed 6 December 2025).
5. The National Center on Addiction and Substance Abuse at Columbia University. Shoveling-up-II-the-impact-of-substance-abuse-on-federal-state-and-local-budgets_0. 2009. Available at: https://cdn-01.drugfree.org/web/prod/wp-content/uploads/2009/05/19202420/Shoveling-up-II-the-impact-of-substance-abuse-on-federal-state-and-local-budgets_0.pdf?_gl=1*w6zjh5*_gcl_au*OTM4MDAxMDYyLjE3NjUwNDkwNjc.*_ga*NjUzNzM4NTQxLjE2ODQzNDY2NDE.*_ga_ECZGQ0GWSZ*czE3NjUwNTIyNjIkbzYkZzAkdDE3NjUwNTIyNjIkajYwJGwwJGgw. Accessed December 6, 2025.
6. Kelly SW, Smith DL, Davis Z, et al. A nationwide analysis of acute pediatric healthcare encounters attributed to substance use before, during, and following the COVID-19 pandemic. J Am Acad Child Adolesc Psychiatry 2026;65(5):712–22.
7. Tanz LJ, Dinwiddie AT, Mattson CL, et al. Drug overdose deaths among persons aged 10–19 years — united States, July 2019–December 2021. MMWR Morb Mortal Wkly Rep 2022;71. https://doi.org/10.15585/mmwr.mm7150a2.
8. Camenga DR, Hammer LD. The Committee on substance use and prevention and C on CHF. Improving substance use prevention, assessment, and treatment financing to enhance equity and improve outcomes among children, adolescents, and young adults. Pediatrics 2022;150(1):e2022057992. https://doi.org/10.1542/peds.2022-057992.

9. SAMHSA. Screening, brief intervention and referral to treatment in behavioral healthcare. 2011. Available at: https://www.samhsa.gov/sites/default/files/sbirtwhitepaper_0.pdf. Accessed February 3, 2026.
10. Levy SJL, Williams JF, Committee on Substance Use and Prevention. Substance use screening, brief intervention, and referral to treatment. Pediatrics 2016; 138(1):e20161211. https://doi.org/10.1542/peds.2016-1211.
11. Ozechowski TJ, Becker SJ, Hogue A. SBIRT-A: adapting SBIRT to maximize developmental fit for adolescents in primary care. J Subst Abuse Treat 2016; 62:28–37.
12. Hadland SE. Filling in the gaps: building the evidence base for SBIRT in adolescents. J Adolesc Health 2022;71(4 Suppl):S1–4.
13. Levy S, Wiseblatt A, Straus JH, et al. Adolescent SBIRT practices among pediatricians in Massachusetts. J Addiction Med 2020;14(2):145.
14. Harris BR, Shaw BA, Sherman BR, et al. Screening, brief intervention, and referral to treatment for adolescents: attitudes, perceptions, and practice of New York school-based health center providers. Subst Abuse 2016;37(1): 161–7.
15. Ragan-Burnett K, Schieber L, Terranella A, et al. Substance use screening, brief intervention, and referral to treatment among youth-serving Clinicians. JAMA Netw Open 2025;8(5):e2511579. https://doi.org/10.1001/jamanetworkopen.2025.11579.
16. Hammond CJ, Parhami I, Young AS, et al. Provider and practice characteristics and perceived barriers associated with different levels of adolescent SBIRT implementation among a national sample of US pediatricians. Clin Pediatr (Phila) 2021;60(9–10):418–26.
17. Monico LB, Mitchell SG, Gryczynski J, et al. Organizational acceptability of implementing SBIRT for adolescents in primary care. Subst Use Misuse 2021;56-(10):1536–42.
18. Farhoudian A, Razaghi E, Hooshyari Z, et al. Barriers and facilitators to substance use disorder treatment: an overview of systematic reviews. Subst Abuse 2022;16:11782218221118462. https://doi.org/10.1177/11782218221118462.
19. Van Hook S, Harris SK, Brooks T, et al. The “six t's”: barriers to screening teens for substance abuse in primary care. J Adolesc Health 2007;40(5):456–61.
20. Palmer A, Karakus M, Mark T. Barriers faced by physicians in screening for substance use disorders among adolescents. PS 2019;70(5):409–12.
21. Kristman-Valente AN, McCarty CA, Walker DD, et al. Barriers to implementing a cannabis focused SBIRT in adolescent primary care. Subst Abuse 2022;16: 11782218221111837. https://doi.org/10.1177/11782218221111837.
22. Wisdom JP, Cavaleri M, Gogel L, et al. Barriers and facilitators to adolescent drug treatment: youth, family, and staff reports. Addiction Res Theor 2011; 19(2):179–88.
23. Berridge BJ, McCann TV, Cheetham A, et al. Perceived barriers and enablers of help-seeking for substance use problems during adolescence. Health Promot Pract 2018;19(1):86–93.
24. Hogue A, Becker SJ, Wenzel K, et al. Family involvement in treatment and recovery for substance use disorders among transition-age youth: research bedrocks and opportunities. J Subst Abuse Treat 2021;129:108402. https://doi.org/10.1016/j.jsat.2021.108402.
25. Chen E, Seely HD, Thurstone C. Reducing barriers to promote engagement and retention in adolescent substance use treatment: results from a quality

improvement evaluation. Front Child Adolesc Psychiatry 2024;3. https://doi.org/10.3389/frcha.2024.1393401.
26. Park E, Sidoti O, Faverio M. Internet, digital device access among US teens, by demographic traits. Pew Research Center. 2025. Available at: https://www.pewresearch.org/internet/fact-sheet/teens-and-internet-device-access-fact-sheet/. Accessed April 26, 2026.
27. The International Telecommunication Union, UN Agency for digital technologies. Facts and figures 2022 - mobile phone ownership. 2022. Available at: https://www.itu.int/itu-d/reports/statistics/2022/11/24/ff22-mobile-phone-ownership. Accessed June 24, 2025.
28. Harris SK, Knight JR, Van Hook S, et al. Adolescent substance use screening in primary care: validity of computer self-administered versus clinician-administered screening. Subst Abuse 2016;37(1):197–203.
29. Treatment C for SA. Appendix E—Assessment instruments for adolescent populations. In: *combining alcohol and other drug abuse treatment with diversion for juveniles in the justice System*. Substance abuse and mental health Services administration (US). 1995. Available at: https://www.ncbi.nlm.nih.gov/books/NBK64476/. Accessed November 20, 2025.
30. Paperny DM, Aono JY, Lehman RM, et al. Computer-assisted detection and intervention in adolescent high-risk health behaviors. J Pediatr 1990;116(3):456–62.
31. Thomas BS. Computer-assisted decision making: a strategy for primary prevention of substance abuse. J Pediatr Health Care 1991;5(5):257–63.
32. Schinke SP, Schwinn TM, Ozanian AJ. Alcohol abuse prevention among high-risk youth: computer-based intervention. J Prev Interv Community 2005;29-(1–2):117–30.
33. Whittaker R, Maddison R, McRobbie H, et al. A multimedia Mobile phone–based youth smoking cessation intervention: findings from content development and piloting studies. J Med Internet Res 2008;10(5):e1007. https://doi.org/10.2196/jmir.1007.
34. Haug S. Mobile phone text messaging to reduce alcohol and tobacco use in young people - a narrative review. Smart Homecare Technol TeleHealth 2013;1:11–9.
35. Mason M, Ola B, Zaharakis N, et al. Text messaging interventions for adolescent and young adult substance use: a meta-analysis. Prev Sci 2015;16(2):181–8.
36. Rodriguez DM, Teesson M, Newton NC. A systematic review of computerised serious educational games about alcohol and other drugs for adolescents. Drug Alcohol Rev 2014;33(2):129–35.
37. Lee S, Kim J, Bockhold S, et al. Game-based digital interventions for enhancing positive development and addressing substance use in adolescents: a systematic review. Children 2024;11(12):12.
38. Weser VU, Duncan LR, Sands BE, et al. Evaluation of a virtual reality E-cigarette prevention game for adolescents. Addict Behav 2021;122:107027. https://doi.org/10.1016/j.addbeh.2021.107027.
39. Prediger C, Helmer SM, Hrynyschyn R, et al. Virtual reality-based alcohol prevention in adolescents: a systematic review. Adolescents 2021;1(2):138–50.
40. Carreiro S, Chai PR, Carey J, et al. mHealth for the detection and intervention in adolescent and young adult substance use disorder. Curr Addict Rep 2018;5(2):110–9.

41. Fucito LM, Ash GI, Wu R, et al. Wearable intervention for alcohol use risk and sleep in young adults: a randomized clinical trial. JAMA Netw Open 2025; 8(5):e2513167. https://doi.org/10.1001/jamanetworkopen.2025.13167.
42. Bergwerff CE, Buisman RSM, Nibbering N, Noordermeer SDS. Using wearables in mental health care for children and adolescents: a scoping review. Res Child Adolesc Psychopathol 2026;54(1):16.
43. Kim S, Kim H, Kim S, et al. Machine learning–based prediction of substance use in adolescents in three independent worldwide cohorts: algorithm development and validation study. J Med Internet Res 2025;27(1):e62805. https://doi.org/10.2196/62805.
44. Han DH, Lee S, Seo DC. Using machine learning to predict opioid misuse among U.S. adolescents. Prev Med 2020;130:105886. https://doi.org/10.1016/j.ypmed.2019.105886.
45. Afzali MH, Sunderland M, Stewart S, et al. Machine-learning prediction of adolescent alcohol use: a cross-study, cross-cultural validation. Addiction 2019;114(4):662–71.
46. Squeglia LM, Ball TM, Jacobus J, et al. Neural predictors of initiating alcohol use during adolescence. Am J Psychiatry 2017;174(2):172–85. Erratum in: Am J Psychiatry. 2017 Jan 1;174(1):80. https://doi.org/10.1176/appi.ajp.2016.1741correction.
47. Deng T, Urbaczewski A, Lee YJ, et al. Identifying marijuana use behaviors among youth experiencing homelessness using a machine learning–based framework: development and evaluation study. JMIR AI 2024;3(1):e53488. https://doi.org/10.2196/53488.
48. Ni Y, Bachtel A, Nause K, et al. Automated detection of substance use information from electronic health records for a pediatric population. J Am Med Inform Assoc 2021;28(10):2116–27.
49. Aneni K, Chen CH, Meyer J, et al. Identifying game-based digital biomarkers of cognitive risk for adolescent substance misuse: protocol for a proof-of-concept study. JMIR Res Protoc 2023;12(1):e46990. https://doi.org/10.2196/46990.
50. Knight JR, Sherritt L, Shrier LA, et al. Validity of the CRAFFT substance abuse screening test among adolescent clinic patients. Arch Pediatr Adolesc Med 2002;156(6):607–14.
51. Kelly SM, Gryczynski J, Mitchell SG, et al. Validity of brief screening instrument for adolescent tobacco, alcohol, and drug use. Pediatrics 2014;133(5):819–26.
52. Levy S, Weiss R, Sherritt L, et al. An electronic screen for triaging adolescent substance use by risk levels. JAMA Pediatr 2014;168(9):822–8.
53. Child Health and Development Interactive System (CHADIS),. CHADIS. Available at: https://site.chadis.com/about-us. Accessed November 13, 2025.
54. Gao C, O'Connell MM, Howard BJ, et al. Does screening mode matter? A repeated cross-sectional study of computer self-administered vs. clinician-administered screening of youth substance use in pediatric primary care. Front Adolesc Med 2025;3. https://doi.org/10.3389/fradm.2025.1694040.
55. Ranginwala M, Greiner MV, Fox K, et al. Reducing bias in substance use detection in adolescents via standardized substance use screening. Pediatrics Open Science 2025;1(1):1–3.
56. Gibson EB, Knight JR, Levinson JA, et al. Pediatric primary care provider perspectives on a computer-facilitated screening and brief intervention system for adolescent substance use. J Adolesc Health 2021;69(1):157–61.

57. CHADIS. Teen substance use summary - online system for primary care to prevent and address teen substance use. CHADIS. Available at: https://site.chadis.com/teen-substance-use-summary. Accessed April 21, 2026.
58. Moyer A, Finney JW, Swearingen CE, et al. Brief interventions for alcohol problems: a meta-analytic review of controlled investigations in treatment-seeking and non-treatment-seeking populations. Addiction 2002;97(3):279–92.
59. Tevyaw TO, Monti PM. Motivational enhancement and other brief interventions for adolescent substance abuse: foundations, applications and evaluations. Addiction 2004;99(s2):63–75.
60. Aneni K, Meyer J, Funaro MC, et al. A systematic review and meta-analysis evaluating the efficacy of stand-alone digital interventions to prevent substance use among adolescents. Curr Addict Rep 2023;10(3):378–95.
61. Monarque M, Sabetti J, Ferrari M. Digital interventions for substance use disorders in young people: rapid review. Subst Abuse Treat Prev Policy 2023;18:13.
62. Tekinbas KS, Zimmerman E. Rules of play: game design fundamentals. The MIT Press; 2003.
63. Deterding S, Dixon D, Khaled R, et al. From game design elements to gamefulness: defining gamification, 11, 2011. p. 15. https://doi.org/10.1145/2181037.2181040.
64. Re-Examining categories of computer-based learning in mathematics education – CITE journal. Available at: https://citejournal.org/volume-3/issue-3-03/mathematics/re-examining-categories-of-computer-based-learning-in-mathematics-education. Accessed February 3, 2026.
65. Lateef F. Simulation-based learning: just like the real thing. J Emergencies, Trauma, Shock 2010;3(4):348–52.
66. Boumparis N, Loheide-Niesmann L, Blankers M, et al. Short- and long-term effects of digital prevention and treatment interventions for cannabis use reduction: a systematic review and meta-analysis. Drug Alcohol Depend 2019;200:82–94.
67. Aneni K, Fernandes CSF, Hoerner LA, et al. A video game intervention to prevent opioid misuse among older adolescents: development and preimplementation study. JMIR Serious Games 2023;11(1):e46912. https://doi.org/10.2196/46912.
68. Boomer T, Hoerner L, Larkin K, et al. A videogame for perceived risk of harm from opioid misuse in adolescents: a randomized controlled trial. Nat Health 2025;1–12. https://doi.org/10.1038/s44360-025-00010-z.
69. Williams C, Griffin KW, Macaulay AP, et al. Efficacy of a drug prevention CD-ROM intervention for adolescents. Subst Use Misuse 2005;40(6):869–78.
70. Walton MA, Chermack ST, Shope JT, et al. Effects of a brief intervention for reducing violence and alcohol misuse among adolescents: a randomized controlled trial. JAMA 2010;304(5):527.
71. Doumas DM, Esp S, Turrisi R, et al. A test of the efficacy of a brief, web-based personalized feedback intervention to reduce drinking among 9th grade students. Addict Behav 2014;39(1):231–8.
72. Stormshak EA, Matulis JM, Nash W, et al. The family Check-Up online: a telehealth model for delivery of parenting skills to high-risk families with opioid use histories. Front Psychol 2021;12. https://doi.org/10.3389/fpsyg.2021.695967.
73. Murry VM, Berkel C, Inniss-Thompson MN, et al. Pathways for African American success: results of three-arm randomized trial to test the effects of technology-based delivery for rural African American families. J Pediatr Psychol 2019;44(3):375–87.

74. Mason MJ, Coatsworth JD, Russell M, et al. Reducing risk for adolescent substance misuse with text-delivered counseling to adolescents and parents. Subst Use Misuse 2021;56(9):1247–57.
75. Newton NC, Chapman C, Slade T, et al. Internet-based universal prevention for students and parents to prevent alcohol and cannabis use among adolescents: protocol for the randomized controlled trial of climate schools plus. JMIR Res Protoc 2018;7(8):e10849. https://doi.org/10.2196/10849.
76. Kemp K, Micalizzi L, Becker SJ, et al. Intervention for marijuana using, court-involved non-incarcerated youth. J Subst Use Addict Treat 2023;152:209100. https://doi.org/10.1016/j.josat.2023.209100.
77. Walton MA, Bohnert K, Resko S, et al. Computer and therapist based brief interventions among cannabis-using adolescents presenting to primary care: one year outcomes. Drug Alcohol Depend 2013;132(3):646–53.
78. Cunningham RM, Chermack ST, Ehrlich PF, et al. Alcohol interventions among underage drinkers in the ED: a randomized controlled trial. Pediatrics 2015;136(4):e783–93.
79. Mason M, Mennis J, Way T, et al. Text message delivered peer network counseling for adolescent smokers: a randomized controlled trial. J Prim Prev 2016;37(5):403–20.
80. Newton NC, Teesson M, Vogl LE, et al. Internet-based prevention for alcohol and cannabis use: final results of the climate schools course. Addiction 2010;105(4):749–59.
81. Hieftje KD, Fernandes CSF, Lin IH, et al. Effectiveness of a web-based tobacco product use prevention videogame intervention on young adolescents' beliefs and knowledge. Subst Abuse 2019;1–7. https://doi.org/10.1080/08897077.2019.1691128.
82. Jiang C, Dietrich T, Durl J, et al. Virtual reality in adolescent alcohol and other drugs education programs: a systematic scoping review. J Adolesc Health 2026;78(3):373–85.
83. Schinke SP, Fang L, Cole KCA, et al. Preventing substance abuse among black and Hispanic adolescent girls: results from a computer-delivered, mother-daughter intervention approach. Subst Use Misuse 2011;46(1):35–45.
84. Griffin KW, Williams C, Botvin CM, et al. Effectiveness of a hybrid digital substance abuse prevention approach combining e-Learning and in-person class sessions. Front Digit Health 2022;4. https://doi.org/10.3389/fdgth.2022.931276.
85. Marsch LA, Moore SK, Grabinski M, et al. Evaluating the effectiveness of a web-based program (POP4Teens) to prevent prescription opioid misuse among adolescents: randomized controlled trial. JMIR Public Health and Surveillance 2021;7(2):e18487. https://doi.org/10.2196/18487.
86. Ho FK, Tung KTS, Wong RS, et al. An internet quiz game intervention for adolescent alcohol drinking: a clustered RCT. Pediatrics 2021;148(6):e2021051005. https://doi.org/10.1542/peds.2021-051005.
87. Haug S, Paz Castro R, Wenger A, et al. A Mobile phone–based life-skills training program for substance use prevention among adolescents: cluster-randomized controlled trial. JMIR mHealth uHealth 2021;9(7):e26951. https://doi.org/10.2196/26951.
88. Jander A, Crutzen R, Mercken L, et al. Effects of a web-based computer-tailored game to reduce binge drinking among Dutch adolescents: a cluster randomized controlled trial. J Med Internet Res 2016;18(2):e29. https://doi.org/10.2196/jmir.4708.

89. Kazemi DM, Li S, Levine MJ, et al. Systematic review of smartphone apps as a mHealth intervention to address substance abuse in adolescents and adults. J Addict Nurs 2021;32(3):180–7.
90. Aneni K, Pegram D, Meyer J, et al. Systematic review: culturally tailored digital substance use prevention interventions for black adolescents. JAACAP Open 2026. https://doi.org/10.1016/j.jaacop.2026.03.007.
91. O'Logbon J, Wickersham A, Williamson C, et al. The effectiveness of digital health technologies for reducing substance use among young people: a systematic review & meta-analysis. J Ment Health 2024;33(5):645–73.
92. Villanueva-Blasco VJ, Eslava D, Olave L, et al. Electronic interventions in primary care to address substance use: a systematic review. Addict Behav 2024;156:108073. https://doi.org/10.1016/j.addbeh.2024.108073.
93. Asuzu K, Matin A, Noord M, et al. Electronically-delivered interventions to reduce cannabis use in adolescents: a systematic review. Adolesc Psychiatry 2018;09. https://doi.org/10.2174/2210676609666181203094249.
94. Karas D, Eggleston L, Goldman W, et al. Substance use screening in a large pediatric primary care network: a quality improvement project. Pediatr Qual Saf 2024;9(4):e745. https://doi.org/10.1097/pq9.0000000000000745.
95. Hargraves D, White C, Frederick R, et al. Implementing SBIRT (screening, brief intervention and referral to treatment) in primary care: lessons learned from a multi-practice evaluation portfolio. Public Health Rev 2017;38:31.
96. Richardson LP, Zhou C, Gersh E, et al. Effect of electronic screening with personalized feedback on adolescent health risk behaviors in a primary care setting: a randomized clinical trial. JAMA Netw Open 2019;2(5):e193581. https://doi.org/10.1001/jamanetworkopen.2019.3581.
97. McCarty CA, Gersh E, Katzman K, et al. Screening and brief intervention with adolescents with risky alcohol use in school-based health centers: a randomized clinical trial of the check yourself tool. Subst Abuse 2019;40(4):510–8.
98. Deluca P, Coulton S, Alam MF, et al. Effectiveness and cost-effectiveness of face-to-face and electronic brief interventions versus screening alone to reduce alcohol consumption among high-risk adolescents presenting to emergency departments: three-arm pragmatic randomized trial (SIPS Junior high risk trial). Addiction 2022;117(8):2200–14.
99. Mello MJ, Baird J, Spirito A, et al. Implementing screening, brief interventions, and referral to treatment at pediatric trauma centers: a step wedge cluster randomized trial. J Pediatr Surg 2024;59(11):161618. https://doi.org/10.1016/j.jpedsurg.2024.07.003.
100. Melcher J, Torous J. Smartphone apps for college mental health: a concern for privacy and quality of current offerings. Psychiatr Serv 2020;71:1114–9.
101. Huckvale K, Torous J, Larsen ME. Assessment of the data sharing and privacy practices of smartphone apps for depression and smoking cessation. JAMA Netw Open 2019;2(4):e192542. https://doi.org/10.1001/jamanetworkopen.2019.2542.
102. Torous JB, Chan SR, Gipson SYMT, et al. A hierarchical framework for evaluation and informed decision making regarding smartphone apps for clinical care. Psychiatr Serv 2018;69(5):498–500.
103. The app evaluation model. Available at: https://www.psychiatry.org:443/psychiatrists/practice/mental-health-apps/the-app-evaluation-model. Accessed December 16, 2025.
104. Agarwal S, Jalan M, Wilcox HC, et al. Framework training guide: framework to assist stakeholders in technology evaluation for recovery (FASTER) to mental

health and wellness framework assessment. In: Evaluation of mental health Mobile applications [Internet]. Agency for Healthcare Research and Quality (US); 2022. Available at: https://www.ncbi.nlm.nih.gov/books/NBK580946/. Accessed February 3, 2026.
105. McCall T, Asuzu K, Oladele CR, et al. A socio-ecological approach to addressing digital redlining in the United States: a call to action for health equity. Front Digit Health 2022;4. Available at: https://www.frontiersin.org/articles/10.3389/fdgth.2022.897250. Accessed July 27, 2022.
106. Hichborn E, Turner A, Moore S, et al. Technology-Based interventions in tobacco use treatment among people who identify as African American/Black, Hispanic/Latina/o, and American Indian/Alaska native: scoping review. J Med Internet Res 2024;26(1):e50748. https://doi.org/10.2196/50748.
107. Moore SK, Boggis JS, Gauthier PR, et al. Technology-based interventions for substance use treatment among people who identify as African American or black, Hispanic or Latino, and American Indian or Alaska native: scoping review. J Med Internet Res 2024;26(1):e53685. https://doi.org/10.2196/53685.
108. Kiselev N, Schaffner R, Csepregi Z, et al. Factors influencing engagement in a digital substance use prevention program: qualitative study using the capability, opportunity, motivation model and theoretical domains framework. JMIR mHealth uHealth 2025;13(1):e64861. https://doi.org/10.2196/64861.
109. Singh KP, Camenga DR, Aneni K, et al. Beyond user-centered design: designing digital health technologies for substance use prevention and treatment in children and youth. In: Wells JL, editor. A clinical lens on pediatric engineering: pioneering science and technology for cutting-edge patient care. Switzerland: Springer Nature; 2025. p. 231–49. https://doi.org/10.1007/978-3-031-84655-7_10.
110. Heather Stringer. New reimbursement pathways have opened doors for using digital therapeutics. Available at: https://www.apaservices.org. Available at: https://www.apaservices.org/practice/business/technology/tech-talk/reimbursement-pathways-digital-therapeutics. Accessed February 4, 2026.
111. Ng S. Navigating adolescent mental health in the age of artificial intelligence. JAACAP Connect 2025. https://doi.org/10.62414/001c.150329. Published online December 8.
112. Booth R, editor RBU technology. Teen killed himself after 'months of encouragement from ChatGPT', lawsuit claims. The Guardian. August 27, 2025. Available at: https://www.theguardian.com/technology/2025/aug/27/chatgpt-scrutiny-family-teen-killed-himself-sue-open-ai. Accessed February 3, 2026.
113. Schinke SP, Schwinn TM, Fang L. Longitudinal outcomes of an alcohol abuse prevention program for urban adolescents. J Adolesc Health 2010;46(5):451–7.
114. Hill ED, Kashyap P, Raffanello E, et al. Prediction of mental health risk in adolescents. Nat Med 2025;31(6):1840–6.
115. Wei S, Van S, Shia C, et al. Psychophysiological Rresponses in virtual reality for assessing current nicotine use and future addiction risk among young adults: protocol for a mixed methods study. JMIR Res Protoc 2026;15:e89382.
116. Dennis ML, Scott CK, Funk RR, et al. A pilot study to examine the feasibility and potential effectiveness of using smartphones to provide recovery support for adolescents. Subst Abuse 2015;36(4):486–92.
117. Russell MA, Gajos JM. Annual research review: ecological momentary assessment studies in child psychology and psychiatry. J Child Psychol Psychiatry 2020;61(3):376–94.

Harm Reduction in Adolescent Substance Use

Brady J. Heward, MD[a,*], Jennifer C. Creedon, MD[b],
Peter R. Jackson, MD[a]

KEYWORDS

- Harm reduction • Substance use • Substance use disorders
- Substance use treatment

KEY POINTS

- Despite being relatively common, no level of substance use is safe in adolescents and substance use is associated with physical, mental, and social harms.
- All youth should be screened for substance use, risky patterns of use, use disorders, and current behavior that may increase or reduce risk of harms.
- Harm reduction includes clinical and public health practices designed to reduce the harm associated with substance use regardless of whether abstinence is the goal or outcome.
- Harm reduction in adolescents can help providers decrease risk of adolescent use through decreased potency, sobriety or tolerance breaks, not using alone, safer settings of use, naloxone, drug test strips, sterile supplies, and other practices.
- Harm reduction messaging should augment not replace messaging on prevention and treatment of substance use in teens.

INTRODUCTION

Substance use prevention for children and adolescents has long been considered a national and international priority. In Article 33 of the Convention of the Rights of the Child, the United Nations calls on all states to "take all appropriate measures... to protect children from the illicit use of... substances."[1] The convention further recognized that children (defined as individuals under the age of 18) "by reason of his physical and mental immaturity, need special safeguards and care including appropriate legal protections."[1] Efforts to protect children from the use and consequences of substances have largely taken the form of prevention.[2] Due to neuro and psychological development, best outcomes for children are most likely with complete abstinence from

[a] Department of Psychiatry, University of Vermont Larner College of Medicine, Burlington, VT, USA; [b] Department of Clinical Psychiatry, Louisianna State University Health New Orleans School of Medicine, New Orleans, LA, USA
* Corresponding author. Department of Psychiatry, University of Vermont Larner College of Medicine, 1 South Prospect Street, Burlington, VT 05401.
E-mail address: bradyjhewardmd@gmail.com

Child Adolesc Psychiatric Clin N Am 35 (2026) 637–653
https://doi.org/10.1016/j.chc.2026.05.002 childpsych.theclinics.com

Abbreviations	
HIV	Human Immunodeficiency Virus
SUD	substance use disorder

substances.[3–5] Efforts at prevention include, among other approaches, limiting access to the drug supply, criminalization of distribution and use, public service announcements/mass media, and school-based education.

While eliminating substance use amongst youth would be ideal, the risk-taking nature of adolescent development can come into conflict with rigid, abstinence-only approaches.[6] Adolescence is associated with heightened reward sensitivity, peer influence, and novelty seeking in the setting of still developing executive function. Recent data show an overall reduction in adolescent substance use over the past 20 years, likely, in part, due to prevention efforts (**Fig. 1**).[7] Despite these efforts, adolescents continue to access and use substances at significant rates.[8–10] An estimated 9.3% and 26.8% of individuals aged 12 to 17 and 18 to 25, respectively, in the United States needed substance use treatment in 2024 as defined by meeting criteria for a use disorder or currently being in treatment.[8] Only 30.2% of adolescents and 11.3% of young adults in need of treatment accessed any care.[8] Some research shows that adolescents and young adults are less likely than any other group to access Medications for Opioid Use Disorder, demonstrating that evidence-based treatments are often last to reach this age group.[11] Availability of treatment resources is not the biggest reason that 69.8% of adolescents in need did not engage; 93.3% of these adolescents did not recognize their own need for treatment.[8] With

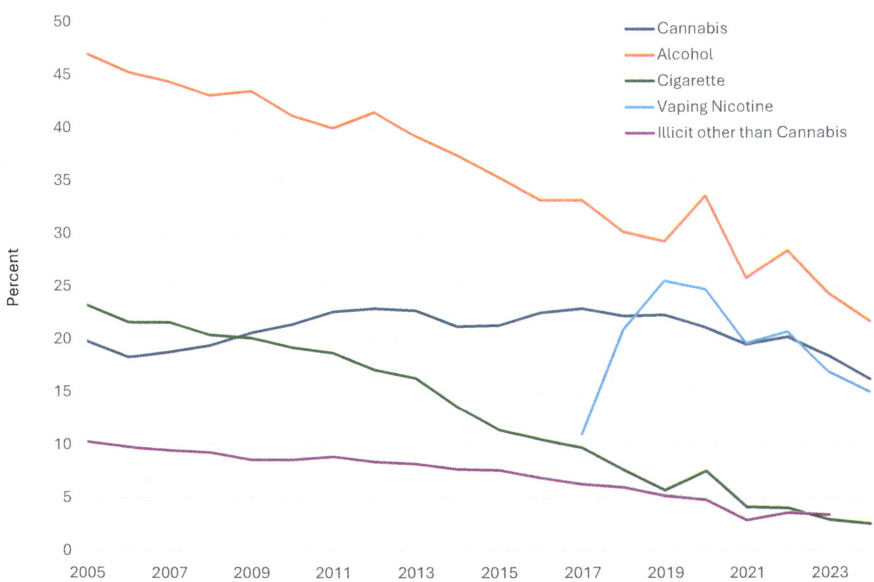

Fig. 1. Past month substance use in US 12th graders. (*Data from* Miech RA, Johnston LD, Patrick ME, et al. Monitoring the Future National Survey Results on Drug Use, 1975–2024: Overview and Detailed Results for Secondary School Students. Institute for Social Research, University of Michigan; 2025. Accessed January 2, 2026. https://monitoringthefuture.org/wp-content/uploads/2024/12/mtf2025.pdf.)

ongoing substance use in youth, limited rates of accessing evidence-based care, expanding beyond prevention and treatment is needed to promote the health and wellbeing of all youth.

The primary focus of this article is to discuss incorporating harm reduction practices into the treatment of adolescent (here defined as under 18) substance use. While the age of majority (18 in the United States) is a legal definition that simplifies policies and procedures, it has led to the exclusion of adolescents from certain evidence-based practices and research within harm reduction that primarily has focused on adults.[2,12,13] This article will prioritize discussing harm reduction practices in adolescents; many of these principles equally apply to young adults (here defined as 18–25) who share many of the same vulnerabilities yet lack the same legal protections and, at times, restrictions.[13] For example, consent laws may limit what an adolescent can access without parental consent and some harm reduction services may only be available to individuals aged 18 years or older.

The Spectrum of Adolescent Substance Use

The age of first substance use often occurs in adolescents with the mean age of first alcohol consumption between 14 and 15 and the first cannabis use at 16.[14–17] The probability of using a new substance after first use of cannabis is 25% by 2 years and between 70% and 80% by 8 years in adolescents.[18] Youth also have high rates of experimentation with multiple substances, with up to 40% of adolescents with past month use using more than one substance.[19] There is a wide range of adolescent substance use ranging from no use, to experimentation, to regular use, to heavy daily use with significant variability in between (**Fig. 2**).[7] Given the variability in use patterns, a wide spectrum of approaches must be considered to help prevent escalation of use and decrease the frequency and harm associated with use.

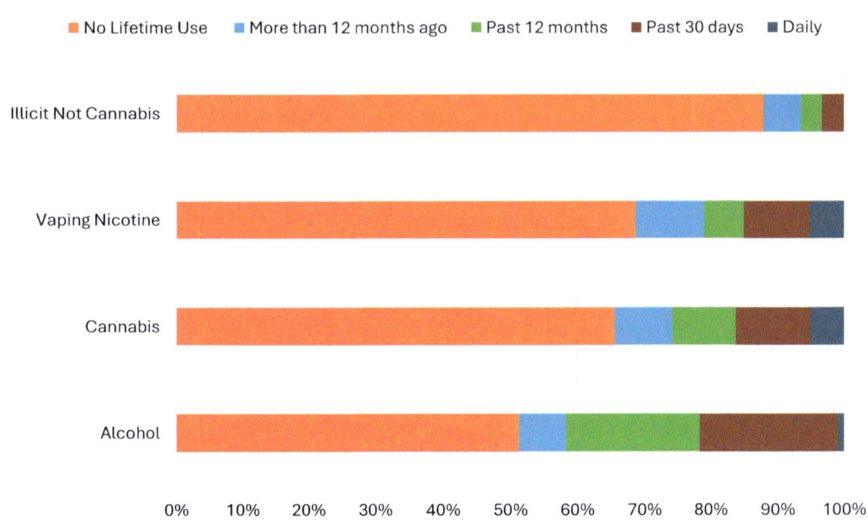

Fig. 2. Frequency of 12th-grader substance use. (*Data from* Miech RA, Johnston LD, Patrick ME, et al. Monitoring the Future National Survey Results on Drug Use, 1975–2024: Overview and Detailed Results for Secondary School Students. Institute for Social Research, University of Michigan; 2025. Accessed January 2, 2026. https://monitoringthefuture.org/wp-content/uploads/2024/12/mtf2025.pdf)

Risks Associated with Adolescent Substance Use

Depending on the substances of use, methods of use, locations of use, sources of the substances, and behaviors associated with use (eg, how substances are obtained, activities engaged in during and after use, use in other high-risk situations), adolescent substance use can be associated with significant harms.[20–24] Notably, overdose mortality has rapidly increased in recent years, increasing more rapidly than in the general population from 2020 to 2021 (20% increase in adolescents 14–18 years of age compared with 11.5% increase in the general population) with a higher rate of fentanyl involvement in adolescents in 2021 (77%–90% compared with 66%).[25,26] Recent DEA data from 2024 indicated almost 50% of seized pressed/counterfeit pills contained potentially lethal amounts of fentanyl, likely contributing to fentanyl associated overdose fatalities in adolescent attempting to use other substances.[25–27] National data from CDC Wonder have shown recent decreases in overdose fatalities in the general population, a trend that has been relatively flat in adolescents (**Fig. 3**).[28]

In addition to overdose fatalities, substance use in adolescents is associated with a variety of other negative physical health, mental health, social, and developmental problems (**Table 1**).[20–24,29–36] While greater risk exists for more frequent and heavier use, even one time use can be associated with negative outcomes including accidents, trauma, social consequences, or overdose given the increasingly adulterated drug supply. Only focusing on adolescents before they first use or on those who are willing to engage in treatment is a missed opportunity to reduce the overall harms associated with all levels of substance use in this age range.

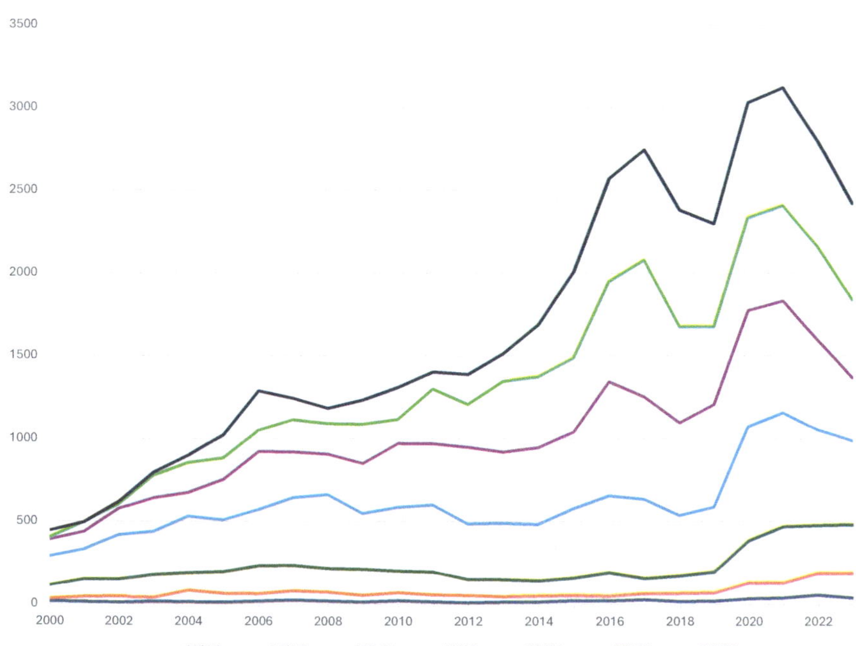

Fig. 3. Overdose fatalities from 2000 to 2023 in 12 to 25 year olds. (*Data from* Centers for Disease Control and Prevention WONDER (Wide-Ranging Online Data for Epidemiologic Research) database. Accessed 12/26/2026.)

Table 1
Potential acute and chronic risks of adolescent substance use

Physical Health (acute and chronic)	**Indirect Impacts**
Infectious diseases (HIV, hep C, hep B, cellulitis, abscesses, etc.)	Accidents (driving, falls, unintentional injuries)
Wounds	Academic achievement
Diseases of solid organs	School suspension/expulsion
Cancers	Loss of employment
Hyperemesis	Legal problems
Anorexia	Loss of positive/protective activities
Mental Health (acute and chronic)	Loss of or strained relationships
Mood disorders	Illegal activities
Anxiety	Risky sexual activities
Psychosis	Trafficking
Cognitive impacts	Fighting
Sleep disorders	Lower socioeconomic outcomes
Suicidality	

Defining Harm Reduction in Adolescents

There have been many efforts to define harm reduction over the years.[13,37–40] Recognizing that prevention and abstinence-based treatment also reduce the harm caused by substance use, Lenton and Single argued for a more narrow definition with the primary goal of "the reduction of drug related harm rather than drug use."[39] Wodak and Saunders differentiated the terms "reduction of harm," which is inclusive of prevention and use reducing interventions from "harm reduction" that seeks to reduce harm without the goal of interfering with consumption.[40] One recent effort to define harm reduction for minors states "Child-centred harm reduction is the study and practice of reducing the health and social harms to those under the age of 18 due to their own use, parental or family drug use, or related laws and policies" and further clarifies harm reduction "neither presupposes nor precludes abstinence as a goal."[13]

For the purposes of this article, harm reduction will include clinical and public health practices designed to reduce the harm associated with use regardless of whether abstinence is the goal or outcome. Harm reduction can be the underlying approach while providers continue to focus on reduction of harm across the use spectrum including through preventing initiation of use, limiting escalation of use, building motivation for decreased use, and engaging in treatment. Providers can be clear that best outcomes occur with no use.

ASSESSMENT OF ADOLESCENT SUBSTANCE USE AND RISK

To reduce the harms associated with substance use (see **Table 1**), an assessment must go beyond simply identifying whether an individual meets criteria for a substance use disorder (SUD). Specific assessment of risk and attention to that risk can strengthen and complement a review of diagnostic criteria. Validated substance use screening tools include both diagnostic and risk components. For example, the CRAFFT screening tool (CRAFFT 2.1 provider manual) includes stepwise screening, risk assessment not directly correlated with diagnostic criteria, asking every adolescent about riding in a car with an intoxicated driver for example, followed by further questions which more directly address diagnostic criteria and predict likelihood of an SUD diagnosis.[41] Higher risk substance use behaviors are often, but not always, correlated with likelihood of SUD diagnosis.

Components of a risk-focused assessment that are not necessarily correlated with or included in diagnostic criteria include route of administration, sourcing and means of obtaining drugs or alcohol, presence of unknown or unpredicted substances in the drug supply, use frequency and volume of use per episode. These and other components are described in **Table 2**.

In our clinical experience it is common that a more in-depth review of risk, including questions about the content in **Table 2**, yields at least some information about areas where adolescents have established boundaries for themselves, desire to reduce their risk and/or have already taken steps to do so. By beginning the risk-focused

Table 2
Risk focused components of substance use assessment

Risk Category	Risk Component	Examples
Contributory Risks	Age of first use and likability	• Patient describes first use at very early age and describes experience as "love at first sight"
	Modeling in the home	• Adolescent observes or is asked to participate in criminal activity • Parent is modeling repeated use of unsterile needles
Sourcing Risks	Drug impurity	• Patient is unaware of adulterants in the drug supply and not informed of the presence of other drug classes in a urine drug screen
	Means of acquiring	• Patient selling/distributing drugs or engaging in other illegal activity • Patient is exchanging sex for drugs • Patients are buying from the dark web
Direct Use Risks	Volume of use per occurrence	• Infrequent alcohol use but drinking to blackout at every occurrence
	Route of administration	• Patient quickly transitioned from oral to intranasal to intravenous use
	Location and presence of others	• Patient is using alone • High-risk environments to use
	Other activities during use	• Use while operating a motor-vehicle • Use while responsible for minor children • Use while swimming or around bodies of water • High-risk sexual activities while high or intoxicated
	Mixing or concurrent use	• Patients are mixing drugs with increased risk (eg, benzos/alcohol and opioids)

components of a substance use assessment with open-ended questions, a provider can more quickly understand where risk-reducing clinical effort might most effectively focus. Such questions can also strengthen therapeutic alliance, reducing likelihood of an adolescent feeling lectured, threatened, or scolded.

Example open-ended questions.

- What do you know or what have you already been taught about the risks of using X?
  - How has that impacted your decisions?
- What steps have you taken to reduce the risk of harm from using X?
  - Why did you choose to try that/take that step/make that change?
  - How did it go/how has it gone?
- What purpose does using X serve in your life?
  - Given what you know about the risks, what potentially safer alternative have you tried or considered to accomplish that purpose?

Expanding understanding through these questions, a provider can better understand risk trajectory. Seeing the course of substance use more broadly, rather than only a single point in time, a provider may even recognize that a patient is already working to protect themself from harm, with a pattern of decreasing risk, even if not yet at zero risk. Consistent with the principles of motivational interviewing and motivational enhancement therapy, providers can reflect back the adolescent's own reasons to reduce harm and steps already taken to do so. Subsequently, less energy and clinical time is spent challenging an adolescent in areas where they do not wish to make change.

HARM REDUCTION PRACTICES

Evidence for Harm Reduction Practices in Adolescents

A portion of adolescents who use substances, particularly those who have come to the attention of mental health professionals, may not identify complete abstinence as their goal or intention. Others may not meet criteria for an SUD but still are at risk for health consequences of use. Expanding the scope of interventions for adolescent substance use to include harm reduction principles can help to mitigate risks of morbidity and mortality associated with use, while meeting the adolescent where they are at, thus increasing the likelihood they will continue to participate honestly in treatment. Clinicians working with adolescents who are using substances are likely incorporating discussion of harm reduction strategies, even if they aren't immediately recognized as such. This can include discussion of using a designated driver or rideshare if drinking alcohol, knowing the signs of alcohol poisoning, reducing potency of THC used, and tapering down on nicotine content in electronic cigarettes.[5]

While there are not yet widely established evidence-based harm reduction interventions targeting adolescent substance use, there are pilot studies of school-based curriculum that show promise for implementation of these interventions on a broader scale. An Australian study of a school-based harm reduction curriculum targeting alcohol use followed over 2300 students assigned to either intervention or control groups. Students in the intervention group received harm minimization curriculum delivered in 2 phases at ages 13 and 14 years. Control groups received standard school-based alcohol education. Students in the intervention group were less likely to drink; those who did drink consumed less alcohol and were less likely to drink at risk levels and experienced less alcohol-related harm than those in the control group.[42]

In a more recent pilot study on the implementation of "Safety First," a school-based harm reduction curriculum, to high school freshmen in New York City and San Francisco, Students demonstrated increased ability to evaluate safety information about various substances and were more knowledgeable in how to manage their own risks after the curriculum. Of students who used substances, they also reported decreased use after the intervention. Despite initial concerns, shifting to a harm reduction curriculum from an abstinence-only approach did not lead to an increase in reported substance use.[43]

As with other clinical situations where adolescent-specific evidence lags behind adult data, clinicians should consider the balance of risks versus benefits for implementing harm reduction strategies with adolescent patients. Considering the reassuring safety profiles of harm reduction interventions (both pharmacological and non-pharmacological) in adults compared with the high risk of morbidity and mortality associated with substance use in adolescence, clinicians are justified in providing guidance around harm reduction with adolescent patients, even while adolescent specific studies are ongoing.

Evidence-Based Harm Reduction Practices for Opioid Use

Studies examining the impact of targeted harm reduction interventions for adolescents who use drugs are lacking; however, evidence from adult populations can be considered for extrapolation to younger populations.

Naloxone

Harm reduction interventions for opioids, particularly overdose prevention strategies, are typically the most widely recognized and accessible. Increasing access to the opioid reversal agent, naloxone, has been a significant harm reduction strategy in the effort to reduce opioid overdose deaths in the United States. Naloxone access laws help to decrease barriers to obtain naloxone for people who use opioids and those who may be positioned to witness an overdose. Such laws include third party prescribing (allowing prescribing of naloxone to individuals not directly assessed by the prescribing physician) standing orders allowing for individuals to obtain naloxone directly from the pharmacy, and naloxone distribution without a prescription. Between 2010 and 2017, all 50 states and Washington, DC, had enacted some form of naloxone access laws. A systematic review of the literature found that naloxone access laws were correlated with increased public access to naloxone, increased opioid-related emergency room visits (suggesting patients were accessing overdose reversal and medical care) and decreased rates of opioid overdose deaths.[44]

Naloxone is FDA-approved for patients 12 years and older, however efforts at increasing access to overdose prevention in adolescents have been sparse. A survey of over 7000 adolescents and young adults found that only 30% could correctly identify the purpose of naloxone, and 14% reported knowing how to administer naloxone.[45]

One argument against expansion of naloxone access for adolescents has been belief that it would lead to an increase in adolescent substance use. However, a review of data from states with expanded naloxone access did not reveal any increase in opioid or intravenous drug use among youth, instead showing slight decreases in both.[46]

There have been calls to implement overdose prevention training and naloxone access in schools in response to the recent increase in deaths by accidental opioid overdose in adolescents.[47] Several proposed congressional acts (School Access to Naloxone Act of 2023, Stop Overdose in Schools Act, Helping Educators Respond to Overdoses Act) would have established federal funding and grants to support overdose prevention education and naloxone access in school settings.[48] The proposals all died in committee.

Drug testing supplies

In response to overdose deaths driven by fentanyl contamination of heroin and other drugs, there have been harm reduction efforts to increase legal access to fentanyl test strips. There is evidence that use of fentanyl test strips is associated with reduced frequency and amount of injected opioid use and increase in other overdose prevention behaviors (supervised use, having naloxone available).[49,50] State laws vary with regards to whether drug testing equipment such as fentanyl test strips are considered "drug paraphernalia," though, increasingly, states have moved to decriminalize possession and distribution of fentanyl test strips.[51] Access to testing supplies is typically focused on adults who use substances. With the disturbing rise in accidental overdose deaths in youth driven by unintended fentanyl exposure, incorporating information about drug testing into overdose prevention education may be an additional tool in reducing overdose deaths in this population.

Sterile supplies

While harm reduction efforts to reduce overdose deaths have received attention over the recent years, syringe exchange programs have operated for several decades. The primary harm reduction goal of syringe exchange programs is to reduce transmission of blood borne pathogens, such as Hepatitis C and Human Immunodeficiency Virus (HIV). Reviews of outcomes have demonstrated that access to syringe exchange programs is associated with reduced rates of HCV and HIV transmission among people who inject drugs.[52,53] Most syringe exchange sites offer additional services, including naloxone access, HIV/HCV testing, needle disposal, and referrals to treatment. There is evidence that individuals who utilize syringe exchange programs are more likely to access treatment for opioid-use disorder.[54] Syringe exchange programs are typically limited to individuals over age 18, so there is a dearth of evidence investigating the utility of these services for minors who use injection drugs.

There are unique issues that arise when considering harm reduction interventions such as naloxone prescribing and recommending safe supply use while working with youth. As with other sensitive topics, issues around parental involvement and confidentiality can arise. While family involvement is vital in the treatment of adolescent SUDs, risks of disclosure should be considered as well. When caregivers are involved, navigating their openness to harm reduction approaches is also necessary to maintain trust and rapport. Aspects of motivational interviewing can be helpful in these conversations, particularly when there is discord between the goals of the family and those of the youth.

Expanding Beyond Harm Reduction for Opioid Use

Recent harm reduction initiatives and research have centered around the opioid crisis due to recent overdose trends and the desire to decrease the risk of death. As previously mentioned, overdose deaths in teens have recently increased without the same level of decreases seen in the national sample (see **Fig. 3**). Despite this, overdose fatalities represent just a fraction of the harms experience by adolescent substance use. It is imperative that we expand harm reduction in teenagers to include more attention on alcohol, nicotine/tobacco, cannabis and other substances.[13] **Table 3** provides a more expansive view of harm reduction strategies in adolescents.[3,5,6,55,56]

Table 3
Harm reduction considerations for adolescents with substance use

Harm Reduction Practices	Considerations When Working with Adolescents
General Strategies	
Education on Options for Treatment and Safety	• Safest course and best outcomes are through no use • While there are many ways to reduce risk, there is no completely safe way to use substances • There are good options to help adolescents reduce and stop • Pair harm reduction practices with information on treatment options and open the door for further discussion, but don't require abstinence for treatment engagement

Location of Use	• Educate on the risks of using in specific locations
	  ○ School—risk of negative consequences such as suspension or expulsion
	  ○ Public—risk of police involvement, legal charges
	• Address potential environmental risks that make using in a location unsafe before, during, or after intoxication (staircases, heights and ledges, exposure to elements, etc.)
	• Review need for additional resources to support health (eg, snacks, water, extra clothing)

Never Use Alone	• Encourage youth to have a trusted individual present who is not using (reduce risks of unexpected substance related outcomes or being victimized) • Provide contact for never use alone hotlines
Drug Source	• Inform about high rates of counterfeit or pressed pills • Encourage youth to consider where the drug is coming from (risk of being counterfeit vs pharmaceutical grade) • Warn against purchasing or taking from untrustworthy sources (dark web, new dealers) • Provide reputable resources adolescents can use to learn about the drugs they use including effects, side effects, and risks
Drug Testing	• Know local trends and educate about high rates of adulterants in drugs • Fentanyl and xylazine test strips can decrease risks of unintentional overdose. Note that, in some jurisdictions, they can be viewed as drug paraphernalia • Review that test doses/very small amount on first use can help perceive potency and unintended risks
Planning/limiting	• Help adolescents decide before on a limit for their use or a maximum amount they will use • Invite adolescents to identify firm boundaries they commit to not cross and why • Ask adolescent how they intend to monitor these self-commitments
Tolerance Breaks	• To reduce tolerance and risk of dependence, discuss options for tolerance or abstinence breaks with teens • Encourage less frequent use and significant time between use

(*continued on next page*)

Table 3
(continued)

Harm Reduction Practices	Considerations When Working with Adolescents
Overdose Prevention	• Discuss overdose prevention with all teens using drugs, regardless of substance, given high rates of adulterants and lethal levels of fentanyl and other contaminants in the drug supply • Provide adolescents with Naloxone, a prescription for Naloxone, or a location where they can get Naloxone and educate about correct administration
Infection Protection Strategies	
Sterile Supplies	• While injection drug use is relatively rare in adolescents, risks associated with use are significant • Help adolescents know the risks of sharing needles • Help teens not willing to stop injecting to identify locations where they can access sterile equipment
Safe Injection Techniques	• Provide instructions on sterile technique for injections to limit spread of diseases and injection site infections
Infectious Disease	• Test for HIV, hepatitis B, hepatitis C, and other infectious diseases associated with their use or other high-risk behaviors • Ask about symptoms and examine injection sites
Immunization	• Ensure that youth have been immunized for hepatitis A and B
Safe Consumption Sites	• Though there are limited sites in the United States, if there is an available site nearby, reach out regarding age restrictions
PrEP	• For those at risk due to injection or sexual activity, provide PrEP that is FDA-approved for use in adolescents who weigh at least 77 pounds
Substance Specific Practices	
Alcohol	• Discuss the importance of having a designated driver • Advise on slower rate of drinking, food intake, alternating with non-alcoholic beverages • Discuss drinking beverages with lower alcohol concentration
Nicotine/Tobacco	• Educate about decreased health risks with vaping and nicotine pouches compared with combustible cigarettes • Discuss increased risk of using cigarettes in those who use other nicotine formulations • Discuss decreasing concentrations of nicotine in products • Encourage tolerance breaks
Cannabis	• Encourage use of lower potency products • Educate on timing of onset of action in different methods of use to prevent overuse (eg, edibles)
Opioids	• Inform on risks of overdose, risks with co-consumption of alcohol, benzodiazepines, stimulants, and other substances • Ensure access to Naloxone • Educate on Good Samaritan Laws • Offer medication for opioid use disorder

(*continued on next page*)

Table 3 (continued)	
Harm Reduction Practices	**Considerations When Working with Adolescents**
Other Substances	• Generally, encourage lower potency, lower risk methods of use, decreased frequency, and limiting co-consumption
Family-Based Strategies	
Parent Involvement	• Encourage open, frequent communication with parents • Ensure that parents have access to Naloxone • Educate parents on harm reduction practices • Help parents see harm-reduction as an immediate goal, but not the only goal
Family Preparation	• Limit access to medications, sharps, guns, or other risky items • Ensure family has access to Naloxone and educate on proper administration

Data from[3,5,6,55,56]

Legal Limits of Harm Reduction Practices in the United States

It is important for those treating youth with SUDs to be aware of relevant legal statutes related to confidentiality, consent, treatment, and harm reduction interventions as these vary by state/territory.[51,57–60] A barrier to uptake of evidence-based harm reduction practices has been concern that items such as naloxone or test strips can be classified as "drug paraphernalia" and lead to legal charges for such. As costs associated with the opioid crisis have risen, both with regards to lives lost and the financial burden of medical sequelae, there has been movement toward decriminalization of the possession of harm reduction supplies. As of August 2025, 47 states, the District of Columbia, and 4 US territories did not criminally penalize possession of at least one form of drug testing equipment (most commonly fentanyl test strips).[51] Twenty-nine states had revised their laws since 2018 to eliminate possession of drug testing equipment from the definition of drug paraphernalia. Similarly, states may vary in whether syringes are considered to be drug paraphernalia. In most cases, there are not specific differences in statutes based on age. In places where legal ambiguity remains, clinicians should have frank discussions with youth and families regarding possible legal risks related to possession of harm reduction supplies, as well as medical and legal risks of continued substance use. Getting familiar with local community harm reduction services can be helpful in providing such guidance.

DISCUSSING HARM REDUCTION WITH PATIENTS AND FAMILIES

Harm reduction messaging can be uniquely tailored with the wellbeing of children and youth in mind.[3,12,13] Harm reduction conversations should be developmentally appropriate. Cognitive development, risk perception, and autonomy vary significantly from early to late adolescence and may influence how harm reduction strategies are discussed and implemented. For example, clinicians working with early adolescents may be particularly attentive to the harms associated with any use, while clinicians working with older adolescents may more strongly recognize limiting harms associated with individual choice. Across all stages, clinicians should be cautious that messaging, including tone and interpersonal engagement, does not inadvertently condone use. Because earlier use predicts higher rates and increased severity of SUDs and perception of risk has been demonstrated to be inversely proportional to frequency of substance use among adolescents, it is important that harm reduction messages are delivered in the greater context of harmfulness of drugs.[7,61] Given the heightened consequences of substance use among youth compared with adults, information on harm reduction resources and approaches should be accompanied by ongoing emphasis on prevention, early intervention and treatment for adolescent SUD.[62]

Substantial research and widely accepted guidelines from national organizations highlight the importance of parent-child communication about substance use generally.[63,64] It follows that accurate parental understanding and parent-child messaging on harm reduction will impact adolescent perspectives. Some studies have shown that providers may be less likely to share harm reduction resources or practices due to concern about parental disapproval.[65] Indeed, parental perceptions on harm reduction practices must be sought and understood in anticipation of making clinical recommendations. Some parents may take a more strict or authoritarian stance on substance use and may initially feel uncomfortable with the idea of reducing harm rather than ceasing use. Such parents may benefit from education that:

- In meeting an adolescent where they're at, the intention is not to leave them where they are at.
- Harm reduction measures can reduce risk while clinicians build rapport and engage in motivational enhancement strategies.
- Harm reduction doesn't stand alone as an intervention and is not a pivot in treatment philosophy, rather is one component of intervention.
- Extensive research on motivational interviewing demonstrates efficacy in a guiding rather than leading or following treatment approach and demonstrates the impact of engaging adolescents in "change talk" while softening and sometimes even not responding to "sustain talk."[66]
- Demanding change in an authoritarian approach can inadvertently lead to opposition and entrenched use.[67]

In contrast, parents with a more permissive perspective on adolescent substance use may benefit from education on current rates of overdose death among adolescents and young adults, adulterants and unpredictability in the current drug supply and the evidence for harm reduction practices described above.

CLINICS CARE POINTS

- Clinical interviews regarding youth substance use can expand beyond standard diagnostic criteria to include robust risk assessment.
- Ask all adolescents using substances open-ended questions about what they are doing or have already done to reduce the risk of harm.
- Pair harm-reduction messaging with prevention, early intervention, and treatment messaging.
- National organizations responsible for adolescent health increasingly advocate for universal education about and access to naloxone for adolescents.
- In addition to overdose reversal medications, there are many other approaches adolescents and providers can use to reduce the harms associated with substance use (**Table 3**).

- Given adolescent's heightened vulnerabilities to substance use, do not equate harm reduction recommendations with condoning use.
- Focus clinical and therapeutic messaging on the desire to keep a youth or adolescent safe, not make drugs safe. The mindset can be person-focused, not drug-focused.
- Inform parents and caregivers that harm reductions measures are often immediate, safety-focused goals, but not the only goals or end goals of clinical work with their children.
- While not holding abstinence as a requirement of engagement, partner harm reduction conversations and interventions with motivational enhancement interventions.

DISCLOSURES

The author has nothing to disclose.

REFERENCES

1. Convention on the Rights of the Child. OHCHR. Available at: https://www.ohchr.org/en/instruments-mechanisms/instruments/convention-rights-child. Accessed December 31, 2025.
2. Watson TM, Strike C, Kolla G, et al. “drugs don't have age limits”: the challenge of setting age restrictions for supervised injection facilities. Drugs Educ Prev Policy 2015;22(4):370–9.
3. Heward BJ, Yule AM, Jackson PR. How should harm reduction strategies differ for adolescents and adults? AMA J Ethics 2024;26(7):534–45.
4. Quigley J, Ryan SA, Camenga D, et al, COMMITTEE ON SUBSTANCE USE AND PREVENTION. Alcohol use by youth. Pediatrics 2019;144(1):e20191356.
5. Winer JM, Yule AM, Hadland SE, et al. Addressing adolescent substance use with a public health prevention framework: the case for harm reduction. Ann Med 2022;54(1):2123–36.
6. Jakub G, Krzysztof O, Katarzyna D, et al. “It'll Never Be Safe, But You Can Limit the Harms”. Exploring Adolescents' strategies to reduce harms associated with psychoactive substance use. Subst Use Misuse 2022;57(3):380–91.
7. Miech RA, Johnston LD, Patrick ME, et al. Monitoring the future National Survey results on drug use, 1975-2024: overview and detailed results for secondary school students. Institute for Social Research, University of Michigan; 2025. Available at: https://monitoringthefuture.org/wp-content/uploads/2024/12/mtf2025.pdf. Accessed January 2, 2026.
8. Substance Abuse and Mental Health Services Administration. Key substance use and mental health indicatorsin the United States: Results from the 2024 National Survey on Drug Use and Health (HHS Publication No.PEP25-07-007, NSDUH Series H-60). Center for Behavioral Health Statistics and Quality, Substance Abuse andMental Health Services Administration. 2025. Available at: https://www.samhsa.gov/data/data-we-collect/nsduh-national-survey-drug-use-and-health/national-releases.
9. Miech RA, Patrick ME, O'Malley PM, et al. Monitoring the future national survey results on drug use, 1975–2025: overview and key findings for secondary school students. Ann Arbor (MI): Institute of Social Research, University of Michigan; 2026.
10. Youthonline.cdc.gov. Available at: https://youthonline.cdc.gov/. Accessed January 13, 2026.

11. Mauro PM, Gutkind S, Annunziato EM, et al. Use of medication for opioid use disorder among US adolescents and adults with need for opioid treatment, 2019. JAMA Netw Open 2022;5(3):e223821.
12. Barrett D, Petersson F, Turner R. Best interests and low thresholds: legal and ethical issues relating to needle and syringe services for under 18s in Sweden. Harm Reduct J 2022;19:15.
13. Barrett D, Stoicescu C, Thumath M, et al. Child-centred harm reduction. Int J Drug Policy 2022;109:103857.
14. Schuckit MA. Alcohol-use disorders. Lancet Lond Engl 2009;373(9662):492–501.
15. Chen CM, Yoon YH. *TRENDS IN UNDERAGE DRINKING IN THE UNITED STATES, 1991–2019*. National Institute on alcohol abuse and alcoholism, division on epidemiology and prevention research, alcohol epidemiologic data system. 2021. Available at: https://www.niaaa.nih.gov/sites/default/files/SR116_Underage_Drinking.pdf. Accessed January 9, 2026.
16. Swendsen J, Burstein M, Case B, et al. Use and abuse of alcohol and illicit drugs in US adolescents: results of the national comorbidity survey–adolescent supplement. Arch Gen Psychiatry 2012;69(4):390–8.
17. Chen X, Yu B, Lasopa SO, et al. Current patterns of marijuana use initiation by age among US adolescents and emerging adults: implications for intervention. Am J Drug Alcohol Abuse 2017;43(3):261–70.
18. Zhang S, Wu S, Wu Q, et al. Adolescent drug use initiation and transition into other drugs: a retrospective longitudinal examination across race/ethnicity. Addict Behav 2021;113:106679.
19. Banks DE, Rowe AT, Mpofu P, et al. Trends in typologies of concurrent alcohol, marijuana and cigarette use among US adolescents: an ecological examination by sex and race/ethnicity. Drug Alcohol Depend 2017;179:71–7.
20. Sultan RS, Zhang AW, Olfson M, et al. Nondisordered cannabis use among US adolescents. JAMA Netw Open 2023;6(5):e2311294.
21. Steinfeld MR, Torregrossa MM. Consequences of adolescent drug use. Transl Psychiatry 2023;13(1):313.
22. Kann L, McManus T, Harris WA, et al. Youth risk behavior surveillance — united States, 2017. MMWR Surveill Summ 2018;67(8):1–114.
23. Alemu BT, Baydoun HA, Olayinka O, et al. Substance use disorders among adolescents in the United States: 2000–2019. South Med J 2024;117(2):80–7.
24. Hansen ER, Kruckow S, Ewing SWF, et al. Adolescent substance use patterns and subsequent risk of mental and behavioural disorders, substance use, and suicidal behaviour: a cohort study. Lancet Public Health 2025;10(7):e578–87.
25. Friedman J, Godvin M, Shover CL, et al. Trends in drug overdose deaths among US adolescents, January 2010 to June 2021. JAMA 2022;327(14):1398–400.
26. Tanz LJ, Dinwiddie AT, Mattson CL, et al. Drug overdose deaths among persons aged 10–19 years — united States, July 2019–December 2021. MMWR Morb Mortal Wkly Rep 2022;71. https://doi.org/10.15585/mmwr.mm7150a2.
27. Pill press resources. Available at: https://www.dea.gov/resources/pill-press-resources. Accessed January 6, 2026.
28. Centers for Disease Control and Prevention. CDC WONDER database. Available at: https://wonder.cdc.gov/. Accessed December 26, 2025.
29. Vergunst F, Chadi N, Orri M, et al. Trajectories of adolescent poly-substance use and their long-term social and economic outcomes for males from low-income backgrounds. Eur Child Adolesc Psychiatry 2022;31(11):1729–38.
30. Carbonneau R, Vitaro F, Brendgen M, et al. Longitudinal patterns of polysubstance use throughout adolescence: association with adult substance use and

psychosocial outcomes controlling for preadolescent risk factors in a male cohort. Soc Psychiatry Psychiatr Epidemiol 2023;58(10):1469–81.
31. Schaefer JD, Hamdi NR, Malone SM, et al. Associations between adolescent cannabis use and young-adult functioning in three longitudinal twin studies. Proc Natl Acad Sci U S A 2021;118(14):e2013180118.
32. Al Ma'ani M, Castillo Diaz F, Hejazi O, et al. The alarming surge of driving under the influence-related motor vehicle crashes. J Surg Res 2025;314:146–52.
33. Terry-McElrath YM, O'Malley PM, Johnston LD. Alcohol and marijuana use patterns associated with unsafe driving among U.S. high school seniors: high use frequency, concurrent use, and simultaneous use. J Stud Alcohol Drugs 2014;75(3):378–89.
34. Hadland SE, Walker LR. Medical comorbidity and complications. Child Adolesc Psychiatr Clin N Am 2016;25(3):533–48.
35. Mason MJ, Aplasca A, Morales-Theodore R, et al. Psychiatric comorbidity and complications. Child Adolesc Psychiatr Clin N Am 2016;25(3):521–32.
36. Adjei BN, Afetor M, Ansong-Aggrey S, et al. Substance use and adolescent injuries: a multi-country analysis of the association and mediating effect of interpersonal violence among 122,945 in-school paediatric populations in 29 countries. Front Public Health 2023;11:1193711.
37. Hawk M, Coulter RWS, Egan JE, et al. Harm reduction principles for healthcare settings. Harm Reduct J 2017;14(1):70.
38. Drucker E, Anderson K, Haemmig R, et al. Treating addictions: harm reduction in clinical care and prevention. J Bioethical Inq 2016;13(2):239–49.
39. Lenton S, Single E. The definition of harm reduction. Drug Alcohol Rev 1998;17(2):213–20.
40. Wodak A, Saunders B. Harm reduction means what I choose it to mean. Drug Alcohol Rev 1995;14(3):269–71.
41. Mitchell SG, Kelly SM, Gryczynski J, et al. The CRAFFT cut-points and DSM-5 criteria for alcohol and other drugs: a re-evaluation and re-examination. Subst Abuse 2014;35(4):376–80.
42. McBride N, Farringdon F, Midford R, et al. Harm minimization in school drug education: final results of the school health and alcohol Harm Reduction Project (SHAHRP). Addiction 2004;99(3):278–91.
43. Fischer NR. School-based harm reduction with adolescents: a pilot study. Subst Abuse Treat Prev Pol 2022;17(1):79.
44. Smart R, Pardo B, Davis CS. Systematic review of the emerging literature on the effectiveness of naloxone access laws in the United States. Addict Abingdon Engl 2021;116(1):6–17.
45. Freibott CE, Vest N, Stein MD, et al. Opioid overdose knowledge among adolescents and young adults. JAMA Pediatr 2024;178(6):618–20.
46. Bruzelius E, Cerdá M, Davis CS, et al. Naloxone expansion is not associated with increases in adolescent heroin use and injection drug use: evidence from 44 US states. Int J Drug Policy 2023;114:103980.
47. Moran M. AMA backs making overdose reversal meds accessible in schools. Washington, DC: Psychiatr News; 2023. https://doi.org/10.1176/appi.pn.2023.08.8.41.
48. Calihan JB, Carney BL, Schmill DM, et al. The call for a school-based approach to opioid overdose prevention. Am J Public Health 2024;114(12):1305–8.
49. Pridgen BE, Bontemps AP, Lloyd AR, et al. U.S. substance use harm reduction efforts: a review of the current state of policy, policy barriers, and recommendations. Harm Reduct J 2025;22(1):101.

50. Kutscher E, Barber Grossi M, LaPolla F, et al. Fentanyl test strips for harm reduction: a scoping review. J Addiction Med 2024;18(4):373–80.
51. Drug checking equipment needles syringes and drug paraphernalia summary of state laws, *Legislative Analysis and Public Policy Association*, 2025, 1-174. Available at: https://legislativeanalysis.org/wp-content/uploads/2025/09/Drug-Checking-Equipment-50-State-Summary-1.pdf (Accessed 9 January 2026).
52. Rossi RM, Brady MJ, Hall ES, et al. Effect of needle exchange program on maternal hepatitis C virus prevalence. Am J Perinatol 2020;37(09):881–9.
53. Ruiz MS, O'Rourke A, Allen ST, et al. Using interrupted time series analysis to measure the impact of legalized syringe exchange on HIV diagnoses in Baltimore and Philadelphia. JAIDS J Acquir Immune Defic Syndr 2019;82(2):S148–54.
54. Jakubowski A, Pappas A, Isaacsohn L, et al. Development and evaluation of a pilot overdose education and naloxone distribution program for hospitalized general medical patients. Subst Abuse 2019;40(1):61–5.
55. Hosek S, Henry-Reid L. PrEP and adolescents: the role of providers in ending the AIDS epidemic. Pediatrics 2020;145(1):e20191743.
56. Witt LB, Greenberg J, Cantone RE. Harm reduction and substance use in adolescents. Prim Care 2024;51(4):629–43.
57. Sharko M, Jameson R, Ancker JS, et al. State-by-State variability in adolescent privacy laws. Pediatrics 2022;149(6):e2021053458.
58. Ford CA, Millstein SG, Halpern-Felsher BL, et al. Influence of physician confidentiality assurances on adolescents' willingness to disclose information and seek future health care. A randomized controlled trial. JAMA 1997;278(12):1029–34.
59. Kerwin ME, Kirby KC, Speziali D, et al. What can parents do? A review of state laws regarding decision making for adolescent drug abuse and mental health treatment. J Child Adolesc Subst Abuse 2015;24(3):166–76.
60. Pathak PR, Chou A. Confidential care for adolescents in the U.S. health care system. J Patient-Centered Res Rev 2019;6(1):46–50.
61. Volkow ND, Han B, Einstein EB, et al. Prevalence of substance use disorders by time since first substance use among young people in the US. JAMA Pediatr 2021;175(6):640–3.
62. Stockings E, Hall WD, Lynskey M, et al. Prevention, early intervention, harm reduction, and treatment of substance use in young people. Lancet Psychiatry 2016;3(3):280–96.
63. Concerned parents. NACoA. Available at: https://nacoa.org/families/concerned-parents/. Accessed January 13, 2026.
64. Why it's important to talk to your child about alcohol & drugs. 2024. Available at: https://www.samhsa.gov/substance-use/prevention/talk-they-hear-you/parent-resources/talk-with-your-child. Accessed January 6, 2026.
65. Welsh JW, Dennis ML, Funk R, et al. Trends and age-related disparities in opioid use disorder treatment admissions for adolescents and young adults. J Subst Abuse Treat 2022;132:108584.
66. Miller WR, Rollnick S. Motivational interviewing: helping people change and grow. New York: The Guilford Press; 2023.
67. Slemon A, Jenkins EK, Haines-Saah RJ, et al. "You can't chain a dog to a porch": a multisite qualitative analysis of youth narratives of parental approaches to substance use. Harm Reduct J 2019;16:26.

Updated Review for the Treatment of Adolescent Nicotine Use Disorders

Jordan Davis, PhD[a], Leila M. Vaezazizi, MD[b],
Pantea Farahmand, MD[a,*]

KEYWORDS

- Nicotine use disorders • Electronic cigarettes • Adolescents • Addictions
- Medication-assisted treatments

KEY POINTS

- Nicotine use is common among adolescents, and nicotine products are more addictive than in previous decades due to higher nicotine concentration products.
- Regular screening of adolescents 10 years and older at every primary care appointment is recommended by American Academy of Child and Adolescent Psychiatry, American Academy of Pediatrics, and American Thoracic Society.
- There are several evidence-based behavioral therapies for the treatment of nicotine use disorders in adolescents.
- Medication-assisted treatments are underutilized and can be used for treatment of adolescent nicotine use disorder.

INTRODUCTION

Tobacco products, consisting of the highly addictive chemical, nicotine, are commonly used in the United States. Chronic nicotine use remains the leading cause of preventable disease and death in the United States.[1] The vast majority of adults with nicotine addiction began using the substance during adolescence.[2] Existing research suggests that adolescents experience increased susceptibility to nicotine addiction.[3]

Nicotine addiction or Tobacco Use Disorder is characterized by clinically significant impairment and distress related to nicotine consumption (DSM-5).[4] Individuals must have at least 2 of 11 symptoms during a 12 month period in order to meet diagnostic criteria (**Box 1**). Symptoms include nicotine cravings, using more than intended, persistent interpersonal problems surrounding nicotine use (eg, conflict with loved

[a] Department of Child and Adolescent Psychiatry, NYU Grossman School of Medicine, NY 10016, USA; [b] Department of Psychiatry, NYU Grossman School of Medicine, NY 10016, USA
* Corresponding author. NYU Langone, Department of Child and Adolescent Psychiatry, One Park Avenue Suite 7, New York, NY 10016.
E-mail address: pantea.farahmand@nyulangone.org

Child Adolesc Psychiatric Clin N Am 35 (2026) 655–675
https://doi.org/10.1016/j.chc.2026.05.006 **childpsych.theclinics.com**
1056-4993/26/

Abbreviations	
AAP	American Academy of Pediatrics
AHA	American Heart Association
CBT	Cognitive Behavioral Therapy
CM	Contingency Management
CRAFT	Community Reinforcement Approach and Family Training
HTPs	heated tobacco products
IARC	International Agency for Research on Cancer
IRR	incidence rate ratio
MAT	medication-assisted treatments
MI	Motivational Interviewing
nAChRs	nicotinic acetylcholine receptors
NYTS	National Youth Tobacco Survey
PAHs	polycyclic aromatic hydrocarbons
PFC	prefrontal cortex
ST	Skills Training
STPs	smokeless tobacco products
TSNAs	tobacco-specific nitrosamines

ones about use), and unsuccessful efforts to reduce use. Individuals may also notice increased tolerance to nicotine, requiring increased amounts of tobacco to achieve the desired effect, and withdrawal symptoms when cessation is attempted. Common nicotine withdrawal symptoms include irritability, anxiety, restlessness, difficulty concentrating, insomnia, increased appetite, and depressed mood. These symptoms are often misinterpreted as worsening mood or behavioral symptoms. The use of

Box 1
DSM-5 diagnostic criteria for tobacco use disorder

A problematic pattern of tobacco use leading to clinically significant impairment or distress, as manifested by at least 2 of the following, occurring within a 12 month period.

- Tobacco is often taken in larger amounts or over a longer period than was intended
- There is a persistent desire or unsuccessful efforts to cut down or control tobacco use
- A great deal of time is spent in activities necessary to obtain or use tobacco
- Craving, or a strong desire or urge to use tobacco
- Recurrent tobacco use resulting in a failure to fulfill major role obligations at work, school, or home
- Continued tobacco use despite having persistent or recurrent social or interpersonal problems caused or exacerbated by the effects of tobacco
- Important social, occupational, or recreational activities are given up or reduced because of tobacco use
- Recurrent tobacco use in situations in which it is physically hazardous
- Tobacco use is continued despite knowledge of having a persistent or recurrent physical or psychological problem that is likely to have been caused or exacerbated by tobacco
- Tolerance, as defined by either (a) a need for markedly increased amounts of tobacco to achieve desired effect, or (b) markedly diminished effect with continued use of the same amount of tobacco
- Withdrawal, as manifested by either (a) the characteristic withdrawal syndrome for tobacco, or (b) tobacco (or a closely related substance) is taken to relieve or avoid withdrawal symptoms

electronic cigarettes (ie, vapes), has become increasingly common over the past decade, particularly for adolescents. In 2020, 1 in 5 high school students and 1 in 20 middle school students used electronic nicotine devices (ie, vapes) in the past month.[5] Nicotine use in adolescence is associated with increased risk of addiction to other substances,[6] higher symptom ratings of suicidal thoughts, depression, anxiety, inattention, and hyperactivity.[7] Nicotine use is also associated with a number of medical complications, including asthma, chronic obstructive pulmonary disease, periodontitis, cardiovascular disease, and stroke.[8] Early identification and treatment is therefore important to mitigate these future risks.

Adolescent Risk Taking

Adolescence is a developmental period associated with an increase in risk-taking behaviors.[9] One reason why adolescents take more risks is brain-based. The prefrontal cortex (PFC) is responsible for decision-making and behavioral control. During adolescence, the PFC is going through its primary development and maturation. The limbic regions of the brain, which are involved with emotional processing and reward seeking, come to full maturity during adolescence. The disparity in maturity of the PFC and the limbic region results in adolescents being less able to inhibit emotional impulses in comparison to adults. This puts teens at high risk of engaging in impulsive decision-making, which is often at play in risk-taking.

The neurotransmitter dopamine, which is associated with feelings of pleasure, reward, and motivation, also plays a role in adolescent risk-taking.[9] In comparison to the adult brain, the adolescent brain has lower levels of dopamine at baseline. This leads teens to feel bored more easily and to seek dopamine via novel experiences. When they engage in novel experiences, adolescents also get a bigger increase in and release of dopamine in comparison to adults. This results in more natural inclination toward seeking novelty during the adolescent years. Risk taking is often in the form of alcohol, nicotine, and other substance use.

In addition to brain-based differences between teens and adults, we know that adolescents rationalize risk and reward differently than adults. More weight is given to emotional experience in the moment—"Am I having fun?" "Are my friends enjoying this?" "Do I want to keep going?"—than to potential consequences. The aforementioned context helps elucidate why adolescents might be particularly at risk of experimenting with nicotine.

Unlike the adult brain, the adolescent brain is particularly vulnerable to the harmful effects of drugs of abuse, including tobacco and nicotine containing products because it is undergoing maturation. Nicotine binds to nicotinic acetylcholine receptors (nAChRs), which are widely distributed throughout the human brain and are critical in neurotransmitter release, brain maturation, reward processing, and cognition. Nicotine exposure during adolescence, therefore, disrupts the normal development, and expression of neuronal nAChRs, which ultimately alters the release of reward-related neurotransmitters and making adolescents more prone to nicotine dependence[10]

EPIDEMIOLOGY OF NICOTINE USE AND DISORDERS

According to annual surveys completed through the University of Michigan's Monitoring the Future Studies, adolescents in the 8th, 10th, and 12th grades have declining prevalence rates of nicotine vaping since 2020 with most recent data collected in 2024 for all 3 grades.[11] 8th, 10th, and 12th grade adolescents have reported declining use of nicotine vapes when asked about over the past 30 day use and annual use. Data collected related to nicotine pouches—collected starting in 2023—have found an increased prevalence over the past year in 10th and 12th grades for daily use, over the past 30 day use and annual use. Prevalence rates for 8th graders were less in 30 day and lifetime use, and unchanged for use in the last 12 months. In another study of those high schoolers and middle schoolers reporting use of nicotine vapes 88.2% and 85.7%, respectively, reported using flavored nicotine vapes, and of those reporting using nicotine pouches 86.1% of high school students and 85.4% of middle school students reported using flavored nicotine pouches.[5] The National Youth Tobacco Survey of 2024 found that 19.0% (5.28 million) of US middle school and high school students reported any tobacco use and 8.1% (2.25 million) reporting current use of any tobacco product.[12,13] Highest prevalence tobacco products reportedly currently being used are nicotine vapes and nicotine pouches: 5.9% and 1.8%, respectively. These rates are down since 2023 in which current use of any tobacco product was reported at 10%, and nicotine vapes at 7.7% when pooled. However, when analyzed separately, middle schooler prevalence rates have been found to have no significant change between 2023 and 2024 for any tobacco product (Appendix 1). These studies highlight that the types of nicotine products being used are shifting despite possible decline.

Evolution of Nicotine Products over Time

Humans began using tobacco over 12,000 years ago.[14] In the United States, a significant increase in tobacco consumption began in 1900 and peaked in the 1960s.[15] Prior to the 1960s, disapproval of tobacco use focused on social and moral concerns. By the late 1970s, tobacco became increasingly recognized as addictive and dangerous to health.[15] Indeed, decreased tobacco consumption in the United States during the past five decades is largely attributable to evidence linking chronic tobacco use to health risks and resulting government regulations.[15]

For many centuries, pipes, chewing tobacco, cigars, and cigarettes were among the most common ways to consume tobacco.[15,16] Heated tobacco products, which heat rather than burn tobacco leaves, were introduced in the late 1980s and have expanded since, though they remain unpopular, particularly in the United States.[16,17] Dissolvable oral nicotine products expanded significantly starting in the early 2000s, and electronic nicotine devices (vapes) launched in 2007.[16,18] Since their introduction, vapes have been growing in popularity and have even been suggested as a form of harm reduction for adults who use cigarettes. However, vapes are many individuals'—particularly adolescents'—first introduction to nicotine.[19] In 2014, vapes overtook cigarettes as the most commonly used nicotine product for adolescents.[5,12,13]

Nicotine Products Used by Adolescents

The landscape of nicotine product use has shifted dramatically over the past decade. According to data from the CDC's 2024 National Youth Tobacco Survey (NYTS), 8.1% of all middle and high school students reported current use of nicotine, with 5.9% reporting e-cigarette use, 1.8% reporting nicotine pouch use, 1.4% reporting use of traditional combustible cigarettes, and 1.2% reporting use of smokeless tobacco products.[12] Cigarette smoking prevalence among high school students peaked in the mid-1990s and was over 35%,[20] but following years of aggressive public health intervention, current cigarette smoking prevalence among this group is at a historic low. However, this progress has been offset by the emergence of other nicotine delivery products such as e-cigarettes and nicotine pouches, which has created new public health challenges. These products differ substantially in their nicotine source, chemical composition, and potential health consequences (**Table 1**).

Table 1
Comparison of nicotine products used by adolescents

Product	Cigarettes	E-cigarettes	Nicotine Pouches
Nicotine Source	Tobacco combustion	Nicotine salt solution (heated aerosol)	Synthetic or tobacco-derived nicotine (oral absorption)
Transfer Efficiency[a]	10%–15%	94%	59%
Time to Peak (Tmax)[b]	10–20 min	5–10 min	30–60 min
Key Substances[c]	Tar, CO, TSNAs, PAHs, heavy metals	Propylene glycol, vegetable glycerin, flavorings, heavy metals	Flavorings, pH adjusters, formaldehyde (trace), heavy metals (trace)

[a] Transfer efficiencies: e-cigarettes: 94%; nicotine pouches: 59% (value is specific to Zyn 6 mg pouch); cigarettes 10% to 15%.
[b] Older and less efficient e-cigarette devices show longer Tmax values.
[c] Substances represent compounds found across product categories; specific formulations vary by manufacturer.

Cigarettes

Combustible cigarettes remain the most extensively studied nicotine delivery system. Cigarette smoke is an aerosol containing over 7000 chemicals, including 70+ known carcinogens, carbon monoxide, heavy metals (including arsenic, cadmium, and lead), tar, and particulate matter. The most harmful carcinogens in cigarette smoke include tobacco-specific nitrosamines (TSNAs), polycyclic aromatic hydrocarbons (PAHs), and aromatic amines. TSNAs are specific to tobacco and are formed during the curing and processing of tobacco leaves.

Over the past 2 decades, marked strides have been made in reducing cigarette use among adolescents. The declining prevalence of cigarette smoking has been accompanied by a dramatic shift toward lighter and non-daily use patterns. Between 1991 and 2021, frequent (defined as $\geq$ 20 days/month) and daily use showed the steepest declines (greater than 15 fold) compared with occasional use (a 7 fold decline). As of 2021, among high school students, occasional cigarette use was 3.8% while frequent use was 0.7% and daily use was 0.6%, indicating that the majority of current adolescent smokers are occasional rather than established daily smokers.[21]

E-cigarettes

E-cigarettes are devices that create a nicotine aerosol using basic components that include a battery, heating element (typically a small metal coil called an atomizer), and a chamber storing the nicotine solution. When the user activates the device, the battery sends power to the coil that rapidly heats to very high temperatures, aerosolizing the nicotine solution for inhalation. E-cigarette devices vary widely and include cig-a-likes (which look like cigarettes), pod systems, tanks, and disposables. Among adolescents, the most commonly used device types have changed over time—previously tanks were most common, but now disposables dominate the market. In 2024, nearly 90% of youth users used flavored products (fruit, candy, or mint); the most common brands were Elf Bar, followed by Breeze, Mr. Fog, Vuse, and JUUL. E-cigarettes mechanistically increase risk for nicotine dependence through nicotine salts, rapid delivery, and high frequency of use features. Higher concentration and increased frequency nicotine hits systems also make withdrawal and treatment options more challenging.

E-cigarettes, in contrast to traditional combustible cigarettes, showed a dramatic increase in uptake among adolescents during the 2010s with a peak prevalence in 2019, when 27.5% of high schoolers reported current use, before declining to 7.8% of high schoolers by 2024.[12] The dominance of high-concentration nicotine salts in modern e-cigarette products enables users to consume substantially more nicotine per day, which has contributed to higher nicotine dependence indicators among youth compared with those using traditional cigarettes. The intensity of e-cigarette use has also markedly increased over time: median use frequency rose from 3 to 5 days/month in 2014 to 2018, to 10 to 19 days/month in 2021; additionally, 10.3% of youth e-cigarette users reported using within 5 minutes of waking up, a hallmark of nicotine dependence. This stands in contrast to youth cigarette users, where 6.1% smoke within 5 minutes of waking up according to available data between 2014 and 2021.[22]

Youth engagement with e-cigarettes extends beyond its manufacturer-intended use—approximately 40% tamper or "hack" their device that is reportedly easily learned from social media or vape shops. This is often done to add flavorings, cannabis products, refill single-use disposables, or alter settings.[23] Further, about 18% of youth e-cigarette users report using their device to vape cannabis products, a practice that is far more common among youth compared with adults.[24] These modification practices introduce additional risks to e-cigarette use from contaminants and burns.

Nicotine pouches and other emerging products

Nicotine pouches are an emerging product which utilize tobacco-derived nicotine salt or synthetic nicotine, packaged in a small pouch that the user then places between their gum and cheek. In contrast with traditional smokeless tobacco products (STPs) like moist snuff and chewing tobacco, these products have significantly lower and often undetectable amounts of cancer-causing TSNAs, though they may contain other carcinogenic chemicals such as formaldehyde and trace amounts of heavy metals.[25] These products have rapidly increased in popularity globally, particularly in Scandinavia where they originated, and are appealing to many users because they are discreet, odorless, available in appealing flavors, and do not require spitting. For adolescents these features also allow for inconspicuous use in the home and near schools. Nicotine pouch use has also grown among adolescents, aided by widespread social-media promotion including by so-called "Zynfluencers." Between 2023 and 2024, prevalence nearly doubled from 3.0% to 5.4% among high school students,[26] with Zyn as the most popular brand, followed by on!, Rogue, and Velo.[5]

YOUTH HEALTH CONSEQUENCES OF NICOTINE USE

As nicotine delivery methods continue to diversify and as the industry moves toward synthetic nicotine and nicotine derived from highly purified tobacco, it becomes increasingly important to understand the risks specifically attributable to nicotine versus tobacco smoke. In the absence of randomized control trials, Mendelian randomization studies provide one of the most rigorous methodologies for disentangling these effects. These studies use genetic variants associated with nicotine metabolism, adjusted for smoking intensity, as a natural experiment to isolate disease risk specific to nicotine exposure. What we learn from those studies are that nicotine itself does not appear to cause the majority of smoking-related diseases such as lung cancer, COPD, stroke, coronary heart disease, or type 2 diabetes; further, there is no evidence from these studies that nicotine alone is carcinogenic.[27]

However, nicotine itself is not without significant risks, and has many side effects, particularly for adolescents who are still in an active neurodevelopmental period.

Nicotine is addictive, may increase the likelihood of transitioning to cigarette use or other substance use, has anxiogenic effects, disrupts sleep, increases heart rate, and negatively impacts fertility. More specifically for adolescents these consequences of use can contribute to worsening mental health. Additionally, the specific delivery method (cigarette, e-cigarettes, STPs, nicotine pouches) introduces its own set of risks beyond nicotine exposure alone.

Addiction Liability and Gateway Concerns

Nicotine, the primary addictive component in e-cigarettes, can be delivered more efficiently than in traditional cigarettes, where the majority of nicotine is burned off during combustion. Youth e-cigarette addiction markers have dramatically worsened between 2014 to 2021; in 2021, 10.3% of e-cigarette users reported using within 5 minutes of waking up (a classic indicator of nicotine dependence) compared with less than 1% in 2014 to 2017. This 2021 rate exceeds the 6.1% rate observed with youth cigarette smokers during the same time period, indicating that addiction markers have worsened and now exceed those of youth cigarette smokers.

There is less data on addiction markers with nicotine pouch, given its relatively recent uptake among youth, but there is reason for concern. Higher potency nicotine pouches can deliver significantly more nicotine compared with a regular cigarette, and the discreetness of pouches enables use outside of the typical constraints of smoking cigarettes. This allows users to maintain elevated levels of nicotine throughout the day, which may accelerate the development of nicotine dependence.

Beyond concerns about nicotine addiction, a major public health question is whether e-cigarettes act as a gateway to other substance use, increasing the risk for later transition to cigarette smoking or cannabis use. While recent prospective longitudinal studies and meta analyses have reported strong associations between e-cigarette use and subsequent cigarette smoking,[28] methodological limitations in these studies, including sample selection biases, make it unclear whether the effect is causal or rather a marker for youth already predisposed to cigarette smoking.[29]

Another concern involves the association between e-cigarette use and later initiation of cannabis use. A recent prospective longitudinal study by Sun and colleagues found strong individual-level effects with an approximately 2 to 3 fold increased risk, yet the question remains as to whether this reflects causality or common liability from shared risk factors.[30] The same authors estimated that even assuming complete causality, changes in e-cigarette use among adolescents would account for less than 1% point change in population prevalence of cannabis use. It is worth noting that despite the rise in adolescent e-cigarette use over the past decade, population prevalence of both cigarette and cannabis use among youth has continued to decline.

An emerging issue is that increasing numbers of youth report uncertainty as to whether they have vaped synthetic cannabinoids, raising questions about the risks of inadvertent exposure and its long-term health implications.[31] What is clear is the addictive risk with nicotine, and informing patient and parents about the ever increasing risk of nicotine addiction with adolescent use is important psychoeducation to provide.

Carcinogenic Liability

Nicotine itself is not carcinogenic nor is it classified as such by the International Agency for Research on Cancer (IARC), but there are carcinogen risks specific to the mode of delivery. The carcinogenic liability of cigarettes is well-understood and has been covered extensively elsewhere; here we focus on the risks of other nicotine products increasingly used by youth including e-cigarettes and nicotine pouches.

E-cigarettes

E-cigarettes contain a number of known carcinogens, but at levels that are substantially lower than traditional cigarettes, with the reduction in specific carcinogens ranging from 9 to 450 fold (not including heavy metals). Importantly, e-cigarettes eliminate 2 major sources of harm from traditional cigarettes including tar, which contains the majority of tobacco carcinogens including PAHs and carbon monoxide.

Among the most important carcinogens related to tobacco use are the TSNAs, and these constituents are vastly reduced in e-cigarettes, showing a 40 to 380× reduction. Formaldehyde and acetaldehyde, on the other hand, are formed in e-cigarettes by heating the e-liquid base (typically propylene glycol and/or vegetable glycerin), but their levels are also significantly reduced compared with cigarettes. Formaldehyde shows a modest 9 fold reduction, while acetaldehyde shows a more substantial 450 fold reduction.[32]

E-cigarettes introduce other carcinogenic exposures through their heating elements, which contain heavy metals including lead, nickel, chromium and cadmium. All 4 are classified as known or probable human carcinogens by the IARC, with nickel, cadmium, and chromium having the strongest evidence for cancer risk. The exposure to heavy metals varies widely between e-cigarette devices, with some devices exceeding exposures with traditional cigarettes for specific metals like nickel and chromium,[33] and with some disposable brands found to have exceedingly high levels of heavy metals compared with older refillable devices.[34]

The clinical significance of these trade-offs in carcinogen exposure remains uncertain. E-cigarettes have a unique profile of carcinogen exposure in that tar and carbon monoxide are eliminated, TSNAs are vastly reduced, as are formaldehyde and to an even greater extent acetaldehyde, but heavy metal exposure (particularly from nickel and chromium)[35] may be higher than what one would encounter with cigarette smoking alone. No epidemiological studies have yet demonstrated an increased cancer risk in e-cigarette users, however tobacco-related cancers have a long latency period and take years to develop; insufficient follow-up times, given the relatively recent introduction of these products, limits their interpretation. However, with early initiation of these highly addictive nicotine products, and use in adolescence there is greater potential for cumulative exposure to carcinogenic elements over time despite lower per exposure carcinogen levels.

Nicotine Pouches

It is not yet known if nicotine pouches cause cancer. Because modern nicotine pouches like Zyn, on!, and Velo use synthetic or tobacco-extracted nicotine that manufacturers claim is purified, they contain significantly reduced or undetectable amounts of carcinogenic TSNAs compared with cigarettes and STPs, like moist snuff or chewing tobacco. TSNAs are the most important carcinogen for assessing oral cancer risk from STPs; however, carcinogens like formaldehyde, and heavy metals like nickel and chromium have been found in pouches.[36] Further, nicotine pouches have been shown to cause white lesions in the mouth associated with high levels of inflammatory biomarkers, which suggests it may increase the risk of oral cancers, though currently there is no epidemiological data on cancer outcomes due to their long latency period.[37] Furthermore, high nicotine concentrations and discreet use may facilitate continuous use throughout the day, which exacerbates risks of addiction and symptoms of withdrawal.

Cognitive and Mental Health Effects

Nicotine use in adolescents differs from adults in that the adolescent brain is actively developing and, in many cases, shows effects distinct from adult users. Acutely, nicotine use can enhance memory and concentration, though in dependent users this may reflect relief from withdrawal symptoms. However, there is strong causal evidence, predominantly from controlled animal studies, that nicotine exposure during adolescence causes persistent deficits in attention, learning and impulsivity in adulthood - even after cessation of nicotine use.[10] The generalizability and clinical magnitude of these effects in humans remains uncertain.

Similarly, there is strong causal evidence from animal studies that nicotine exposure during adolescence causes persistent increases in anxiety- and depression-like symptoms, even following cessation.[10,38] Cross-sectional survey data from NYTS support these findings, showing that in a study of over 60,000 US adolescents, those using nicotine products had significantly higher odds for experiencing anxiety and depression, with dual users of e-cigarettes and traditional cigarettes being at the highest risk showing a 1.6 to 1.9 fold increased odds for these mental health outcomes.[39] E-cigarette use is of particular concern, given that they deliver nicotine more efficiently than cigarettes and can contain higher nicotine concentrations, enabling youth to achieve higher nicotine exposure levels than they would with traditional cigarettes. Systematic reviews of Mendelian randomization studies show robust bidirectional causal associations between smoking and mental health conditions in adults, though these studies examine lifetime exposure and do not isolate adolescent-specific risks.[40] While the clinical magnitude of these effects in adolescents remains unclear, converging evidence from multiple methodologies suggests that adolescent nicotine use is causally linked to later development of mental health problems, and preventative counseling is warranted.

Cardiopulmonary Effects

E-cigarettes are the most commonly used nicotine products by adolescents, followed by nicotine pouches. The American Heart Association (AHA) acknowledges that e-cigarettes are touted as a safer alternative to combustible cigarettes, but emphasize the unknown long-term risks from components of e-cigarette aerosol that have known cardiopulmonary toxicity, including flavoring agents, heavy metals, and thermal degradation components.[41,42] Prospective data from the PATH study demonstrated respiratory risks from e-cigarettes independent of cigarette smoking, with an incidence rate ratio (IRR) of approximately 1.3 for composite respiratory diseases (COPD, chronic bronchitis, emphysema, and asthma), and an IRR of 1.7 for emphysema alone[43]—the latter being of particular concern given its alignment with animal data showing emphysematous changes from e-cigarette exposure.[44]

The AHA further outlines the cardiac risks of e-cigarette use, noting that acute effects include systemic inflammation, endothelial dysfunction, elevated blood pressure, and heart rate, and that these changes herald the development of cardiovascular disease in middle age, though long-term data are lacking. Though these data are from adults, the cardiopulmonary effects of e-cigarette use in adolescents remain largely unstudied despite this being the primary user demographic.

Nicotine pouches, the second most commonly used nicotine products by adolescents and young adults, deliver nicotine transmucosally without inhalation or combustion, bypassing direct pulmonary toxicity. The AHA notes that despite the growing popularity of these products, no data are currently available on the long-term health risks of these products.[45] Studies on the acute effects of nicotine pouches demonstrate an increase in heart rate (~10 BPM using 6 mg pouches) and arterial stiffness, with nicotine doses comparable to or exceeding traditional cigarettes.[46,47] The lack of long-term data, combined with documented acute cardiovascular effects, raises concern given the rapid recent uptake of these products among youth.

TREATMENT RECOMMENDATIONS

Guidelines from the American Academy of Child and Adolescent Psychiatry, American Academy of Pediatrics (AAP), and American Thoracic Society recommend routine screening for all adolescents aged 10 to 18 years for use of nicotine products including cigarettes, electronic cigarettes, smokeless tobacco, nicotine pouches, cigars and hookahs (**Table 2**).[13,55–57] AAP advises for screening at every clinical encounter, and for those who screen positive for nicotine use disorders to set a quit date within 2 weeks. All academies recommend referral to empirically tested and evidence based behavioral and medication treatments. Medication-assisted treatments (MAT) such as nicotine replacement therapies, varenicline, and bupropion are limited by lack of clinical trials exploring the use of these medications in adolescent populations. However, clinical experience and the studies that have been done show benefit from prescribing MAT after a review of the risks and benefits with clients. Currently the strongest evidenced MAT is varenicline, which has been found to reduce nicotine in the short term with continued benefit after discontinuation of the medication (**Table 3**); however individualized recommendations should be made and all medications tried depending on tolerability and effect noted. MAT can be initiated early, concurrently or in lieu of behavioral interventions.

Behavioral Interventions: DBT/Parent Work/Harm Reduction

Most middle and high schoolers who vape are interested in quitting. Data collected in 2020 found that 63.9% of students who reported current vape use had a desire to quit, and 67.4% reported attempting to quit in the past year.[69] However, resources, particularly for teen vape users, continue to be minimal. There are currently no randomized controlled trials for the treatment of vaping in adolescents [**Table 2**].[70]

Cognitive behavioral therapy (CBT),[71] contingency management (CM),[72,73] and motivational interviewing (MI)[74,75] are 3 common behavioral treatments implemented with individuals striving for nicotine cessation. Research on the effectiveness of the aforementioned interventions demonstrates generally positive outcomes,[13,72–76] though, the quality of current evidence for the efficacy of nicotine use treatment is considered to be weak.[13] Emerging research suggests the existence of novel approaches that may be effective for treating nicotine use in adolescents.

Dialectical Behavior Therapy

Though it was initially developed for use in individuals with Borderline Personality Disorder, Dialectical Behavior Therapy (DBT) has in recent years been identified as a transdiagnostic treatment.[77,78] DBT is a comprehensive treatment, often including weekly individual therapy, weekly group therapy, and 24/7 phone coaching. The treatment uses principles of acceptance and change to address emotion dysregulation, suicidality, and self-injurious behaviors.

There have been several adaptations of DBT, including one for the treatment of Substance Use Disorders,[79] as well as one focused specifically on teaching the core skills of DBT—DBT-Skills Training (ST). For individuals who struggle with addiction, DBT-SUD increases emotion regulation skills and skills specific to substance use to encourage moderation of use or abstinence.[79] Though research has not evaluated the effectiveness of DBT-SUD and DBT-ST for the treatment of nicotine use in adolescents, positive outcomes have been seen for general substance use,[80,81] particularly with regard to improved emotion regulation[80,81] and decreased substance use.[81,82]

Parent-involved treatment

Research suggests that incorporating parents into adolescent nicotine use treatment may improve treatment outcomes.[83] Research has identified a number of associations

Table 2
Screening tools for adolescent nicotine use

Tool Name	Age Range	Brief Notes
CRAFFT 2.1+N[48]	12–21 y	• Only validated screen that explicitly screens for vaping with 80%–94% sensitivity/ specificity • Includes 10 item Hooked On Nicotine Checklist • Cut point ≥ 2 indicates high risk for substance use disorder • Available as clinician interview or self-administered
Hooked on Nicotine Checklist[49]	12+ years	• 10 item questionnaire • Any "yes" response indicates nicotine dependence • Number of items endorsed indicates severity • High internal consistency (α = 0.90) and test-retest reliability (ICC = 0.88) • Brief, clear, and easy-to-understand • Any score > 0 indicates loss of autonomy over nicotine use
Screening to Brief Intervention[50]	12–17 y	• Triages into 3 risk levels: no use, lower risk, higher risk • One frequency question per substance • When updated to include "vaping," identifies 92% of nicotine vaping • Area under curve values near or equal to 1 for nicotine use disorders • Self-administered or provider-administered
Brief Screener for Tobacco, Alcohol, and other Drugs[51]	12–17 y	• One question per substance from NIDA • Provides risk level based on responses • When updated with vaping examples, identifies 100% of nicotine vaping • Adequate psychometric properties for tobacco/nicotine use disorders • Shorter administration time than TAPS
Tobacco, Alcohol, Prescription medication, and other Substance use[52]	Adolescents	• Two-part tool: TAPS-1 (screening) + TAPS-2 (brief assessment) • Contains more questions than S2BI or BSTAD • Longer administration time • Similar psychometric properties to shorter tools • Validated for adolescents
Fagerström Test for Nicotine Dependence[53]	Adolescents	• Adult measure adapted for youth • Associated with quantity/frequency of smoking, quit behaviors, and urine cotinine • Assesses nicotine dependence severity • Traditional cigarette-focused tool
E-cigarette Fagerström Test[54]	Adolescents	• Modified version specifically for e-cigarette users • Assesses dependence on electronic nicotine delivery systems • Adaptation of traditional FTND for vaping

Table 3
Evidence for medication-assisted treatments

Medication	Number of Studies (*N*)	Dosing	Study Duration	Safety and Tolerability	Outcomes	Notes
Nicotine Replacement Therapies (NRT)[58–61]	4 (575)	variable	6–12 wk	Positive	Significant benefit < 4 wk Not sustained after 4 wk	Week 1–2: Significant benefit of abstinence 50% vs 26%; 31.9% vs 21.3%
Bupropion SR[62–65]	4 (679)	150–300 mg	6–9 wk	Positive	Benefit noted from 300 mg dosing Relapse common after discontinuation	
Varenicline[62,66–68]	4 (693)	0.5-1 mg BID	12–14 wk	Positive	Sustained benefit demonstrated in multiple studies	• Low-dose: Weeks 9–24 (P = .034) and 9–52 (P = .012) higher abstinence vs placebo • High-dose: Weeks 18 and 26 higher abstinence (RR = 1.82, $P < .05$) • E-cigarettes: 51% vs 14% abstinence weeks 9–12 (aOR = 6.5, $P < .001$); sustained at 24 wk: 28% vs 7%

between parent-controlled factors and reduced nicotine initiation and use. Given these findings, parent-centered treatment goals should include improving parent-child communication,[83,84] strengthening the parent child relationship,[83–87] increasing positive parent-child social interaction,[88] establishing clear rules around smoking,[89–92] monitoring adolescents' adherence to rules,[84,87,93] and consistently applying predetermined consequences for rule-breaking.[87,91]

Parents would also benefit from education about the authoritative parenting style, which has been associated with lower rates of adolescent substance use.[84,92,94,95] An authoritative parenting style is associated with high warmth and responsiveness, with clear, consistent expectations and limits.[94,96,97] Clinicians will benefit from assessing both parent and teen perception of various facets of the parent-child relationship, as some research suggests that the teen's perspective of the relationship is more predictive of nicotine use than the parent's perspective.[93]

Overall, parents would do well to approach rather than avoid conversations about nicotine and other substances with their adolescents.[83] Across multiple studies, the quality of parent–child communication was identified as more important than the quantity of communication.[83,98] Effective parent–child communication is 2 sided, with equal participation on the adolescent's end—parents should avoid lecturing their teens about nicotine use.[98]

Challenges specific to engaging adolescents in nicotine treatment, including low perceived risk, normalization of vaping within peer groups, and concealability of modern nicotine products. Parents who are experiencing a particularly difficult time managing their relationship with their adolescent in the context of nicotine use, may benefit from Community Reinforcement Approach and Family Training (CRAFT).[99] The core goals of CRAFT include, increasing self-care for family members, improving the relationship between substance-using individuals and their family members, effectively encouraging harm reduction using positive reinforcement and natural consequences, and encouraging individuals to engage in substance use treatment.[99]

Harm reduction strategies

In recent years, middle and high school students have been caught vaping on school campuses—often in bathrooms—with increasing frequency. Adolescents may be missing classwork and/or adaptive socialization with peers if they are frequently smoking in the bathroom. They may also be getting in trouble with school staff when caught, which may result in meaningful consequences within the school setting and increased conflict between teens and parents. Harm reduction, aimed at reducing negative consequences like those mentioned above, offers a possible pathway to nicotine use treatment in adolescents. In this population, harm reduction may focus on decreasing time spent using nicotine, reducing money spent on nicotine, and decreasing the effects of nicotine use on various domains of life (eg, home, school, relationships).

There is a dearth of research on the efficacy of harm reduction in adolescent nicotine use treatment; however, somewhat more is known about using these strategies with adults. In one study, implementing nicotine replacement therapy in individuals with no intention to quit smoking helped to reduce the number of cigarettes smoked and even led to eventual nicotine cessation for some.[100] In another study, adults with co-occurring nicotine and opioid use saw increased attempts to quit smoking, increased smoke-free days, and overall reductions in number of cigarettes smoked following completion of a DBT-ST protocol.

Regardless of which treatment option is utilized, clinicians, adolescents, and parents would do well to exercise patience during nicotine cessation treatment. Relapse is a typical part of addiction treatment. When working with adolescents, clinicians would benefit from reminding them that multiple attempts at nicotine cessation will be necessary before they are able to quit completely.[101]

CONCLUDING THOUGHTS

The rising popularity of vaping and other novel nicotine delivery systems among adolescents raises a number of serious health concerns. Effective treatment for adolescents using nicotine is necessary to reduce and/or eliminate the life-long health consequences associated with nicotine use.[4,7,8] Though the overall quality of the evidence for the efficacy of nicotine use treatment has been found to be weak,[13] research indicates that CBT, CM, and MI may all be helpful to reduce nicotine consumption.[71,74] Alternative treatment paths, including DBT-ST, DBT-SUD, harm reduction, and parent-involved interventions[81,82,98] may also be helpful. Additional research on effective nicotine treatments for adolescents is needed, particularly robustly designed and well-powered randomized controlled trials.

CLINICS CARE POINTS

- Addiction risk is heightened in adolescents who use nicotine productions.
- There are numerous mental health and physical risks associated with adolescent exposure to nicotine products.
- Parents and adolescents can be counseled on the risks associated with nicotine and offered MAT concurrently or in lieu of behavioral interventions.

DISCLOSURE

The authors have nothing to disclose.

REFERENCES

1. CDC Tobacco Free. Burden of tobacco use in the U.S. Centers for Disease Control and Prevention; 2024. Available at: https://www.cdc.gov/tobacco/campaign/tips/resources/data/cigarette-smoking-in-united-states.html. Accessed November 15, 2025.
2. CDC. E-cigarette use among youth. Smoking and tobacco use. 2024. Available at: https://www.cdc.gov/tobacco/e-cigarettes/youth.html. Accessed November 15, 2025.
3. Winickoff JP, Evins AE, Levy S. Vaping in youth. JAMA 2024;332(9):749.
4. American Psychiatric Association. (2013). Diagnostic and statistical manual of mental disorders (5th ed). https://doi.org/10.1176/appi.books.9780890425596.
5. Park-Lee E, Jamal A, Cowan H, et al. Notes from the field: e-cigarette and nicotine pouch use among middle and high school students — united States, 2024. MMWR Morb Mortal Wkly Rep 2024;73(35):774–8.
6. Levine A, Huang Y, Drisaldi B, et al. Molecular mechanism for a gateway drug: epigenetic changes initiated by nicotine prime gene expression by cocaine. Sci Transl Med 2011;3(107). https://doi.org/10.1126/scitranslmed.3003062.
7. Tervo-Clemmens B, Gilman JM, Evins AE, et al. Substance use, suicidal thoughts, and psychiatric comorbidities among high school students. JAMA Pediatr 2024;178(3):310.

8. Glantz SA, Nguyen N, Oliveira Da Silva AL. Population-based disease odds for e-cigarettes and dual use versus cigarettes. NEJM Evid 2024;3(3). https://doi.org/10.1056/EVIDoa2300229.
9. National Academies of Sciences, Engineering, and Medicine. In: Kahn NF, Graham R, editors. Promoting positive adolescent health behaviors and outcomes: thriving in the 21st century. National Academies Press; 2019. Available at: https://www.ncbi.nlm.nih.gov/books/NBK554988/.
10. Yuan M, Cross SJ, Loughlin SE, et al. Nicotine and the adolescent brain. J Physiol 2015;593(16):3397–412.
11. Miech RA, Johnston LD, Patrick ME, et al. Monitoring the future national survey results on drug use, 1975–2024: overview and detailed results for secondary school students. Monitoring the future monograph series. Ann Arbor (MI): Institute for Social Research, University of Michigan; 2025.
12. Jamal A, Park-Lee E, Birdsey J, et al. Tobacco product use among middle and high school students — national youth tobacco survey, United States, 2024. MMWR Morb Mortal Wkly Rep 2024;73(41):917–24.
13. Bauer SE, Macrea M, Casey A, et al. Treatment of nicotine use in adolescents under 18 years of age: an official American Thoracic Society clinical practice guideline. Am J Respir Crit Care Med 2025;211(9). https://doi.org/10.1164/rccm.202507-1577ST.
14. Nuwer R. Mammoths roamed when humans started using tobacco at least 12,300 years ago. Sci Am 2021. Available at: https://www.scientificamerican.com/article/mammoths-roamed-when-humans-started-using-tobacco-at-least-12-300-years-ago/. Accessed November 15, 2025.
15. Courtney R. The health consequences of smoking—50 years of progress: a report of the Surgeon General. 2014. Available at: http://www.surgeongeneral.gov/library/reports/50-years-of-progress/. Accessed November 15, 2025.
16. O'Connor R, Schneller LM, Felicione NJ, et al. Evolution of tobacco products: recent history and future directions. Tob Control 2022;31(2):175–82.
17. Simonavicius E, McNeill A, Shahab L, et al. Heat-not-burn tobacco products: a systematic literature review. Tob Control 2019;28(5):582–94.
18. Breland A, Soule E, Lopez A, et al. Electronic cigarettes: what are they and what do they do? Ann N Y Acad Sci 2017;1394(1):5–30.
19. Butler AR, Lindson N, Livingstone-Banks J, et al. Interventions for quitting vaping. Cochrane Central Editorial Service. Cochrane Database Syst Rev 2025; 2025(1). https://doi.org/10.1002/14651858.CD016058.pub2.
20. Centers for Disease Control and Prevention. Tobacco use among high school students — united States, 1997. MMWR Morb Mortal Wkly Rep 1998;47(12): 229–33.
21. Mejia MC, Adele A, Levine RS, et al. Trends in cigarette smoking among United States adolescents. Ochsner J 2023;23(4):289–95.
22. Glantz S, Jeffers A, Winickoff JP. Nicotine addiction and intensity of e-cigarette use by adolescents in the US, 2014 to 2021. JAMA Netw Open 2022;5(11): e2240671.
23. Kong G, Lee J, Ouellette RR, et al. Modification of electronic nicotine delivery systems among adolescents and young adults. Pediatrics 2024;154(1): e2023063984.
24. Morean ME, Kong G, Camenga DR, et al. High school students' use of electronic cigarettes to vaporize cannabis. Pediatrics 2015;136(4):611–6.
25. Back S, Masser AE, Rutqvist LE, et al. Harmful and potentially harmful constituents (HPHCs) in two novel nicotine pouch products in comparison with regular

smokeless tobacco products and pharmaceutical nicotine replacement therapy products (NRTs). BMC Chem 2023;17(1):9.

26. Han D, Harlow AF, Miech RA, et al. Nicotine pouch and e-cigarette use and co-use among US youths in 2023 and 2024. JAMA Netw Open 2025;8(4):e256739.
27. Khouja J, Sanderson E, Wootton R, et al. Estimating the health impact of nicotine exposure by dissecting the effects of nicotine versus non-nicotine constituents of tobacco smoke: a multivariable Mendelian randomisation study. PLoS Genet 2024;20. https://doi.org/10.1371/journal.pgen.1011157.
28. Soneji S, Barrington-Trimis JL, Wills TA, et al. Association between initial use of e-Cigarettes and subsequent cigarette smoking among adolescents and young adults: a systematic review and meta-analysis. JAMA Pediatr 2017;171(8):788–97.
29. Dautzenberg B, Legleye S, Underner M, et al. Systematic review and critical analysis of longitudinal studies assessing effect of E-Cigarettes on cigarette initiation among adolescent never-smokers. Int J Environ Res Publ Health 2023;20-(20):6936.
30. Sun R, Mendez D, Warner KE. Use of electronic cigarettes among cannabis-naive adolescents and its association with future cannabis use. JAMA Netw Open 2022;5(7):e2223277.
31. Chung J, Lim CCW, Stjepanović D, et al. Adolescent cannabis vaping trends (2021-2023): delta-9-tetrahydrocannabinol, cannabidiol, and synthetic cannabinoids. Am J Prev Med 2025. https://doi.org/10.1016/j.amepre.2025.107655.
32. Goniewicz ML, Knysak J, Gawron M, et al. Levels of selected carcinogens and toxicants in vapour from electronic cigarettes. Tob Control 2014;23(2):133–9.
33. Aherrera A, Lin JJ, Chen R, et al. Metal concentrations in E-Cigarette aerosol samples: a comparison by device type and flavor. Environ Health Perspect 2023;131(12):127004.
34. Salazar MR, Saini L, Nguyen TB, et al. Elevated toxic element emissions from popular disposable e-cigarettes: sources, life cycle, and health risks. ACS Cent Sci 2025;11(8):1345–54.
35. Fowles J, Barreau T, Wu N. Cancer and non-cancer risk concerns from metals in electronic cigarette liquids and aerosols. Int J Environ Res Publ Health 2020;17(6):2146.
36. Travis N, Warner KE, Goniewicz ML, et al. The potential impact of oral nicotine pouches on public health: a scoping review. Nicotine Tob Res 2025;27(4):598–610.
37. Rungraungrayabkul D, Gaewkhiew P, Vichayanrat T, et al. What is the impact of nicotine pouches on oral health: a systematic review. BMC Oral Health 2024;24(1):889.
38. Jobson CLM, Renard J, Szkudlarek H, et al. Adolescent nicotine exposure induces dysregulation of mesocorticolimbic activity states and depressive and anxiety-like prefrontal cortical molecular phenotypes persisting into adulthood. Cerebr Cortex 2019;29(7):3140–53.
39. Abdulhay N, Wiener RC, Wen S, et al. Mental health outcomes associated with electronic cigarette use, combustible tobacco use, and dual use among U.S. adolescents: insights from the National Youth Tobacco Survey. PLOS Ment Health 2025;2(7):e0000370.
40. Treur JL, Munafò MR, Logtenberg E, et al. Using Mendelian randomization analysis to better understand the relationship between mental health and substance use: a systematic review. Psychol Med 2021;51(10):1593–624.

41. Rose JJ, Krishnan-Sarin S, Exil VJ, et al. Cardiopulmonary impact of electronic cigarettes and vaping products: a scientific statement from the American heart Association. Circulation 2023;148(8):703–28.
42. Wold LE, Tarran R, Crotty Alexander LE, et al. Cardiopulmonary consequences of vaping in adolescents: a scientific statement from the American heart Association. Circ Res 2022;131(3):e70–82.
43. Xie W, Kathuria H, Galiatsatos P, et al. Association of electronic cigarette use with incident respiratory conditions among US adults from 2013 to 2018. JAMA Netw Open 2020;3(11):e2020816.
44. Rodriguez-Herrera AJ, de Souza ABF, Castro TF, et al. Long-term e-cigarette aerosol exposure causes pulmonary emphysema in adult female and male mice. Regul Toxicol Pharmacol 2023;142:105412.
45. Dennison Himmelfarb CR, Benowitz NL, Blank MD, et al. Impact of smokeless oral nicotine products on cardiovascular disease: implications for policy, prevention, and treatment: a policy statement from the American heart Association. Circulation 2025;151(1):e1–21.
46. Lunell E, Fagerström K, Hughes J, et al. Pharmacokinetic comparison of a novel non-tobacco-based nicotine pouch (ZYN) with conventional, tobacco-based Swedish snus and American moist snuff. Nicotine Tob Res 2020;22(10):1757–63.
47. Mallock-Ohnesorg N, Rabenstein A, Stoll Y, et al. Small pouches, but high nicotine doses-nicotine delivery and acute effects after use of tobacco-free nicotine pouches. Front Pharmacol 2024;15:1392027.
48. Knight JR, Sherritt L, Shrier LA, et al. Validity of the CRAFFT substance abuse screening test among adolescent clinic patients. Arch Pediatr Adolesc Med 2002;156(6):607–14.
49. DiFranza JR, Savageau JA, Fletcher K, et al. Measuring the loss of autonomy over nicotine use in adolescents: the DANDY (Development and Assessment of Nicotine Dependence in Youths) study. Arch Pediatr Adolesc Med 2002; 156(4):397–403.
50. Levy S, Weiss R, Sherritt L, et al. An electronic screen for triaging adolescent substance use by risk levels. JAMA Pediatr 2014;168(9):822–8.
51. Kelly SM, Gryczynski J, Mitchell SG, et al. Validity of brief screening instrument for adolescent tobacco, alcohol, and drug use. Pediatrics 2014;133(5):819–26.
52. Gryczynski J, McNeely J, Wu LT, et al. Validation of the TAPS-1: a four-item screening tool to identify unhealthy substance use in primary care. J Gen Intern Med 2017;32(9):990–6.
53. Heatherton TF, Kozlowski LT, Frecker RC, et al. The fagerström Test for nicotine dependence: a revision of the fagerström tolerance questionnaire. Br J Addict 1991;86(9):1119–27.
54. Morean ME, Krishnan-Sarin S, O'Malley SS. Comparing cigarette and e-cigarette dependence and predicting frequency of smoking and e-cigarette use in dual-users of cigarettes and e-cigarettes. Addict Behav 2018;87:92–6.
55. American Thoracic Society. Clinical practice guideline: treatment of tobacco and nicotine use in children and adolescents. Am J Respir Crit Care Med 2024;209(4):388–406.
56. Walley SC, Wilson KM, Winickoff JP, et al, Section on Tobacco Control. A public health crisis: electronic cigarettes, vape, and JUUL. Pediatrics 2019;143(6): e20182741.
57. Jenssen BP, Walley SC, Groner JA, et al. E-cigarettes and similar devices. Pediatrics 2019;143(2):e20183652.

58. Hanson K, Allen S, Jensen S, et al. Treatment of adolescent smokers with the nicotine patch. Nicotine Tob Res 2003;5(4):515–26.
59. Moolchan ET, Robinson ML, Ernst M, et al. Safety and efficacy of the nicotine patch and gum for the treatment of adolescent tobacco addiction. Pediatrics 2005;115(4):e407–14.
60. Scherphof CS, van den Eijnden RJ, Engels RC, et al. Long-term efficacy of nicotine replacement therapy for smoking cessation in adolescents: a randomized controlled trial. Drug Alcohol Depend 2014;140:217–20.
61. Smith TA, House RF Jr, Croghan IT, et al. Nicotine patch therapy in adolescent smokers. Pediatrics 1996;98(4 Pt 1):659–67.
62. Gray KM, Carpenter MJ, Lewis AL, et al. Varenicline versus bupropion XL for smoking cessation in older adolescents: a randomized, double-blind pilot trial. Nicotine Tob Res : official journal of the Society for Research on Nicotine and Tobacco 2012;14(2):234–9.
63. Killen JD, Robinson TN, Ammerman S, et al. Randomized clinical trial of the efficacy of bupropion combined with nicotine patch in the treatment of adolescent smokers. J Consult Clin Psychol 2004;72(4):729–35.
64. Muramoto ML, Leischow SJ, Sherrill D, et al. Randomized, double-blind, placebo-controlled trial of 2 dosages of sustained-release bupropion for adolescent smoking cessation. Arch Pediatr Adolesc Med 2007;161(11):1068–74.
65. Niederhofer H, Huber M. Bupropion may support psychosocial treatment of nicotine-dependent adolescents: preliminary results. Pharmacotherapy 2004;24(11):1524–8.
66. Evins AE, Cather C, Reeder HT, et al. Varenicline for youth nicotine vaping cessation: a randomized clinical trial. JAMA 2025;333(21):1876–86.
67. Faessel H, Ravva P, Williams K. Pharmacokinetics, safety, and tolerability of varenicline in healthy adolescent smokers: a multicenter, randomized, double-blind, placebo-controlled, parallel-group study. Clin Ther 2009;31(1):177–89.
68. Gray KM, Baker NL, McClure EA, et al. Efficacy and safety of varenicline for adolescent smoking cessation: a randomized clinical trial. JAMA Pediatr 2019;173(12):1146–53.
69. Zhang L, Gentzke A, Trivers KF, et al. Tobacco cessation behaviors among U.S. middle and high school students, 2020. J Adolesc Health 2022;70(1):147–54.
70. Adams ZW, Kwon E, Aalsma MC, et al. Treatment of adolescent e-cigarette use: limitations of existing nicotine use disorder treatment and future directions for e-cigarette use cessation. J Am Acad Child Adolesc Psychiatry 2021;60(1):14–6.
71. Cavallo DA, Krishnan-Sarin S. Nicotine use disorders in adolescents. Pediatr Clin North Am 2019;66(6):1053–62.
72. Cavallo DA, Cooney JL, Duhig AM, et al. Combining cognitive behavioral therapy with contingency management for smoking cessation in adolescent smokers: a preliminary comparison of two different cbt formats. Am J Addict 2007;16(6):468–74.
73. Krishnan-Sarin S, Duhig AM, McKee SA, et al. Contingency management for smoking cessation in adolescent smokers. Exp Clin Psychopharmacol 2006;14(3):306–10.
74. Barnett E, Sussman S, Smith C, et al. Motivational interviewing for adolescent substance use: a review of the literature. Addict Behav 2012;37(12):1325–34.
75. Rollnick S, Miller WR. What is motivational interviewing? Behav Cogn Psychother 1995;23(4):325–34.

76. Laude JR, Bailey SR, Crew E, et al. Extended treatment for cigarette smoking cessation: a randomized control trial: extended CBT for smoking cessation. Addiction 2017;112(8):1451–9.
77. Bedics J, editor. Handbook of dialectical behavior therapy: theory, research, and evaluation. San Diego: Academic Press; 2020. p. 393.
78. Ritschel LA, Lim NE, Stewart LM. Transdiagnostic applications of DBT for adolescents and adults. APT 2015;69(2):111–28.
79. Dimeff L, Linehan MM. Dialectical behavior therapy for substance abusers. Addict Sci Clin Pract 2008;4(2):39–47.
80. McCall MH, Boyd CT, Kerr ND, et al. Dialectical behavior therapy skills training as a brief intervention for cigarette smoking by patients with cancer: a scoping review and narrative synthesis of related literature. Psychooncology 2025;34(1):e70074.
81. Warner N, Murphy M. Dialectical behaviour therapy skills training for individuals with substance use disorder: a systematic review. Drug Alcohol Rev 2022;41(2):501–16.
82. Cooperman NA, Rizvi SL, Hughes CD, et al. Field test of a dialectical behavior therapy skills training–based intervention for smoking cessation and opioid relapse prevention in methadone treatment. J Dual Diagn 2019;15(1):67–73.
83. Levy SA, Westin AM, Reamy AM, et al. Communication about smoking between depressed adolescents and their parents. Nicotine Tob Res 2010;12(3):191–7.
84. McLaughlin A, Campbell A, McColgan M. Adolescent substance use in the context of the family: a qualitative study of young people's views on parent-child attachments, parenting style and parental substance use. Subst Use Misuse 2016;51(14):1846–55.
85. Harakeh Z, Scholte RHJ, Vermulst AA, et al. Parental factors and adolescents' smoking behavior: an extension of the theory of planned behavior. Prev Med 2004;39(5):951–61.
86. Mahabee-Gittens EM, Khoury JC, Huang B, et al. The protective influence of family bonding on smoking initiation in adolescents by racial/ethnic and age subgroups. J Child Adolesc Subst Abuse 2011;20(3):270–87.
87. Mahabee-Gittens EM, Xiao Y, Gordon JS, et al. The role of family influences on adolescent smoking in different racial/ethnic groups. Nicotine Tob Res 2012;14(3):264–73.
88. Cohen DA, Richardson J, LaBree L. Parenting behaviors and the onset of smoking and alcohol use: a longitudinal study. Pediatrics 1994;94(3):368–75.
89. Andersen MR, Leroux BG, Bricker JB, et al. Antismoking parenting practices are associated with reduced rates of adolescent smoking. Arch Pediatr Adolesc Med 2004;158(4):348.
90. Emory K, Saquib N, Gilpin EA, et al. The association between home smoking restrictions and youth smoking behaviour: a review. Tob Control 2010;19(6):495–506.
91. Skinner ML, Haggerty KP, Catalano RF. Parental and peer influences on teen smoking: are white and Black families different? Nicotine Tob Res 2009;11(5):558–63.
92. Stanton CA, Highland KB, Tercyak KP, et al. Authoritative parenting and cigarette smoking among multiethnic preadolescents: the mediating role of anti-tobacco parenting strategies. J Pediatr Psychol 2014;39(1):109–19.
93. Sartor CE, Ye F, Simon P, et al. Youth perceptions of parental involvement and monitoring, discrepancies with parental perceptions, and their associations

with first cigarette use in black and white girls. J Stud Alcohol Drugs 2020;81(2): 180–9.
94. Piko BF, Balázs MÁ. Authoritative parenting style and adolescent smoking and drinking. Addict Behav 2012;37(3):353–6.
95. White HR, Johnson V, Buyske S. Parental modeling and parenting behavior effects on offspring alcohol and cigarette use: a growth curve analysis. J Subst Abuse 2000;12(3):287–310.
96. Calafat A, García F, Juan M, et al. Which parenting style is more protective against adolescent substance use? Evidence within the European context. Drug Alcohol Depend 2014;138:185–92.
97. Kaliamurthy S, Camenga DR. Clinical approach to the treatment of e-cigarette use among adolescents. Curr Probl Pediatr Adol Health Care 2022;52(6): 101203.
98. Carver H, Elliott L, Kennedy C, et al. Parent–child connectedness and communication in relation to alcohol, tobacco and drug use in adolescence: an integrative review of the literature. Drugs 2017;24(2):119–33.
99. Meyers RJ, Miller WR, Hill DE, et al. Community reinforcement and family training (CRAFT): engaging unmotivated drug users in treatment. J Subst Abuse 1998;10(3):291–308.
100. Lindson-Hawley N, Hartmann-Boyce J, Fanshawe TR, et al. Interventions to reduce harm from continued tobacco use. Cochrane Tobacco Addiction Group. Cochrane Database Syst Rev 2016;2016(12). https://doi.org/10.1002/14651858.CD005231.pub3.
101. Upadhyaya H, Deas D, Brady K. A practical clinical approach to the treatment of nicotine dependence in adolescents. J Am Acad Child Adolesc Psychiatr 2005; 44(9):942–6.

APPENDIX: MONITORING THE FUTURE RESULTS: ELECTRONIC CIGARETTE (NICOTINE VAPES)

Daily Use

Interval	Grade	2020	2021	2022	2023	2024
Daily	8th	0.8	1.1	1.2	1.4	0.8
Daily	10th	3	2.5	3.3	2.4	2.7
Daily	12th	5.2	5.4	6.2	5.8	5.2

30 Day Use

Interval	Grade	2020	2021	2022	2023	2024
30 day	8th	10.5	7.6	7.1	7	5.7
30 day	10th	19.9	19.3	14.2	11.9	9.8
30 day	12th	24.7	19.6	20.7	16.9	15

12 Month Use

Interval	Grade	2020	2021	2022	2023	2024
12 month	8th	16.6	12.1	12	11.4	9.6
12 month	10th	30.7	19.5	20.5	17.6	15.4
12 month	12th	34.5	26.6	27.3	13.2	21

Nicotine Pouches
30 Day Use

Interval	Grade	2023	2024
30 day	8th	0.4	0.2
30 day	10th	1.1	1.8
30 day	12th	1.4	3.5

12 Month Use

Interval	Grade	2023	2024
12 month	8th	0.6	0.6
12 month	10th	1.9	3.4
12 month	12th	2.9	5.9

Lifetime Use

Interval	Grade	2023	2024
Lifetime	8th	1.2	0.8
Lifetime	10th	2.6	4.1
Lifetime	12th	3.6	6.8

Adolescent Opioid Use Disorder

Assessment, Treatment, and Overdose Prevention

Sivabalaji Kaliamurthy, MD, FASAM[a,b,c,d,*],
Prianka Kumar, MD, MPH[e]

KEYWORDS

• Opioid use disorder • Overdose prevention • MOUD • Nasal naloxone

KEY POINTS

- Adolescent overdose deaths have risen dramatically, requiring expansion of prevention and treatment approaches that specifically address widespread fentanyl exposure in youth drug supplies.
- Illicitly manufactured fentanyl is now the primary driver of unintentional overdose mortality among adolescents, reflecting shifts in drug markets and increased potency of available substances.
- Expanding access to overdose prevention strategies, particularly widespread naloxone distribution and education, is an urgent public health priority for protecting adolescents at risk.
- Early identification of opioid use disorder, timely access to medications for OUD, and meaningful family engagement are essential components for improving treatment outcomes among youth.
- Emerging adolescent-focused care models include long-acting injectable medications, school-based interventions, and peer recovery support to enhance engagement and continuity of care.

INTRODUCTION AND BACKGROUND

Over the past decade, the epidemiology of adolescent opioid use has changed. Although the overall prevalence of adolescent substance use has declined or

[a] Division of Psychiatry, Children's National, Washington, DC, USA; [b] Department of Psychiatry and Pediatrics, The George Washington University, Washington, DC, USA; [c] Department of Psychiatry, Howard University, Washington, DC, USA; [d] Yale University, New Haven, CT, USA; [e] Department of Psychiatry, University of California San Diego, San Diego, CA, USA
* Corresponding author. Children's National, Division of Psychiatry, 6833 4th street NW, Washington, DC, 20012.
E-mail address: Skaliamurt@childrensnational.org

Child Adolesc Psychiatric Clin N Am 35 (2026) 677–691
https://doi.org/10.1016/j.chc.2026.05.008 **childpsych.theclinics.com**
1056-4993/26/

Abbreviations	
A-CRA	Adolescent Community Reinforcement Approach
BSFT	brief strategic family therapy
CBT	cognitive behavioral therapy
COWS	Clinical Opiate Withdrawal Scale
DSM-5	Diagnostic and Statistical Manual of Mental Disorders, Fifth Edition
IMF	illicitly manufactured fentanyl
IOP	intensive outpatient programs
MDFT	multidimensional family therapy
MOUDs	medication for opioid use disorder
MST	multisystemic therapy
NSDUH	National Survey on Drug Use and Health
OUD	opioid use disorder
PHP	partial-hospitalization program
UDS	urine drug screen
XR-NTX	extended-releast naltrexone

stayed the same depending on the substance, opioid-related mortality has surged, largely driven by the proliferation of illicitly manufactured fentanyl (IMF) and counterfeit pills.[1] This trend has contributed to a broader increase in pediatric mortality, most pronounced in adolescents aged 15 to 19 years.[1] Despite this alarming pattern, adolescent overdose deaths have often been underrepresented in the national discussions of the opioid crisis, which have focused primarily on adult populations. This omission is concerning, as population-level analyses demonstrate that the rate of increase in opioid overdoses rose more sharply for adolescents in 2020 compared to the overall population (adults and adolescents combined).[2] IMF, a highly potent synthetic opioid distributed in powder and pill form, is now implicated in the majority of opioid-related overdose deaths. Among opioid overdose deaths in adolescents, 83.9% have involved IMFs; yet, only 35% of decedents had documented opioid use history,[3] consistent with reported higher rates of ‘unintentional’ exposure. Compounding this risk, many nonopiate counterfeit pills (such as benzodiazepines, stimulants, among others) can be contaminated with IMFs, which puts adolescent patients at high risk for overdoses.[4] Parallel to these trends, national survey data from the National Survey on Drug Use and Health (NSDUH) demonstrate a significant increase in past-year opioid use disorder (OUD) diagnosis in adolescents age 12 to 25.[5]

Adolescent’s interactions with opioids can be broadly conceptualized across 3 overlapping but nonmutually exclusive groups, as outlined in a recent review paper of the overdose crisis.[6] The first includes adolescents who experiment with substances, do not meet criteria for OUD, and may be unaware of the risks associated with fentanyl. The second group includes adolescents with mental health or trauma history who may seek substances as a way of coping or managing symptoms. The third group is adolescents diagnosed with an opioid use disorder, who may be knowingly or unknowingly using fentanyl. Importantly, adolescents within all 3 categories face high risk of mortality and other opioid-related sequelae.

Historically, opioids have been accessible to adolescents through prescriptions written for parents or other adults in the household. However, adolescents increasing access to nonprescribed drugs from illicit sources now have an additional risk of contamination from illicitly manufactured fentanyl. Even legitimate opioid exposure is not benign; one study estimated that adolescents who are prescribed an opioid for any reason have a 33% increased risk for misuse compared to their peers.[7] Adult data demonstrate decreases in injection and increases in smoking and intranasal opioid administration.[8] We can hypothesize that trends in adolescent populations mirror this pattern.

Despite the rising burden of opioid-related morbidity and mortality among adolescents, a substantial treatment gap persists for youth at risk for opioid use disorder and related harms. A recent study found that 41% of adolescents who died of an overdose between July 2019 and Dec 2021 had a known mental health problem or history of receiving mental health care, but only 11% had a history of receiving substance use treatment.[3] This disparity highlights the missed opportunities for early identification and intervention within the health care systems adolescents already access. Barriers to care include limited availability to adolescent specific addiction services, regulatory and logistic challenges, and provider discomfort with addressing substance use in pediatric health care settings. Medications for opioid use disorder such as buprenorphine, methadone and naltrexone have been studied to have a mortality benefit in adults with OUD,[9] but the literature is not as robust for adolescents, given the challenges with performing large-scale studies in this age group. Nonetheless, emerging data suggest that treatment with these medications is feasible and lifesaving in younger populations and should be routinely considered as part of the treatment plan for adolescents who are diagnosed with OUD.[10–12]

Clinical Presentation and Evaluation

Patient Vignette: A 16-year-old girl presents to the emergency room requesting help to stop using M 30 pills (**Fig.1**). *She reports recent onset of rhinorrhea, myalgias, diarrhea, and restlessness, and expresses concern that she may have influenza or COVID-19. Urine toxicology is negative for all substances tested. (This case is fictitious and presented solely for illustrative purposes; no real patient data were used).*

Evaluation of an adolescent with suspected opioid use must begin with an assessment of their clinical risk and determination of appropriate treatment setting (eg, inpatient, outpatient, residential and so on). Adolescents may present with signs of acute opioid withdrawal, symptoms consistent with opioid use disorder (OUD), or manifestations of a co-occurring psychiatric condition. Presentations are often complicated by overlapping medical, psychological and social stressors, including trauma exposure, housing instability and exploitation. Determining the appropriate level of care requires understanding he acuity of substance use and the severity of psychiatric comorbidity.

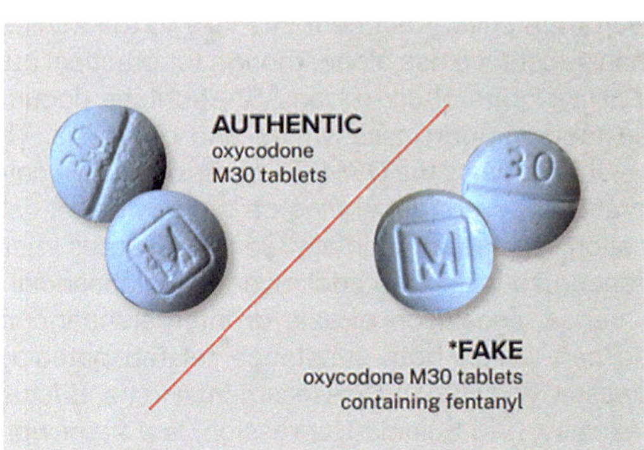

Fig. 1. *Counterfeit *M30* oxycodone tablets containing fentanyl are visually indistinguishable from authentic oxycodone.

In contrast to adults, adolescents often present with rapidly evolving risk for overdose, legal involvement, trafficking, poor engagement and retention in treatment in addition to co-occurring psychiatric illness, family dependence, and developmental vulnerability, all of which must be incorporated into placement decisions. The *American Society of Addiction Medicine (ASAM) Criteria for adolescents* 4th *edition*[13] provides a standardized, multidimensional framework for determining level of care and are increasingly applied to adolescent populations with substance use disorders.

The ASAM Criteria assess 6 core dimensions: (1) acute intoxication, withdrawal, and addiction medications, (2) biomedical conditions, (3) psychiatric and cognitive concerns, (4) substance use-related risks, and (5) recovery environment interactions. In adolescents, particular emphasis is placed on withdrawal risk, suicidality or severe psychiatric symptoms, family supervision, housing stability, and exposure to exploitation or violence. Using these dimensions, clinicians can match youth to an appropriate continuum of care ranging from outpatient treatment (ASAM Level 1), intensive outpatient or partial hospitalization (Level 2), residential treatment (Level 3), or medically managed inpatient services (Level 4).[14]

In practice, adolescents with mild opioid use disorder as defined by *Diagnostic and Statistical Manual of Mental Disorders, Fifth Edition* (DSM 5), stable psychiatric symptoms, and a supportive recovery environment may be safely treated in outpatient or intensive outpatient settings with close follow-up. In contrast, those presenting with moderate to severe withdrawal, polysubstance use, suicidality, unstable housing, or limited caregiver supervision often require higher levels of care, including treatment and evaluation in the emergency department, followed by inpatient stabilization, or residential treatment. Importantly, level-of-care determinations should remain dynamic, with respect to family supervision, housing stability, and reassessment as clinical status evolves.

To further refine placement decisions, Yule and colleagues have proposed a complementary four-quadrant framework for adolescents based on the relative severity of substance use and co-occurring psychiatric illness.[7] Adolescents with low severity in both domains (Quadrant I) may benefit from early intervention and outpatient care, whereas those with high psychiatric severity but lower substance use severity (Quadrant II) are best managed in psychiatric settings with integrated substance use expertise. Adolescents with high substance use severity and lower psychiatric severity (Quadrant III) may benefit from substance-focused programs, while those with high severity in both domains (Quadrant IV) typically require integrated inpatient or residential dual-diagnosis care. When used along with the ASAM Criteria, this model highlights the importance of matching treatment intensity to the adolescent's full clinical complexity rather than substance use alone, though for practical purposes, insurance reimbursements for clinical care often rely on ASAM criteria documentation.

Several structured tools support assessment and diagnosis. The standard diagnostic framework for OUD remains the *DSM-5 Text Revision* (*TR*) criteria, which stratify OUD as mild, moderate, or severe depending on the number of criteria met. Beyond diagnostic classification, a developmentally sensitive assessment is essential to contextualize substance use within the adolescent's psychosocial environment. Behaviors such as tolerance, escalation of use, or interpersonal conflict may emerge rapidly in youth and can reflect both substance related pathology and normative developmental processes. The HEADSS assessment (Home, Education/Employment, Activities, Drugs, Sexuality, and Suicide/Depression) is a framework originally developed in 1991 as a structured way to explore domains in adolescent psychosocial functioning.[15] While this is not a diagnostic tool, the HEADSS assessment can help clinicians understand the impact of substance use on key developmental domains such as school performance, peer relationships, and family functioning. Integrating findings from the HEADSS interview with DSM-5 diagnostic criteria allows clinicians to assess for a more nuanced evaluation of severity and functional impairment, which in turn informs the level of care and engagement strategies.

Assessment of acute opioid withdrawal should be systematic and guided by instruments such as the Clinical Opiate Withdrawal Scale (COWS) which is clinician-administered and the Subjective Opiate Withdrawal Scale, which is completed by patients.[16,17] These tools may also be particularly useful in adolescents, in whom withdrawal symptoms maybe misattributed to viral illnesses, anxiety or other medical conditions, as illustrated in the clinical vignette. Objective measurement of withdrawal severity also informs time-frame for initiation of opioid agonist therapy, particularly buprenorphine, while reducing the risk of precipitated withdrawal.

In addition to clinical assessment, laboratory and toxicology testing can play a role in the evaluation of adolescents with suspected opioid use but results must be interpreted cautiously. A urine drug screen (UDS) is often the first step, but clinicians should be aware that standard immunoassay panels frequently fail to detect synthetic opioids such as fentanyl and its analogs. As a result, a negative UDS does not exclude recent opioid exposure or withdrawal. Expanded or confirmatory testing using gas chromatography–mass spectrometry or liquid chromatography–tandem mass spectrometry can confirm the presence of fentanyl and identify other emerging substances, but these assays often require several days to result,[18] so rarely guide initial management.

Given the evolving drug supply, clinicians should consider targeted testing for adulterants such as xylazine, nitazenes, and benzodiazepine analogs (if these tests are available) in cases of unexplained sedation, prolonged withdrawal, or toxidromes discordant with reported use or UDS. Recognition of these limitations is essential to avoid false reassurances, delays in treatment and inappropriate discharge decisions.

Adjunctive laboratory evaluation is an important but often ignored component of assessment of adolescents with suspected opioid exposure or opioid use disorder. In addition to toxicology, evaluation should include assessment of hepatic and renal function, infectious disease screening (hepatitis B and C, human immunodeficiency virus [HIV], and sexually transmitted infections), and pregnancy testing for female adolescents of reproductive potential. These results inform medication choice and support comprehensive, developmentally appropriate care planning with attention to confidentiality, consent, and state specific regulations.

Regardless of treatment setting, adolescents diagnosed with OUD should be offered medications for opioid use disorder as early as clinically feasible, with careful attention to withdrawal severity, medical comorbidities, and caregiver involvement.

Patient Vignette: In the clinical vignette presented earlier, the patient's negative urine toxicology, withdrawal symptoms mimicking viral illness, and urgency to leave the emergency department illustrate common challenges in adolescent opioid evaluation. Despite limited objective confirmation, integration of clinical findings and psychosocial risk factors supports timely escalation of care and initiation of evidence-based treatment.

Pharmacologic management

Pharmacologic treatment is a central component of effective care for adolescents with opioid use disorder and opioid withdrawal and should be integrated with psychosocial interventions across treatment settings. Medications serve 2 key functions: alleviating symptoms associated with withdrawal and reduce symptoms of cravings and relapse risk. Selection and timing of pharmacologic interventions should be guided by severity of illness, level of care, co-occurring psychiatric and medical conditions, and the adolescent's developmental context, family involvement and capacity for follow-up. Methadone and Buprenorphine are 2 Medication for Opioid Use Disorders (MOUDs) that serve the function of treating acute opioid withdrawal symptoms and OUD. We will discuss the nuances of using these medications along with adjunctive supportive medications in the following sections.

Management of acute opioid withdrawal

Management of acute opioid withdrawal should focus on symptom relief, stabilization, and facilitation of engagement in ongoing treatment. While opioid withdrawal is rarely life threatening, untreated symptoms can be highly distressing and may precipitate lack of engagement in treatment or return to opioid use. Symptom-targeted pharmacotherapy is therefore an important component of care, especially in the hospital setting.

Adjunctive medications such as clonidine for autonomic symptoms, antiemetics for nausea and vomiting, antidiarrheals, nonopioid analgesics, and agents for anxiety or insomnia should be used to improve comfort during withdrawal (**Table 1**). These medications do not treat OUD itself but can reduce suffering and support retention until initiation of definitive treatment of OUD. These medications can be used concurrently while starting MOUD to target specific symptoms.

Medication for Opioid Use Disorder

MOUD is the cornerstone of effective treatment of OUD and significantly reduces the risk of overdose, relapse and all-cause mortality. Despite this evidence, adolescents remain vastly undertreated: fewer than 5% receive any medication for OUD[19]

Table 1
Opioid withdrawal management

Symptom	Medication	Dosing
Nausea/vomiting	Ondansetron	4 mg PO q6h PRN
Nausea/vomiting/anxiety	Prochlorperazine	10 mg PO q6h PRN
Abdominal cramping	Dicyclomine	20 mg PO q6h PRN
Diarrhea	Loperamide	4 mg PO once, then 2 mg PO q6h PRN
Sympathetic activation/ agitation	Clonidine[a]	0.1 mg PO q4h if triggered by COWS score Taper: 0.2 mg PO q6h for 4 d 0.1 mg PO q6h for 2 d 0.05 mg PO q12 h for 1 d
Pain/myalgia	Acetaminophen Ibuprofen	650 mg PO q6h PRN 400 mg PO q6h PRN
Anxiety	Hydroxyzine	25 mg PO q6h PRN

Abbreviation: PO, by mouth; PRN, as needed; q6h, every 6 h.

[a] Monitor blood pressure. Hold for blood pressure lower than 90 systolic and 60 diastolic.

Adapted from Erstad BL, Quaye AN, Hellwege ME, et al. Nonopioid medications for managing opioid withdrawal in acute care settings: A scoping review. *Am J Health Syst Pharm*. 2025;82(16):898–905. https://doi.org/10.1093/ajhp/zxae371

compared with nearly 25% of adults.[20] Barriers to access include limited prescriber comfort, regulatory barriers, and misconceptions regarding safety and appropriateness in younger populations. Recent policy changes including the elimination of the federal Drug Enforcement Administration (DEA) X-waiver requirement have expanded the pool of eligible prescribers and provided an opportunity to close this treatment gap.

Three medications are Food and Drug Administration (FDA) approved to treat OUD in adults, buprenorphine, methadone, and naltrexone, but only Buprenorphine is currently approved for individuals younger than 18 years (>16 and older), and has been used-off label in people aged less than 16 to treat OUD (State specific laws may prohibit off label use of Buprenorphine). Hence, buprenorphine is the most widely used and evidence-supported option in adolescents, with multiple studies demonstrating feasibility, safety, and treatment retention (**Table 2**).[10,21]

EXTENDED RELEASE NALTREXONE

Extended-releast Naltrexone (XR-NTX) remains an option for highly motivated adolescents who have completed detoxification and prefer an antagonist-based approach. Existing studies have demonstrated the feasibility in using naltrexone for adolescents

Table 2
Medication for opioid use disorder

Medication	Mechanism/ Type	Common Formulations	Key Considerations in Adolescents
Buprenorphine	Partial μ-opioid receptor agonist/ κ-antagonist	Sublingual tablets or films (buprenorphine/ naloxone), monthly or weekly extended-release injections	Strong evidence base; flexible dosing; can be initiated in outpatient, ED, or inpatient settings; may be used off-label in <16 y with guardian consent if state laws allow.
Methadone	Full μ-opioid receptor agonist	Daily oral liquid via certified OTP	Effective but limited by regulatory barriers; not available in all states; in states it is available, for adolescents <18 y, often requires 2 failed prior treatments and OTP waiver.
Naltrexone	μ-opioid receptor antagonist	• Oral daily tablets (Not FDA approved for OUD in adults, can be used off label); • Monthly extended-release injection	Requires full detoxification before initiation; adherence challenges; best suited for highly motivated youth with strong support systems. Used off-label in patients younger than 18.

Abbreviation: OTP, opioid treatment program

Adapted from: Camenga DR, Colon-Rivera HA, Muvvala SB. Medications for Maintenance Treatment of Opioid Use Disorder in Adolescents: A Narrative Review and Assessment of Clinical Benefits and Potential Risks. *J Stud Alcohol Drugs*.2019;80(4):393–402.

with OUD in a community treatment model, and preliminary data suggests XR-NTX maybe comparable in effectiveness to other medications for OUD.[22,23] Upon completion of detoxification from opioids, and no earlier than 7 days after last use, adolescents may safely initiate Naltrexone. Although oral Naltrexone is not FDA approved for OUD, it is recommended that adolescents are transitioned to oral naltrexone first and tolerability is established before transition to XR-NTX. Although there are no standardized pediatric guidelines for transitioning adolescents from oral naltrexone to XR-NTX, a commonly used clinical approach is to establish tolerability with oral naltrexone over 7 days, often beginning with 25 mg daily for 3 days followed by 50 mg daily for 4 days before XR-NTX administration. While adult studies demonstrate efficacy comparable to buprenorphine in preventing relapse, youth studies remain limited and highlight challenges related to initiation, injection-site discomfort, and retention.[24]

BUPRENORPHINE INITIATION

If chosen as the MOUD, initiation of buprenorphine should occur once moderate withdrawal is established (COWS $\geq$ 8–12) to avoid precipitated withdrawal. Induction can be safely performed in a variety of settings, including the emergency department, inpatient units, or outpatient clinics, depending on risk level and available supports. Careful patient and family education regarding the induction process is essential particularly for adolescents with limited prior treatment exposure.

For adolescents using fentanyl or high-potency synthetic opioids, traditional induction strategies may be poorly tolerated. In these cases, drawing on research in adults with OUD, microinduction (*low-dose initiation*) strategies maybe a safe and tolerable approach depending on situation.

Patient vignette: For the adolescent described in the vignette, objective signs of withdrawal and disclosure of counterfeit pill use would support buprenorphine initiation in the ED or inpatient hospital setting, with careful counseling and linkage to outpatient follow-up.

MAINTENANCE AND MONITORING

Following induction, buprenorphine dosing should be titrated to suppress cravings and withdrawal symptoms, with typical daily maintenance doses ranging from 8 to 16 mg of buprenorphine (sublingual) and higher doses as needed up to a maximum of 32 mg per day total. (Doses toward the higher end of this range may be required for patients regularly using fentanyl). Treatment duration should not be time-limited; evidence supports sustained maintenance to prevent relapse. Regular monitoring should include urine drug testing, assessment of treatment adherence, side effects, and co-occurring mental health symptoms. Integration of family involvement and psychosocial interventions enhances adherence and long-term outcomes.

TRANSITION AND COORDINATION OF CARE

Medication initiation should be viewed as the beginning of treatment engagement rather than a discrete intervention. Adolescents frequently transition between inpatient, residential, and outpatient settings and lapses in medication access during transition can be a major risk for return to substance use and overdose. Active coordination among addiction medicine, psychiatry, and primary care providers is key to ensure continuity of care. Collaboration with family members and caregivers is essential to ensure medication continuity and to address stigma, which remains a major barrier to adherence.

EMERGING THERAPIES

Advances in pharmacologic treatment of OUD are increasingly focused on improving adherence, safety, and accessibility, especially for younger populations. Several extended-release and alternative delivery systems are under investigation or in early clinical use, offering promising strategies to address developmental and systemic barriers to ongoing care.

Extended-release buprenorphine has garnered particular interest as a mechanism to enhance engagement and reduce the risks associated with daily dosing and diversion. Weekly and monthly injectable formulations provide stable plasma concentrations, minimize fluctuations in craving and withdrawal, and reduce medication-related stigma by eliminating the need for visible daily administration.[25] Early experience in adolescent populations suggests these formulations are well tolerated and highly acceptable, particularly when paired with supportive family or peer engagement models. Emerging evidence also suggests that extended release (ER) formulations are efficacious in patients using fentanyl.[26]

These innovations, alongside integrated psychosocial interventions, represent a shift toward sustained, low-burden, and youth-friendly treatment approaches that may redefine the standard of care for adolescent OUD in the coming decade.

PSYCHOSOCIAL INTERVENTIONS

Patient vignette: Following discharge on buprenorphine, the adolescent described earlier attended her initial outpatient visit but missed subsequent appointments, citing school stress, family conflict, and difficulty navigating transportation. These are common barriers to treatment retention after MOUD initiation. Her caregiver expressed uncertainty about how to support recovery while managing concerns about trust and safety at home. These challenges prompted referral to structured psychosocial treatment, including family-based intervention.

Although they should not replace MOUD, psychosocial interventions should be considered as an essential component of care along with the medication options described earlier. Even when adolescents are able to access pharmacologic treatment, retaining them in care remains a significant challenge.[27] Substance use in adolescence often results in lost developmental opportunities, including disruptions in education, peer relationships, and family functioning, as well as co-occurring mental and physical health conditions. Psychosocial interventions are essential for helping adolescents reengage with their developmental trajectory by supporting treatment adherence, addressing co-occurring psychiatric symptoms, and promoting long-term recovery. These interventions include peer mentoring, prosocial support groups, recovery-oriented high schools, individual and group therapy, intensive outpatient and partial hospitalization programs, and in-home services.

The intensity and setting of psychosocial treatment should be matched to illness severity and level of care, consistent with ASAM Criteria and complementary frameworks described earlier. Standard options for mental health treatment of adolescents include partial-hospitalization programs (PHP), intensive outpatient programs (IOP), residential/inpatient treatment, and dual-diagnosis programs. Some of these options are not specifically tailored for youth with substance use disorders but can still play a role in addressing psychosocial needs and treating co-occurring mental health symptoms. Those who are more medically stable and not acutely at risk of self-harm are appropriate to treat in a PHP, which allows for higher intensity therapeutic interventions. IOPs provide increased flexibility for adolescents that are more stable and can be completed while maintaining school/work responsibilities.

Across treatment settings, there are some key evidence-based therapies that can and should be integrated into care. Several studies support the use of cognitive behavioral therapy (CBT), mindfulness-oriented recovery enhancement, and motivational interviewing in treating adolescents with OUD.[28] CBT functions to help correct maladaptive thought patterns and promote coping and resilience. It is often administered in parallel with physician appointments by licensed therapists. CBT can be administered in both individual and group formats and can be at any of the aforementioned care settings. Motivational interviewing or motivational enhancement therapy is used in the early stages of treatment, with the goal of enhancing a patient's readiness to change. This therapy can be administered in short time-periods, during both intake and follow-up appointments, and is well-regarded for its ability to improve treatment outcomes for all substance use disorders. Mindfulness-based interventions can be used as adjunctive methods alongside the earlier treatments and help build distress tolerance skills and awareness.

Beyond these individual level interventions, it is equally important to involve the family/supportive persons when caring for adolescent with OUD. Strong relationships encourage healthy development in adolescents and allow for support outside the clinic/hospital setting. One treatment modality that leverages family involvement is the Adolescent Community Reinforcement Approach (A-CRA). A-CRA is an evidence-based method with its foundations in CBT, which has demonstrated efficacy in patients with OUD and cannabis use disorder. It involves individual sessions with patients to identify their needs and goals, individual sessions with caregivers to work on problem solving and communication skills, and joint sessions to integrate these skills into the family unit. Studies have demonstrated the feasibility of A-CRA and its potential to improve treatment engagement among patients with opioid use by leveraging the involvement of concerned significant others (CSOs).[29] In the literature, CSOs are typically caregivers, but can also include other family members, friends or partners of patients. A narrative review conducted on the relationship between young adults and CSOs identified that these relationships helped to motivate treatment and recovery, and that the CSOs experienced their own personal benefits through engaging with care.[30] The involvement of CSOs can happen as early as the intake visit, but should be encouraged at any point along a patient's treatment course.

Another evidence-based family intervention relevant to adolescents with opioid use disorder is the brief strategic family therapy (BSFT). BSFT is a manualized, family-based intervention grounded in structural and strategic family therapy principles that targets maladaptive family interaction patterns contributing to adolescent substance use. BSFT is delivered through structured sessions involving adolescents and caregivers, with a focus on strengthening parental leadership, improving communication, and reducing conflict by actively restructuring family interactions. Clinical trials demonstrate that BSFT is feasible in outpatient and community settings and is associated with improved treatment engagement, retention, family functioning, and reductions in adolescent substance use.[31] BSFT is particularly well suited for adolescents whose substance use occurs in the context of family conflict, disengagement, or inconsistent supervision.

Interventions targeting support persons, such as Community Reinforcement and Family Training (CRAFT), also play an important role. CRAFT is a structured, evidence-based approach that equips family members and other CSOs with skills to identify environmental triggers and reinforcers that influence a patient's substance use. The model emphasizes reinforcing nonsubstance-using and treatment-seeking behaviors while withdrawing reinforcement for substance use, without relying on punishment, confrontation, or shaming. Through CRAFT, support persons are trained in nonjudgmental communication strategies, recognizing *windows of opportunity* to encourage engagement in treatment, and principles of harm reduction. Multiple randomized and observational studies have demonstrated that individuals with substance use disorders are significantly more likely to enter treatment when CRAFT-based interventions are used compared with traditional approaches such as confrontational methods or Al-Anon facilitation.[32,33] When structured approaches are not accessible, providers can use principles of family systems approach or to speak to parents in clinic.[34] Providers can also integrate principles from other evidence-based modalities for adolescent substance use that leverage family and broader social systems, such as multisystemic therapy (MST)[35] and multidimensional family therapy (MDFT).[36] MST is an intensive, home- and community-based intervention that targets the multiple systems including family, peers, school, and neighborhood, by addressing risk factors and strengthening protective supports. MDFT is a family-centered treatment that works simultaneously with adolescents, caregivers, and relevant systems to improve family functioning, communication, and problem-solving while reducing substance use and associated behavioral and mental health problems.

Together, these psychosocial interventions complement pharmacologic treatment by addressing the behavioral, emotional, and relational dimensions of opioid use disorder. When integrated with MOUD and delivered in developmentally appropriate setting, these interventions enhance retention, support recovery, and improve long term outcomes for adolescents.

CHALLENGES

Despite growing recognition of the need for evidence-based treatment of adolescent opioid use disorder, multiple barriers continue to limit access and continuity to care. Patients only benefit from MOUD initiation in the hospital, home, or clinic if they can continue to access the medications in the community. There are several geographic and systemic barriers that can limit access to MOUD, including availability of prescribers, location of clinics, and insurance coverage. Relatively few physicians regularly prescribe MOUD to adolescents, and patients may need to travel far distances to see these providers. Families may face additional logistical challenges, including difficulty with transportation or missing work for recurring appointments. An assessment of these potential barriers should be made at the intake appointment, and relevant social resources should be provided to patient and parent.

Regulatory and systems level barriers further complicate care. If the patient/provider selects methadone for treatment, there are additional challenges as methadone is only dispensed at designated OTPs. Before 2024, federal regulations required adolescents to have 2 failed attempts at abstinence-based treatments for OUD before being permitted to initiate methadone. Though this requirement has now been lifted, access to OTPs based on geography and timing/missing school are still barriers to ongoing care.[37]

Legal considerations related to minor consent and confidentiality laws are another important challenge. Minor consent laws for substance use disorders vary from state to state. Some states allow minors to consent for substance use disorder treatment without parental approval, but others require parental approval. Even in states where minors can consent for MOUD themselves, the age of consent may vary (12–16), and insurance claims/explanation of benefits sent for the medication can disclose a substance use disorder diagnosis to parents unintentionally. While parental involvement is often a key component of effective treatment, in some cases legal confidentiality requirements can result in adolescents avoiding care. All providers should verify their state-specific laws and policies before initiating treatment and engaging in discussion with adolescents and their caregivers.

Finally, stigma remains a pervasive barrier at multiple levels, including individual, familial, institutional, and provider-related stigma. Studies have demonstrated that health care providers often have more negative attitudes and weaker treatment efficacy for patients with substance use disorders compared to other stigmatized conditions.[38] Adolescents may internalize stigma related to substance use or medication treatment through interactions at school including disciplinary action and peer labeling. Caregivers and clinicians may harbor misconceptions regarding safety, appropriateness, or prognosis. A survey conducted on young adults age 19 to 29 revealed that they had moderate levels of stigma toward opioid use, which was negatively correlated for support for policies favorable for people with OUD.[39] Addressing stigma through education, nonjudgmental communication, and normalization of MOUD as standard medical care is essential to improving access and outcomes for adolescents with opioid use disorder.

OVERDOSE PREVENTION

Overdose education and distribution of naloxone is a public health strategy with proven benefits in the adult population in reducing opioid-related mortality[40]; however, fewer data exist for adolescents and their implementation in the adolescent population has lagged. Among the youth who died from an overdose between 2019 and 2021, naloxone was only used 33% of the time.[3] This signals an important opportunity for the prevention of overdose by screening at-risk youth and providing overdose education and naloxone. One study found that for every one naloxone prescription dispensed for youths, nearly 96 were dispensed for adults.[41] This disparity persists despite increasing evidence that adolescent are at high risk of unintentional overdose, particularly in the context of fentanyl-contaminated counterfeit pills.

Traditional risk-based approaches to overdose prevention may be insufficient for adolescents. While evidence-based screening for substance use in adolescent exists, there are no universally accepted method to screen youth for potential high-risk substance use, and with the introduction of counterfeit pills into the recreational market, any/all substance use has the potential to be fatal. As a result, overdose risk cannot be reliably inferred from self-reported substance use patterns or diagnostic thresholds alone.

In this context, universal overdose education and naloxone distribution represents a developmentally appropriate, preventive approach to adolescent care. This recommendation also makes it easier to navigate specific challenges with confidentiality and disclosure that arise when treating youth. Many adolescents may not disclose substance use even when they are screened, and those who do may face legal/parental consequences. Therefore, naloxone distribution and overdose prevention education should be provided as a standard of care and justified as a proactive safety measure that emphasizes preparedness. Parents can be reassured that naloxone is meant as a safety precaution, not because overdose is expected, but because the current drug supply is unpredictable. Providing more widespread access to this education not only saves lives but also helps shift community attitudes and reduce the stigma attached to carrying naloxone.

Patient vignette: As part of discharge planning from the hospital, the adolescent and her caregiver received overdose education and naloxone, framed as a universal safety measure given the fentanyl-contaminated drug supply. Although the patient initially resisted broader family involvement, she agreed to limited caregiver engagement focused on safety planning and medication continuity. This approach balanced autonomy with protection and illustrates how universal overdose prevention can be implemented even amid diagnostic uncertainty, evolving engagement, and confidentiality concerns.

CLINICS CARE POINTS

- *Medications for Opioid Use Disorder (MOUD) are the standard of care for adolescents with (Opioid Use Disorder) OUD* and should be offered across clinical settings including, Emergency departments, inpatient settings and outpatient clinics.
- *Universal overdose education and naloxone distribution should be incorporated into adolescent care,* as overdose risk cannot be reliably predicted based on disclosure, diagnosis, or perceived substance type.
- *Psychosocial interventions should be integrated with, not substituted for, pharmacologic treatment,* with emphasis on engagement, retention, and sustained adherence rather than abstinence alone.
- *Family involvement enhances treatment engagement and outcomes* and should be encouraged when safe and appropriate, using developmentally informed and trauma-sensitive approaches.

DISCLOSURE

S. Kaliamurthy has previously provided consulting services through Tranquil Clinical Research and Consulting Services LLC (completed). S. Kaliamurthy receives research funding and salary support from the District of Columbia Department of Behavioral Health (Opioid Abatement Funds and State Opioid Response Grant), Howard University Department of Psychiatry, Children's National Division of Psychiatry, and the AAAP/SAMHSA Opioid Response Network. These relationships are unrelated to the content of this manuscript. P. Kumar has nothing to disclose.

REFERENCES

1. Gaither JR. National trends in pediatric deaths from fentanyl, 1999-2021. JAMA Pediatr 2023;177(7):733.
2. Friedman J, Godvin M, Shover CL, et al. Trends in drug overdose deaths among US adolescents, January 2010 to June 2021. JAMA 2022;327(14):1398.
3. Tanz LJ, Dinwiddie AT, Mattson CL, et al. Drug overdose deaths among persons aged 10–19 years — united States, July 2019–December 2021. MMWR Morb Mortal Wkly Rep 2022;71(50):1576–82.
4. Wightman RS, Chadronet T, Volpe B, et al. Substances in counterfeit prescription pills seized by law enforcement, 2017-2022. JAMA 2024;331(21):1860.
5. NSDUH. Key substance use and mental health indicators in the United States: results from the 2023 National Survey on drug use and health. Center for Behavioral Health Statistics and Quality, Substance Abuse and Mental Health Services Administration; 2024. Available at: https://www.samhsa.gov/data/report/2023-nsduh-annual-national-report.
6. Friedman J, Hadland SE. The overdose crisis among U.S. adolescents. N Engl J Med 2024;390(2):97–100.

7. Yule AM, Lyons RM, Wilens TE. Opioid use disorders in adolescents-updates in assessment and management. Curr Pediatr Rep 2018;6(2):99–106.
8. Karandinos G, Unick J, Ondocsin J, et al. Decrease in injection and rise in smoking and snorting of heroin and synthetic opioids, 2000–2021. Drug Alcohol Depend 2024;263:111419.
9. Larochelle MR, Bernson D, Land T, et al. Medication for opioid use disorder after nonfatal opioid overdose and Association with mortality: a cohort study. Ann Intern Med 2018;169(3):137–45.
10. Kaliamurthy S, Straton E, Kumar P, et al. Brief report on outpatient treatment of adolescent opioid use disorder. J Addict Med 2025;19(2):230–2.
11. Ryan SA, Gonzalez PK, COMMITTEE ON SUBSTANCE USE AND PREVENTION. Medication-assisted treatment of adolescents with opioid use disorders. Pediatrics 2016;138(3):e20161893.
12. Kaliamurthy S, Straton E, Kumar P. Home initiation of buprenorphine in adolescents with opioid use disorder: a preliminary feasibility study. J Child Adolesc Psychopharmacol 2026;36(4):235–9.
13. American Society of Addiction Medicine. The ASAM Criteria: 4th Edition, Clinical Practice Guideline, Volume 2: Adolescents and Transition-Aged Youth. 2026.
14. The American Society of Addiction Medicine. The ASAM Criteria: treatment criteria for addictive, substance-related, and co-occurring conditions (4th edition). In: Hazelden; 2023.
15. Cohen E, Mackenzie RG, Yates GL. HEADSS, a psychosocial risk assessment instrument: implications for designing effective intervention programs for runaway youth. J Adolesc Health 1991;12(7):539–44.
16. Wesson DR, Ling W. The Clinical Opiate Withdrawal Scale (COWS). J Psychoactive Drugs 2003;35(2):253–9.
17. Gossop M. The development of a short opiate withdrawal scale (SOWS). Addict Behav 1990;15(5):487–90.
18. Marchei E, Ferri MA, Torrens M, et al. Ultra-high performance liquid chromatography-high resolution mass spectrometry and high-sensitivity gas chromatography-mass spectrometry screening of classic drugs and new psychoactive substances and metabolites in urine of consumers. Int J Mol Sci 2021;22(8):4000.
19. Hadland SE, Bagley SM, Rodean J, et al. Receipt of timely addiction treatment and Association of Early Medication treatment with retention in care among youths with opioid use disorder. JAMA Pediatr 2018;172(11):1029.
20. Dowell D, Brown S, Gyawali S, et al. Treatment for opioid use disorder: population estimates — united States, 2022. MMWR Morb Mortal Wkly Rep 2024;73(25):567–74.
21. Hadland SE, Kimmel SD, Yan S, et al. Buprenorphine treatment duration and adherence among youth and subsequent health outcomes. Pediatrics 2025;156(6):e2025071147.
22. Fishman MJ, Winstanley EL, Curran E, et al. Treatment of opioid dependence in adolescents and young adults with extended release naltrexone: preliminary case-series and feasibility. Addiction 2010;105(9):1669–76.
23. Mitchell SG, Fletcher JB, Monico LB, et al. Comparing outcomes of extended-release naltrexone in adolescents and young adults with opioid use disorder. J Subst Use Addict Treat 2024;163:209162.
24. Lee JD, Nunes EV, Novo P, et al. Comparative effectiveness of extended-release naltrexone versus buprenorphine-naloxone for opioid relapse prevention

(X:BOT): a multicentre, open-label, randomised controlled trial. Lancet 2018;391(10118):309–18.
25. Lintzeris N, Dunlop AJ, Haber PS, et al. Patient-reported outcomes of treatment of opioid dependence with weekly and monthly subcutaneous depot vs daily sublingual buprenorphine: a randomized clinical trial. JAMA Netw Open 2021;4(5): e219041.
26. Shiwach R, Le Foll B, Alho H, et al. Comparison of extended-release buprenorphine doses for treating high-risk opioid use: a randomized clinical trial. JAMA Netw Open 2025;8(12):e2548043.
27. Mintz CM, Presnall NJ, Sahrmann JM, et al. Age disparities in six-month treatment retention for opioid use disorder. Drug Alcohol Depend 2020;213:108130.
28. Welsh JW, Mataczynski MJ, Nguyen MD, et al. A review of behavioral therapies in adolescents with opioid use disorder. Harv Rev Psychiatry 2020;28(5):305–15.
29. Godley MD, Passetti LL, Subramaniam GA, et al. Adolescent community reinforcement approach implementation and treatment outcomes for youth with opioid problem use. Drug Alcohol Depend 2017;174:9–16.
30. Porter NP, Dunnsue S, Hammond C, et al. Lessons learned from concerned significant others: a qualitative analysis on involvement in services for young adult opioid use disorder. Front Public Health 2025;13:1512529.
31. Robbins MS, Szapocznik J, Horigian VE, et al. Brief strategic family therapy for adolescent drug abusers: a multi-site effectiveness study. Contemp Clin Trials 2009;30(3):269–78.
32. Roozen HG, De Waart R, Van Der Kroft P. Community reinforcement and family training: an effective option to engage treatment-resistant substance-abusing individuals in treatment. Addiction 2010;105(10):1729–38.
33. Meyers RJ, Miller WR, Smith JE, et al. A randomized trial of two methods for engaging treatment-refusing drug users through concerned significant others. J Consult Clin Psychol 2002;70(5):1182–5.
34. Horigian VE, Anderson AR, Szapocznik J. Family-based treatments for adolescent substance use. Child Adolesc Psychiatr Clin N Am 2016;25(4):603–28.
35. Van Der Stouwe T, Asscher JJ, Stams GJJM, et al. The effectiveness of Multisystemic Therapy (MST): a meta-analysis. Clin Psychol Rev 2014;34(6):468–81.
36. Liddle HA. Multidimensional family therapy: evidence base for transdiagnostic treatment outcomes, change mechanisms, and implementation in community settings. Fam Process 2016;55(3):558–76.
37. Amiri S, McDonell MG, Denney JT, et al. Disparities in access to opioid treatment programs and office-based buprenorphine treatment across the rural-urban and area deprivation continua: a US nationwide small area analysis. Value Health 2021;24(2):188–95.
38. Parish CL, Feaster DJ, Pollack HA, et al. Healthcare provider stigma toward patients with substance use disorders. Addict Abingdon Engl 2025;120(10): 2005–19.
39. Adams ZW, Taylor BG, Flanagan E, et al. Opioid use disorder stigma, discrimination, and policy attitudes in a national sample of U.S. young adults. J Adolesc Health 2021;69(2):321–8.
40. Razaghizad A, Windle SB, Filion KB, et al. The effect of overdose education and naloxone distribution: an umbrella review of systematic reviews. Am J Public Health 2021;111(8):e1–12.
41. Terranella A, Guy G, Mikosz C. Naloxone dispensing to youth ages 10–19: 2017–2022. Pediatrics 2024;154(4):e2023065137.

From Clinic to Capitol

Advocacy Skills for Child and Adolescent Psychiatrists Addressing Adolescent Substance Use Disorders

Debra E. Koss, MD, DFAACAP, DFAPA[a,*], Falisha Gilman, MD[b]

KEYWORDS

- Substance use disorders in adolescents • Advocacy • Legislative advocacy
- Health policy • Advocacy education • Residency training • Professionalism
- Physician advocacy

KEY POINTS

- Adolescents who use substances are at risk for developing a use disorder and therefore require access to screening and early intervention.
- Adolescents with substance use disorders face significant barriers to care due to structural, financial, and workforce limitations.
- Child and adolescent psychiatrists play a critical advocacy role, using clinical expertise to influence policy.
- Effective advocacy requires teachable core skills—persuasive communication, systems navigation, coalition building, and strategic leadership—and should be taught during training and professional development.

INTRODUCTION

Substance use disorders (SUDs) in adolescence are a major public health concern associated with acute and long-term morbidity and mortality. Early onset substance use is associated with increased risk for co-occurring psychiatric disorders, medical problems, neurocognitive impairment, poor academic performance, accidental injuries, and death.[1,2] According to Kaiser Family Foundation reporting of absolute counts, adolescent overdose fatalities declined slightly from 721 in 2022 to 708 in 2023; however, the number remains more than twice as high as prepandemic levels, 282 deaths in 2019.[3] Research has advanced the understanding of adolescent substance use including information on prevalence, neurobiology, risk factors, prevention,

[a] Department of Psychiatry, Rutgers Robert Wood Johnson Medical School, Piscataway, NJ, USA; [b] Department of Psychiatry, Yale University School of Medicine, New Haven, CT, USA
* Corresponding author. 270 Sparta Avenue, Suite 104, PMB 144, Sparta, NJ 07871.
E-mail address: dekoss6@gmail.com

Child Adolesc Psychiatric Clin N Am 35 (2026) 693–706
https://doi.org/10.1016/j.chc.2026.05.003 **childpsych.theclinics.com**
1056-4993/26/

Abbreviations	
AACAP	American Academy of Child and Adolescent Psychiatry
ACGME	Accreditation Council for Graduate Medical Education
ASAM	American Society of Addiction Medicine
CAPs	child and adolescent psychiatrists
CoCM	Collaborative Care Model
PAC	political action committees
SUD	substance use disorders

screening, and treatment, yet adolescents continue to experience difficulty accessing care. In 2024, among individuals aged 12 or older who were classified as needing substance use treatment in the past year, only about 1 in 5 received substance use treatment.[4] Barriers to care include stigma, limited resources, cost of treatment, lack of mental health parity, and work force shortages.

FRAMING THE ISSUE: WHY ADVOCACY IS ESSENTIAL IN ADOLESCENT SUBSTANCE USE CARE

Solutions to these barriers must be informed by scientific research and may be delivered via novel health care policies that result in transformation in health care systems. Clinicians, researchers, policy makers and people living with SUDs all play a critical role in identifying and advocating for these solutions. Child and adolescent psychiatrists (CAPs) are uniquely positioned to contribute to these advocacy initiatives. Medical education and residency and fellowship training provide CAPs with a comprehensive understanding of the neurobiological and psychosocial underpinnings of SUDs, evidence-based prevention and treatment strategies, and an awareness of evidence gaps. CAPs can share this knowledge with stakeholders and decision-makers in an accessible and relatable way, promoting positive beliefs about mental health and substance use, correcting myths and misconceptions that are associated with stigma, and advocating for research to expand our knowledge base to ensure policies are well-informed.

Advocacy is central to the professional identity of CAPs. Like all physicians, we have a duty to address the health and well-being of individual patients as well as the broader populations we serve. Guidance regarding this professional duty is provided by our professional medical organizations. For example, the American Medical Association Declaration of Professional Responsibilities reaffirms a physician's commitment to *advocate for the social, economic, educational, and political changes that ameliorate suffering and contribute to human well-being*.[5] This principle has also been supported by the American Psychiatric Association. 6[6] In addition, the American Academy of Child and Adolescent Psychiatry (AACAP) Code of Ethics outlines in Principle IX that *child and adolescent psychiatrists...[are] urged and encouraged to advocate for provision of appropriate care and services for all youths*.[7] With these principles guiding our advocacy initiatives, we understand that the needs of patients are the priority.

As CAPs, we recognize that mental health and SUDs outcomes are shaped by upstream systems, such as education, housing, and community infrastructure. Improving these through systemic interventions can improve care outcomes, therefore these interventions become the targets for legislative advocacy. Addressing upstream factors in this way shifts focus toward prevention and early intervention, alongside treatment. To maximize population level improvements in pediatric health outcomes, CAPs must step into the legislative arena, interact with lawmakers at the local, state or federal level, and contribute to the development and implementation of health care policies, laws, and regulations. Legislative solutions require bipartisan support; therefore, our advocacy will include discourse with lawmakers from both political parties. Our talking points should be grounded in scientific research and clinical experience, focusing on improving patient outcomes while not being derailed by partisan politics. One need only look to the impact of naloxone distribution programs to understand the impact of legislative advocacy on health outcomes.

CLINICAL VIGNETTE: STATE-LEVEL NALOXONE ACCESS

A 16-year-old with opioid use disorder presents to the emergency room after a nonfatal overdose. The ER psychiatrist prescribes naloxone, but the pharmacy is out of stock, and even if available, the copay is unaffordable. The family returns home full of fear another overdose might occur. His parents are aware that another overdose could occur at any moment. Even if they had access to naloxone, they are unsure about how to use it in an emergency. The patient expresses relief of not having to carry naloxone, embarrassed by the stigma attached to his diagnosis. These gaps in availability, affordability, knowledge, and acceptance leave the family and patient vulnerable, despite clear medical guidance.

This vignette illustrates how gaps in naloxone availability, affordability, education, and stigma can persist despite appropriate clinical care, and will be revisited to demonstrate how state-level policy advocacy can address these barriers.

CORE ADVOCACY SKILLS FOR PSYCHIATRISTS

Mapping Clinical Competencies to Advocacy Skills

The clinical skill sets CAPs use daily—assessment, treatment planning, therapeutic communication, and collaboration—are readily translatable to advocacy. Advocacy specific skill sets, including strategic leadership, persuasive communication, systems navigation, and coalition building, closely parallel these familiar competencies, positioning CAPs to be highly effective advocates. Recognizing this connection can lower barriers to engagement, highlighting that we are applying expertise we already possess rather than learning entirely new skills. **Table 1** illustrates how these core advocacy skill sets map directly onto clinical competencies.

Choosing Your Advocacy Priority

Each of these four core advocacy skill sets, strategic leadership, persuasive communication, systems navigation, and coalition building, can be applied across a range of advocacy topics, such as expanding access to SUD treatment to enforcing mental health parity. Before implementing these skills, choose an advocacy priority that you are passionate about. Advocacy is often a long-term effort, and sustained commitment is easier when you remain motivated by an issue you care about. Once a priority is chosen, the next step is to apply strategic leadership—setting clear goals, prioritizing actions, and guiding efforts over time to maximize impact.

Strategic Leadership

Strategic leadership, a concept often applied in business to guide organizations toward long-term goals, refers to *the ability to anticipate, envision, maintain flexibility, and empower others to create strategic change as necessary.*[8] In the context of advocacy, strategic leadership provides the vision needed to sustain advocacy, ensuring that each step aligns with the broader advocacy goal rather than short-term fixes.

Table 1
Mapping clinical competencies to advocacy skills

Clinical Skill	Parallel Advocacy Skill	Example
Treatment planning, clinical decision-making, and mentorship	Strategic leadership	Provide resident supervision in clinic → mentor next generation of advocacy champions.
Therapeutic communication	Persuasive communication	Discuss confidentiality with teen → write op-ed on importance of adolescent privacy laws for SUD care.
Patient assessment and care coordination	Systems navigation	Identify access issues for patients in rural areas → participate in federal grant application for accessible, affordable internet.
Multidisciplinary collaboration	Coalition building	Coordinate with a social worker to address a patient's housing need → partner with juvenile justice & community youth groups to decriminalize homelessness.

Vision must be present at the start of an advocacy campaign. Without clear advocacy goals, disorganization ensues, advocacy skills are ineffective, and success becomes challenging. Time is a limiting factor for CAPs to get started in advocacy, and a lack of focus can make engagement feel overwhelming and unproductive. Starting with a clear goal, such as making naloxone available in all schools, helps protect valuable time by ensuring that every advocacy step is productive.

Resilience[9] is essential, since advocacy often meets resistance, whether from stigma or legislative gridlock. Efforts to secure parity enforcement for adolescent SUD treatment may stall repeatedly in the state legislature, requiring CAPs to refine strategies and persist over years. *Decision-making* enables psychiatrists to allocate limited resources effectively and prioritize high-impact strategies. For example, deciding to advocate for a state policy that reimburses telepsychiatry at parity for adolescents in rural counties, allows focus on a single, achievable intervention rather than attempt to address every rural access barrier at once. *Strategizing* involves organizing efforts to guide the advocacy, both in the short and long term. This might mean timing advocacy for school-based prevention funding around the release of state education budgets.[9]

Finally, *mentorship* allows for advocacy sustainability, ensuring that the knowledge, skills, and persistence required for effective change are passed on to the next generation of CAPs. By actively training residents and fellows in advocacy and modeling engagement with legislative initiatives, mentors lay the groundwork to expand the physician-advocate workforce. Building on this principle, it is essential to examine how psychiatry training programs can systematically cultivate advocacy skills, provide experiential opportunities, and create structured pathways for CAPs to grow into confident, effective advocates. Additionally, professional development programs, whether in academia or professional organizations, should prioritize advocacy education, support mentorship programs, and reward engagement in advocacy. These efforts build upon the foundation laid in training and invite those no longer in training to engage in this professional responsibility.

Persuasive Communication

At the core of advocacy is persuasive communication, translating our clinical experiences into compelling messages that inspire others to act. This is a skill CAPs use with patients through motivational interviewing. In advocacy, it involves applying the same principles to engage decision-makers, such as legislators or community leaders. This starts with *message framing*, the process of using *underlying moral, psychological, and cognitive factors to form convincing messaging about an issue*.[9] This is accompanied by the *advocacy ask*—a specific, actionable request made to a decision-maker. Knowing your audience is key, as it shapes the content and tone of the message and the ask. For instance, asking a US Senator to support a state bill would be unproductive, since they lack authority over state legislation. It is also helpful to anticipate potential opposition so you can address counterarguments effectively and identify areas where negotiation can help move your shared goals forward.

When translating clinical experiences into persuasive communication, *storytelling* is one of the most effective strategies, especially when the narrative connects to local challenges. Stories stick, making abstract policy issues tangible and memorable. As Holly Amaya, cofounder of Story Imprinting, emphasizes, psychiatrist-advocates should ask: Where are the narrative opportunities? What do you want your audience to know, feel, and do?[10] For example, when discussing Collaborative Care Model (CoCM) with a state legislator, a psychiatrist, who is a constituent and practices in his district, might describe a 17-year-old with co-occurring depression and cannabis use disorder whose primary care pediatrician lacked timely psychiatric support. Delays in medication adjustments and therapy referrals led to missed school and worsening symptoms. Implementing CoCM would provide real-time psychiatric input, enabling faster care and improved outcomes—making the policy issue relatable to the legislator. To protect patient confidentiality, such stories should be composites of multiple clinical encounters and never disclose protected health information.

Message framing, storytelling, and the advocacy ask are all key to effective written and oral communication. *Written communication*, such as op-eds, policy briefs, or professional social media posts can raise awareness and mobilize support. A well-timed op-ed in a local newspaper can draw attention to a topic, such as long emergency room wait times for inpatient psychiatric beds, and inspire action, for example, encouraging readers to contact their legislators to support increased Medicaid funding. Increasingly, professional use of social media platforms (eg X, LinkedIn) allow psychiatrists to reach broad audiences to highlight needs in real time, such as trends on fentanyl contamination, and amplify the voices of individuals with lived experiences. *Oral communication*, including elevator pitches, public testimony, or presentations to community groups, allows direct engagement with decision-makers and can have an immediate impact. A 30-s pitch to a legislator on prior authorization delays, providing public testimony on a scope-of-practice bill, and speaking to a school board about the need for substance use prevention curriculum are examples of how direct contact with a decision-maker can have meaningful impact.

Systems Navigation

Systems navigation enables psychiatrists to turn clinical insights into systemic change. First, psychiatrists must have *systems knowledge*,[9] an understanding of the systems that their patients interact with, including health care, education, child welfare, and juvenile justice systems, as well as knowledge of legislative processes, funding streams, and regulatory levers.

Once systems knowledge is acquired, it helps to inform the practice of *structural competency, the trained ability to discern how a host of issues defined clinically as symptoms, attitudes, or diseases ... also represent the downstream implications of a number of upstream decisions about such matters as healthcare and food delivery systems, zoning laws, urban and rural infrastructures, medicalization, or even about the very definitions of illness and health.*[11] This practice frames stigma and injustice within a broader conceptualization, recognizing that forces outside of individual patient encounters shape health outcomes. Structural competency moves beyond identifying the systems that influence clinical presentation to envisioning—and ultimately implementing—structural interventions. Advocacy is the mechanism through which these interventions become reality.

Clinical experiences uniquely position CAPs to identify system shortcomings, such as unnecessary prior authorization requirements. Once a shortcoming has been identified, CAPs can *translate clinical experiences* into advocacy actions using systems knowledge and practicing structural competency. For instance, a CAP treating a teen with alcohol use disorder who is frequently missing school may need to understand how the education system handles absenteeism and how insurance prior authorizations affect access to injectable naltrexone. Having identified gaps in treatment, the psychiatrist proposes potential solutions at 2 levels: at the school level, implement excused absences for treatment appointments; at the state level, advocate for streamlined prior authorization policies to reduce delays in care. Through the lens of structural competency, the psychiatrist identified upstream systemic factors impacting individual care outcomes, which guided advocacy interventions. This approach not only improves individual patient care but also the broader system, shifting the focus from solely treatment to prevention and early intervention.

Coalition Building

Coalition building is the process of forming an alliance for shared action and recognizes that meaningful change cannot happen in isolation. The structure and composition of a coalition should be guided by the advocacy priority, proposed intervention, and intended audience. Let's use the example of an advocacy campaign aimed at improving SUD treatment access in rural areas through a state statute that ensures permanent pay parity for telehealth services.

The process of coalition building begins with *formation*—thoughtfully recruiting members who share the coalition's vision while bringing complementary perspectives and expertise.[12] In our example, this could include state medical societies, rural health providers, and patient advocacy groups. Once the coalition is established, members should *define roles* and responsibilities based on available resources.[12] For instance, the state medical society has grant funding for printed materials, a rural health provider writes an op-ed to raise awareness of the issue, and patient advocacy groups mobilize constituents to contact their legislators.

Next, coalitions work to *amplify their advocacy goals* through partnerships with others.[12] In our example, a state legislator who has championed other telehealth bills agrees to sponsor the legislation and provides guidance on delivering effective oral testimony at a public hearing.

Throughout this process, it is essential to regularly *evaluate* progress and identify opportunities to deepen impact.[12] The coalition organizes a *Rural Telehealth Day* event, bringing together stakeholders and local media to highlight gaps in care, share patient stories, and demonstrate broad support. Legislators attending the event gain real patient examples of rural access challenges and receive clear recommendations from the coalition on how to address the problem.

From skills to impact

In summary, these 4 skill sets create a foundation for effective advocacy that amplifies impact beyond individual clinical encounters (**Table 2**).

These advocacy skills develop over time and can be strengthened through available resources including *A Psychiatrist's Guide to Advocacy*, the AACAP's Advocacy Toolkit, and the APA's Action Center. Psychiatrists can also seek mentorship from an advocacy champion in their clinic, health system, or state to start, sustain, and

Table 2
Core advocacy skills illustrated through subskills and key actions

Skill Set	Subskills	Key Actions
Strategic Leadership	Vision	Define advocacy objectives, monitor progress, and maintain long-term focus.
	Resilience	Maintain persistence, manage setbacks constructively, and sustain advocacy efforts.
	Decision-making	Allocate resources effectively, focus on strategies with the greatest impact.
	Strategizing	Plan, prioritize, and guide collective efforts for maximum impact.
	Mentorship	Train colleagues, cultivate advocacy champions, and share knowledge and opportunities.
Persuasive Communication	Message Framing	Stay solution-focused, know your audience, and anticipate counterarguments.
	The Advocacy Ask	A clear, actionable request to the decision-maker.
	Storytelling	Humanize policy issues with clinical experiences to make messages memorable.
	Written	Draft compelling op-eds, policy briefs, testimony, and professional social media content.
	Oral	Deliver concise, persuasive messages with an ask during elevator pitches and testimony.
Systems Navigation	Systems Knowledge	Understand health care, education, child-welfare, and justice systems; know legislative processes, funding streams, and regulatory levers.
	Translating Clinical Experience	Use real-world examples to develop actionable solutions.
	Structural Competency	Recognize and respond to upstream social, economic, and environmental factors that impact health.
Coalition Building[12]	Formation	Connect with organizations, build alliances, and negotiate priorities.
	Define Roles	Delegate tasks based on resources and expertise.
	Amplify Goals	Partner with outside agencies to further impact.
	Evaluation	Assess progress, refine roles, and expand coalition.

expand their impact. Additionally, once an advocacy priority is identified, physician-advocates may find it useful to turn to an organization focused solely on that specific issue. For instance, CAPs wishing to address substance use in youth may find useful resources at the American Society of Addiction Medicine (ASAM), the American Academy of Addiction Psychiatry, and the Community Anti-drug Coalitions of America.

POLICY EXAMPLES

Building on the earlier discussion of choosing an advocacy priority, the core skill sets outlined in **Table 2** can be applied across a range of topics. While advocacy education emphasizes skill development over focusing on specific issues, this article takes the opportunity to highlight key policies relevant to adolescent SUDs, recognizing that readers are inherently interested in this topic.

Table 3 highlights key policies that CAPs can engage in advocacy on to improve adolescent SUD prevention and treatment. Included are opportunities for advocacy, as well as relevant resources and coalition partners, to support these efforts. The information included here demonstrates the importance of coordinated action at federal, state, and community levels to strengthen access, equity, and quality of care. While this is not an exhaustive list, it provides a practical starting point to guide advocacy efforts.

TRAINING FUTURE PSYCHIATRIST-ADVOCATES

Although there has been some improvement in the attention to advocacy training during general psychiatry and child and adolescent psychiatry in recent years, both specialties still lag behind the commitment to advocacy training established by pediatrics. Furthermore, a disconnect exists between guidance provided by professional medical organizations such as the AMA, APA, and AACAP, emphasizing advocacy as a core professional responsibility, and the core competencies as outlined by the Accreditation Council for Graduate Medical Education (ACGME).[13–16]

- The ACGME program requirements for graduate medical education in child and adolescent psychiatry note that "fellows must demonstrate an awareness of and responsiveness to the larger context and system of healthcare, including the social determinants of health, as well as the ability to call effectively on other resources to provide optimal healthcare" but do not specifically use more directed language for advocacy training.
- The ACGME program requirements for graduate medical education in psychiatry include language regarding *accountability to patients, society, and the profession*, *knowledge of legal aspects of psychiatric practice*, *advocating for quality patient care and optimal patient care* systems, and *advocating for the promotion of mental health and the prevention of mental disorders*. However, programs are not required to provide an advocacy training experience.
- The ACGME program requirements for graduate medical education in pediatrics includes language regarding *competence in advocating for quality patient care and optimal patient care systems* and modular learning in advocacy, including *a minimum of 5 educational units of ambulatory experiences, including (Core) ambulatory experiences to include elements of community pediatrics and child advocacy*.

In order to be effective in achieving advocacy goals, we must commit to developing an advocacy workforce. Physicians require skills and mentorship to become competent and confident health advocates. Leaders in medical education have a

Table 3
Examples of policies and advocacy initiatives addressing adolescent substance use

Policy	Advocacy Focus	Resources & Coalition Partners
Mental Health Parity and Addiction Equity Act (MHPAEA, 2008)	Federal legislation requiring insurance plans to cover mental health and SUD treatment on equal terms with medical care is not routinely enforced.	APA Parity Resource Center (includes how to file complaint); APA Model Parity Legislation; ASAM Parity Toolkit; state branches of medical associations; The Kennedy Forum
Regulation of Flavored E-Cigarettes	FDA restricts many flavored e-cigarettes to curb youth vaping, however loopholes and inconsistent enforcement allow flavored products to remain widely available.	AAP Policy Statement; AACAP Policy Statement on Vaping and Electronic Cigarettes; Regulations by state; The Campaign for Tobacco Free Kids; Hazelden Betty Ford Foundation
Medicaid/CHIP Protection and Expansion	Inconsistent provision of substance use screening and early intervention among adolescents due to lack of insurance coverage.	AAP Resources; Medicaid.gov/chip; state coalitions; community organizations
CoCM Implementation	Lack of reimbursement and implementation of CoCM, which improves early identification and treatment of adolescent SUDs in primary care.	APA Model Legislation
Confidentiality Laws for Adolescent Care	Federal and state confidentiality laws impact adolescents' ability to seek SUD treatment without parental consent.	AAP Policy Statement
State Cannabis Legalization Statutes	Legalization frameworks without youth protections: potency limits, packaging restrictions, marketing bans, and prevention funding.	NCSL Database; APA Policy Statement; Smart Approaches to Marijuana (learnaboutsam.org); Legal Action Center Policy Recommendations
Telemedicine	Barriers to reimbursement and cross-state licensure for telehealth delivery of adolescent SUD treatment.	APA Model Legislation; APA district branches and state medical societies; Center for Connected Health Policy; AACAP Telepsychiatry Resources
Safe Workforce Expansion	Limited workforce to provide high-quality substance use treatment.	AACAP's Solutions Infographic; AACAP regional organizations and state medical societies

responsibility to prioritize advocacy education for medical students, psychiatry residents and CAP fellows. We can look to our colleagues in pediatrics to identify sample learning objectives, model curricula, and tools for assessing effective advocacy training programs. A 2014 study in *Pediatrics* by Minkovitz and colleagues suggests that when trainees are exposed to advocacy during residency, the positive effects continue post residency and *may lead to a more engaged workforce.*[17]

Training programs may encounter challenges as they begin to develop advocacy training initiatives, including time constraints and lack of faculty with advocacy expertise. Collaboration between medical schools, training programs and professional organizations may result in shared resources and responsibilities. The American Psychiatric Association Resource Document: Advocacy Teaching in Psychiatry Residency Training Programs provides a summary of advocacy curricula with 7 sample residency programs.[18] The appendix provides useful details regarding educational goals and objectives, lecture series information, and sample legislative advocacy projects.

Professional organizations also have a responsibility to prioritize advocacy education as part of professional development for CAPs throughout their careers. In this setting, physician advocacy is rewarding and effective as efforts are part of a coordinated call to action. For instance, AACAP hosts an annual Legislative Conference, bringing together CAPs and family advocates to meet with lawmakers and their staff in Washington D.C. AACAP and the APA are also members of the Mental Health Liaison Group a nonprofit coalition of over 100 national organizations representing individuals with mental illness and SUDs, family members, clinicians, and other stakeholders committed to strengthening access to mental health and substance use care. These organizations set advocacy agendas that address a multitude of issues, including adolescent substance use, with the strength of a collective voice.

Additionally, AACAP provides unique experiential learning opportunities in Washington D.C. The AACAP Resident Advocacy Scholar is a 4-week elective experience for current or rising CAP fellows to experience political, legislative and regulatory factors impacting on patient care, working in conjunction with AACAP's Government Affairs and Clinical Practice Department.

There are also opportunities for psychiatrists who have completed training to build their advocacy skills and experiences. The AACAP Congressional Fellowship is a 10-month fellowship in Washington DC for one CAP with significant interest in mental health advocacy to work in a congressional office.

AACAP also invites AACAP regional organizations to apply for a 1-year Advocacy & Collaboration Grant, awards of up to $5000 to help support new advocacy work and improve collaboration with allied organizations at the state level. Past grant recipients have used this award to support advocacy training initiatives.

RETURNING TO THE CLINICAL VIGNETTE

The 16-year old with opioid use disorder presents to follow-up with his parents. They shared that they were unable to access naloxone and described their concerns even if they had been able to have it at home. The outpatient CAP realized that the appropriate clinical care was undermined by systems failures including gaps in naloxone availability, education, and policy implementation.

Using *strategic leadership*, she developed her *vision* and set a clear goal: expand statewide access to low-cost naloxone for adolescents and ensure families are educated on its use. Recognizing the magnitude of this goal, and the importance of strategically using her times, she contacted her AACAP regional organization and asked about any organized state level advocacy initiatives addressing this clinical need. She learned that the state medical society had recently hosted a meeting of providers to discuss this pressing clinical concern and the group was *building a coalition* of physicians with experience in this field to help develop an advocacy plan. Learning that most meetings would be held virtually, she opted to join the coalition and offer her advocacy skills.

A few months into their work, the state medical society coalition *evaluated* their progress, which was minimal. They identified gaps in membership representation that seemed to be preventing extension of their reach. They invited parent advocacy groups, the state chapter of AACAP, and school administrators to join the coalition. *Roles and responsibilities were defined* based on expertise and capacity. The state medical society coordinated legislative meetings, parent groups mobilized community support through letters and emails, and school administrators provided data on local student mental health needs. Together, the coalition coordinated messaging and prioritized engagement with legislators most likely to champion the policy to *amplify their advocacy goals*.

The state medical society hosted a state advocacy day at the capitol, during which the CAP learned about the importance of developing relationships with her legislators. She reviewed AACAP's State Advocacy Toolkit, including Tips on Effective State Legislative Advocacy, which demystified the legislative process and helped her identify key points where she could be involved. She scheduled a meeting with her state representative, who was pleased to hear about an issue impacting his constituents from a subject matter expert. During her meeting, she used *persuasive communication*, sharing a patient story and highlighting how gaps in pharmacy stocking and insurance coverage place adolescents at risk of preventable overdoses. The representative proposed a bill in the state legislature and encouraged her to provide oral testimony at the public hearing where the bill would be discussed. In preparation for providing *oral testimony*, she consulted with the AACAP Government Affairs Staff and reviewed AACAP's OUD Treatment Policy Statement. She delivered her testimony before the state health committee, blending clinical data with a *patient story* to humanize the policy need. She made a clear *ask*: for each member of the committee to support the proposed bill. The bill was passed out of committee and was to be voted on by the state legislature.

Throughout this process she *mentored* a trainee who was interested in adolescent substance use policy and legislative advocacy. She invited the trainee to join her at the coalition meetings. He volunteered to craft *social media posts* and published an *op-ed* in the local paper to raise public awareness and generate constituent support for the legislative action.

The trainee was inspired by the coalition, and decided to assemble a smaller scale *coalition* with the goal of educating trainees on the importance of contacting their legislators. Working with the Graduate Medical Education Office at his hospital system, he invited trainees of all specialties to attend a virtual meeting during which he demonstrated how to find their state representatives on the legislature's website and provided a sample letter for them to email their legislators, using the proposed bill that would expand naloxone access.

The state medical society arranged for their advocacy chair and the trainee to meet with their representative. In preparation for their meeting, they discovered that the legislator had previously argued that easier access to naloxone could encourage opioid use. Knowing this information, they were able to *frame their message*, sharing evidence that naloxone saves lives without increasing drug use and supplemented this data with a memorable *patient story*. They ended with their *advocacy ask*: for the representative to support the bill. He was grateful for their expertise that helped him understand how this issue was a concern of his constituents. He shared that he would be voting in support of the bill when it came to the floor of his chamber.

After months of work, these advocacy efforts were successful. The bill to expand statewide access to low-cost naloxone for adolescents passed both chambers of the state legislature and was signed into law by the governor. The coalition was invited to attend the bill signing, where legislators recognized the role of clinical expertise and advocacy in shaping policy.

By integrating *strategic leadership*, *persuasive communication*, *systems navigation*, and *coalition-building skills* the psychiatrist and trainee worked as part of a team that transformed a single clinical encounter into a statewide legislative campaign that not only improved access to life-saving medication but also demonstrated how psychiatrists can leverage their expertise to create meaningful, systemic change.

In this example, both the attending physician and the trainee were highly involved in this effort. However, advocacy accommodates smaller levels of engagement—such as voting, signing up for advocacy-focused communications, following social media accounts for state and national organized psychiatry bodies, and supporting professional political action committees (PACs) such as the APA-PAC or AACAP-PAC.[19] All levels of engagement are valuable; our collective voice is louder and stronger than any one individual alone.

A CALL TO ACTION

Integrate advocacy into your clinical practice, mentorship, and professional development. Identify issues you are passionate about, engage with coalitions or professional organizations, and use your clinical insights to inform solutions. Small steps today can lead to meaningful systemic improvements in the care of adolescents with substance use disorders. Every action contributes to collective impact.

CLINICS CARE POINTS

- Adolescents with substance use disorders face persistent barriers to care, including stigma and fragmented systems of care; identifying these barriers in clinical practice can help inform advocacy priorities.
- Child and adolescent psychiatrists are uniquely positioned to translate clinical expertise and scientific evidence into advocacy efforts that improve access to prevention, treatment, and recovery services for youth.
- Strategic leadership, persuasive communication, systems navigation, and coalition building are core advocacy skills that build upon competencies already used in everyday psychiatric practice.
- Advocacy must be integrated into clinical work, mentorship, and professional organizations, allowing psychiatrists to influence systems-level change that improves outcomes for adolescents with substance use disorders.

DISCLOSURE

The authors have no conflicts of interest to disclose.

REFERENCES

1. Adams ZW, Dellucci TV, Agley J, et al. Estimated prevalence of substance use disorders among US adolescents and emerging adults by substance class, severity, and age, 2022. JAACAP Open 2025;3(4):959–71.

2. Gray K, Squeglia LM. Squeglia. Research review: what have we learned about adolescent substance use? JCPP (J Child Psychol Psychiatry) 2018;59(6): 618–27.
3. Panchal N, Zitter S. Teens, drugs, and overdose: contrasting pre-pandemic and current trends. KFF. 2024. Available at: https://www.kff.org/mental-health/teens-drugs-and-overdose-contrasting-pre-pandemic-and-current-trends/. Accessed November 11, 2025.
4. SAMHSA releases annual national survey on drug use and health. SAMHSA. 2025. Available at: https://www.kff.org/mental-health/teens-drugs-and-overdose-contrasting-pre-pandemic-and-current-trends/. Accessed November 11, 2025.
5. AMA declaration of professional responsibilities. 2001. Available at: https://www.ama-assn.org/public-health/prevention-wellness/ama-declaration-professional-responsibility. Accessed November 11, 2025.
6. American Psychiatric Association. The principles of medical ethics with annotations especially applicable to psychiatry. 2013 edition. Arlington, VA: American Psychiatric Association; 2013. Available at: https://www.psychiatry.org/getmedia/3fe5eae9-3df9-4561-a070-84a009c6c4a6/2013-APA-Principles-of-Medical-Ethics.pdf. Accessed November 11, 2025.
7. AACAP code of ethics. 2023: page 14. Available at: https://www.aacap.org/App_Themes/AACAP/docs/about_us/transparency_portal/AACAP_Code_of_Ethics_2023.pdf. Accessed November 11, 2025.
8. Bentley University. What is strategic leadership? 2025. Available at: https://www.bentley.edu/news/what-strategic-leadership. Accessed November 17, 2025.
9. Vance MC, Kennedy KG, Wiechers IR, et al, editors. A psychiatrist's guide to advocacy. Washington, DC: American Psychiatric Association Publishing; 2020. p. 158–9.
10. Amaya H. Importance of storytelling in advocacy. Washington, DC: Presented at: American Psychiatric Association's Federal Advocacy Conference; 2025.
11. Metzl JM, Hansen H. Structural competency: theorizing a new medical engagement with stigma and inequality. Soc Sci Med 2014;103:126–33. Available at: https://pmc.ncbi.nlm.nih.gov/articles/PMC4269606/. Accessed November 17, 2025.
12. Shah S. Going farther by going together: collaboration as a tool in advocacy. Pediatr Clin North Am 2023;70(1):181–91. Accessed November 17, 2025.
13. Sagot A, Flugard A. Advocacy training in residency and addressing needs in child and adolescent psychiatry: a 30 year review. J Am Acad Child Adolesc Psychiatry 2024;63(4):468–73.
14. Accreditation Council for Graduate Medical Education. ACGME program requirements for medical education in child and adolescent psychiatry. Available at: https://www.acgme.org/globalassets/pdfs/milestones/childandadolescentpsychiatry milestones.pdf. Accessed November 11, 2025.
15. Accreditation Council for Graduate Medical Education. ACGME program requirements for medical education in psychiatry. Available at: https://www.acgme.org/globalassets/pdfs/milestones/psychiatrymilestones.pdf. Accessed November 11, 2025.
16. Accreditation Council for Graduate Medical Education. ACGME program requirements for medical education in pediatrics. Available at: https://www.acgme.org/globalassets/pdfs/milestones/pediatricsmilestones.pdf. Accessed November 11, 2025.
17. Minkovitz C, Goldshore M, Solomon B, et al, Community Pediatrics Training Initiative Workgroup. Five-year Follow-up of community pediatrics training initiative. Pediatrics 2014;134(1):83–90.

18. Kennedy K, Vance M. APA resource DocumentAdvocacy teaching in psychiatry residency training programs. 2018. Available at: https://www.psychiatry.org/FileLibrary/Psychiatrists/Directories/Library-and-Archive/resource_documents/2018-Resource-Document-Advocacy-Teaching-in-Psychiatry-Residency-Training.pdf. Accessed November 11, 2025.
19. Ho PA, Hawkes A. The C-L psychiatrist's practical guide to legislative advocacy skills—and why it is imperative for C-L psychiatrists to utilize these skills. J Acad Consult Liaison Psychiatry 2025;66(3):261–5. Accessed November 17, 2025.

Navigating Consent and Confidentiality in Adolescent Substance Use Treatment

Sabihul Alam, MD, JD[a,*], Sivabalaji Kaliamurthy, MD, FASAM[b,c,d,e]

KEYWORDS

- Adolescent substance use • Consent • Confidentiality • Minor consent laws

KEY POINTS

- Consent and confidentiality are central to clinical interventions in adolescent substance use care.
- Authority to consent to treatment and access to health information are related but legally distinct; consent to care does not necessarily confer access to medical records.
- Rising adolescent overdose deaths elevate the importance of harm reduction strategies like naloxone distribution, requiring an understanding of consent and confidentiality laws for effective implementation.
- Health systems and policies must evolve to support confidential, equitable adolescent care including how electronic medical records are designed.

INTRODUCTION

Adolescent substance use over the past decade has shown a paradoxic trend: while self-reported rates of use of many of the substances have stabilized or declined, substance use disorders (SUDs) and overdose mortality have risen sharply.[1] Drug overdoses and poisonings are now among the leading causes of death for US children and adolescents.[2] Beginning in 2019, overdose deaths increased rapidly and continued to climb through the fentanyl era, driven less by the prevalence of use than by the lethality of an increasingly contaminated drug supply.[3,4]

[a] Division of Behavioral Health, Riverside University Health System, Riverside, CA, USA; [b] Division of Psychiatry, Children's National, Washington, DC, USA; [c] Department of Psychiatry and Pediatrics, The George Washington University, Washington, DC, USA; [d] Department of Psychiatry, Howard University, Washington, DC, USA; [e] Yale University, New Haven, CT, USA
* Corresponding author. Riverside University Health System - Behavioral Health, 9890 County Farm Road, Building 1, Riverside, CA 92503.
E-mail address: alam.sabihul@gmail.com

Child Adolesc Psychiatric Clin N Am 35 (2026) 707–721
https://doi.org/10.1016/j.chc.2026.05.009 **childpsych.theclinics.com**
1056-4993/26/

Abbreviations	
HIPAA	Health Insurance Portability and Accountability Act
SUD	substance use disorder

Illicitly manufactured fentanyl has substantially modified the risk landscape of adolescent substance use. Between 2019 and 2021, fentanyl involvement in adolescent overdose deaths increased sharply, accounting for the majority of fatal overdoses.[2,4] By 2021, fentanyl was implicated in over three-quarters of adolescent overdose deaths, underscoring how even intermittent or experimental substance use now carries a markedly higher risk of fatality.[2] This shift from chronic morbidity to acute mortality reframes adolescent substance use as an urgent safety issue, requiring clinicians to recalibrate real-time decisions regarding confidentiality, parental involvement, and overdose prevention strategies, including naloxone distribution.

Substance use among adolescents remains a persistent and evolving public health concern. Early initiation is associated with increased risk for progression to SUDs, psychiatric comorbidity, and poorer long-term psychosocial outcomes.[5] Despite advances in evidence-based screening and treatment, many adolescents who use substances do not engage consistently in care.[5] A critical yet often underrecognized determinant of engagement is whether adolescents trust that disclosures will be handled with respect, transparency, and confidentiality.[6] When confidentiality feels uncertain, adolescents withhold information, avoid care altogether, or disengage during periods of highest risk.

Developmental Vulnerability

Adolescents face a unique neurobiological vulnerability driven by asynchronous brain maturation. The limbic reward system matures early, heightening sensitivity to dopamine and novelty, while the prefrontal cortex governing impulse control does not fully mature until the mid-20s.[7] This *accelerator without brakes* dynamic leaves youth highly susceptible to impulsive use and long-term neurotoxic damage during a critical window of plasticity.[7] In the era of illicitly manufactured fentanyl, this vulnerability has taken on lethal urgency, as the developmental propensity for experimentation now carries the immediate risk of fatal overdose.

These neurobiological vulnerabilities underscore the critical importance of early intervention. Adolescents who initiate substance use before age 14 face significantly higher lifetime risk of developing a SUD, making early treatment essential to interrupt progression from experimentation to dependence.[5,8] Yet a substantial treatment gap persists. In 2023, less than one in 5 of the 2.2 million adolescents with SUDs received any treatment, with disparities most pronounced among youth from marginalized communities.[9,10] Together, these patterns highlight the urgency of identifying modifiable factors that influence whether adolescents seek care, disclose risk and remain engaged in treatment.

Addressing the treatment gap in adolescent substance use requires careful attention to confidentiality and informed consent, which function as legal and ethical gatekeepers to care for minors. These constructs shape whether adolescents seek help, disclose risk, and remain engaged in treatment, particularly in high-stakes contexts such as overdose risk, psychiatric comorbidity, and harm reduction interventions.[6] In this context, developmentally appropriate confidentiality functions as a clinical intervention, increasing the likelihood that adolescents disclose risk and engage in care during a critical window of neuroplastic vulnerability, when early intervention can interrupt the trajectory from experimentation to disorder. Mastery of these concepts is therefore not ancillary to clinical practice but central to it. The sections that follow examine informed consent and confidentiality as distinct but interdependent concepts, and analyze how their interaction influences access to care, therapeutic alliance, and clinical outcomes across outpatient, emergency, and inpatient settings.

Key Frameworks

Consent and confidentiality occupy a uniquely complex space in the care of adolescents with substance use concerns. Adolescence is characterized by evolving decisional capacity, increasing autonomy, and heightened sensitivity to perceived breaches of trust, factors that directly shape willingness to disclose substance use and related risk. At the same time, clinicians must navigate parental involvement, legal requirements, and safety obligations related to self-harm, overdose risk, and child welfare. These tensions are additionally amplified for adolescents with co-occurring psychiatric illness, whose care often spans multiple systems, which include schools, emergency departments, inpatient units, and the juvenile justice system, each with distinct expectations regarding information sharing and disclosure.

Consent

Informed consent is the legal and ethical process through which a patient authorizes a clinical intervention after receiving adequate information and making a voluntary decision.[11] In adolescent health care, however, the threshold question is whether the adolescent has legal authority to consent at all, which varies by age, jurisdiction, clinical context, and type of service.[12,13] Unlike adults, whose consent authority is presumed, adolescents' ability to consent is conditional and context-dependent, shaped by developmental maturity and specific statutory exceptions. When adolescents are legally permitted to consent, such as for certain substance use or mental health services, informed consent rests on 3 core elements: disclosure, understanding, and voluntariness.[11,14] Disclosure requires that clinicians explain the risks, benefits, reasonable alternatives, and potential consequences of declining care. Understanding entails the adolescent's ability to comprehend and appreciate this information in light of their developmental and emotional capacity.[15,16] Voluntariness requires that decisions be made free from coercion, undue pressure, or implicit threats, including fear of punitive disclosure.[11] In the context of adolescent substance use, fear of mandatory parental notification may significantly constrain voluntariness, shaping whether adolescents disclose high-risk behaviors such as fentanyl exposure, experimental use, or impaired driving, thereby distorting clinical risk assessment. Together, these elements operationalize respect for autonomy within the constraints of adolescent development and the legal framework governing minor consent.

Confidentiality

Confidentiality is the legal and ethical duty to protect patients' health information by limiting access to identifiable information to authorized individuals.[17] Its ethical foundation, grounded in respect for autonomy and privacy, promotes trust and creates a safe environment for disclosure of sensitive information without fear of stigma, punishment, or unintended exposure.[6] In adolescent care, confidentiality takes on particular significance, as concerns about parental notification or institutional reporting can strongly influence whether youth seek care or disclose substance use and related risks.[6] Unlike informed consent, which governs authorization for treatment, confidentiality governs control over information and is often conditional for minors. It may be expanded or narrowed depending on legal authority, clinical setting, and safety considerations. In practice, this requires clinicians to continually weigh the benefits of preserving confidentiality against the risks of nondisclosure in situations involving overdose risks or imminent harm. Understanding confidentiality as a distinct yet interdependent concept is critical to supporting disclosure, engagement, and ethical decision-making in adolescent substance use treatment.

Limitations and laws

Informed consent and confidentiality are distinct yet fundamentally interdependent doctrines in adolescent substance use care. Informed consent requires disclosing confidentiality limits, including circumstances requiring disclosure without the adolescent's permission, such as mandatory reporting or imminent risk of harm. Simultaneously, confidentiality is a prerequisite for voluntariness in consent. Adolescents who fear disclosure to caregivers, schools, courts, or law enforcement may withhold information, decline care, or disengage entirely, rendering consent nominal rather than meaningful. Thus, consent and confidentiality operate reciprocally: informed consent requires transparency about confidentiality boundaries, while authentic consent depends on sufficient confidentiality protections to support voluntary decision-making. The legal framework governing these issues in adolescent substance use care is fragmented and frequently misunderstood. State laws vary widely regarding minors' authority to consent to substance use and mental health treatment, while federal privacy regulations add additional layers of complexity.[12,17] Consequently, clinicians are often required to make real-time decisions in ambiguous clinical situations, balancing ethical obligations to promote autonomy and safety against institutional policies and perceived legal risk. In practice, this frequently involves rapid decisions about whether to preserve or breach confidentiality in high-risk situations such as overdose, acute intoxication, or psychiatric crises.

This article aims to provide a practical, clinically grounded framework for navigating consent and confidentiality in the care of adolescents who use substances. Drawing on ethical principles, published literature, developmental considerations, and current legal standards, we focus on common clinical scenarios across outpatient, emergency, and inpatient settings. Particular attention is given to youth with co-occurring psychiatric illness, the role of family engagement, and emerging care models such as peer recovery support. By reframing consent and confidentiality as dynamic components of clinical care rather than static legal hurdles, we aim to support clinicians in fostering trust, engagement, and safe, effective treatment of adolescents and their families.

APPROACH TO LITERATURE REVIEW AND CONCEPTUAL FRAMEWORK

This article is informed by a targeted narrative review of the literature combined with clinical experience in adolescent substance use treatment. This approach does not employ systematic review methods. A structured search of PubMed was conducted using key terms including *substance-related disorders*, *adolescents*, and *confidentiality*, with inclusion of peer-reviewed studies, professional guidelines, and relevant policy and legal sources. Search results were refined through manual review, with Rayyan software used to assist in screening and organization of references. Additional sources, including legal statutes, federal regulations, and professional guidance documents, were identified through manual searches outside of PubMed to ensure comprehensive coverage of consent and confidentiality frameworks relevant to adolescent care.

Sources were included if they addressed confidentiality, consent, or privacy in the context of minors or substance-related disorders. Articles focused primarily on sexually transmitted infections (eg, human immunodeficiency virus [HIV]), abuse or neglect, or specific adolescent subpopulations with distinct confidentiality frameworks (such as lesbian, gay, bisexual, transgender, queer, and other sexual and gender minority [LGBTQ+]–specific care) were excluded to maintain focus on substance use treatment. Rather than aiming for exhaustive synthesis, the review prioritized clinically relevant literature to support a developmentally informed, practice-oriented framework applicable across outpatient, emergency, and inpatient settings.

WHY CONSENT AND CONFIDENTIALITY ARE UNIQUE IN ADOLESCENTS

Legal and ethical approaches to adolescent consent and confidentiality present unique challenges. Unlike adults, who are presumed competent, or young children, who are presumed incompetent, adolescents inhabit a *transitional* status based on their evolving cognitive capacity, increasing autonomy, and incomplete psychosocial maturation.[15,16,18] This creates a disparity between their chronologic age, which determines legal status, and their neurobiological development, which determines decision-making capacity.[7,16] As a result, legal frameworks governing adolescent health care must balance respect for emerging autonomy with the need for protection during a period of heightened vulnerability.

Decisional capacity does not emerge at a single point in development but evolves incrementally across childhood and adolescence.[15,18] Developmental research identifies broad neurocognitive stages that inform clinical judgment regarding assent, consent, and the appropriate scope of confidentiality.[15]

Early Childhood (≈0–7 years)

Children in early childhood lack cognitive skills for meaningful consent or assent. Their thinking is concrete and egocentric, steered by preoperational logic.[11] Accordingly, medical decisions are made entirely by parents based on the child's best interests.[15]

Middle Childhood (≈7–11 years)

During this period, competence begins to emerge as children enter the concrete operational thinking stage with improved logical reasoning, memory, and attention.[18] Research suggests that children can meaningfully assent around age 7, demonstrating an understanding of basic treatment goals.[19] However, their difficulty with long-term consequences and abstract concepts precludes the capacity for full legal consent.[15,19] Empirical studies using the MacArthur Competence Assessment Tool identify a critical transitional period between ages 9.6 and 11.2 years.[18] Although focused on consent to participate in research, these findings remain salient for developmental competence. Children aged less than 9.6 rarely demonstrate capacity, while around 11.2, a *changeover* point emerges where children begin to show adult-like decision-making abilities.[18]

Early Adolescence (≈11–14 years)

Early adolescence marks rapid cognitive expansion as youth enter Piaget's *formal operational* stage, where they gain the capacity for abstract reasoning and hypothetical thinking.[20,21] However, the limbic reward system matures earlier than the prefrontal cortex, creating heightened sensation-seeking with immature impulse control.[7] As a result, youth may reason effectively in calm, structured settings yet become impulsive in emotionally charged or peer-influenced situations—a distinction with important implications for consent, confidentiality, and risk assessment in substance use care.[7]

Mid-to-Late Adolescence (≥15 years)

By mid-to-late adolescence, many youth demonstrate cognitive capacities for informed consent comparable to adults, with adult-like reasoning and risk appraisals emerging around ages 15 to 16.[16] However, psychosocial maturity continues to lag into the mid-20s, leaving adolescents vulnerable to impulsivity, peer influence, and emotionally driven decision-making.[16] This developmental dissonance supports legal exceptions granting minor consent in many jurisdictions while necessitating caution, given the emotional and social drivers of substance use.

Adolescents' unique developmental position, distinct from both children and adults, has profound implications for consent and confidentiality. Legal frameworks address this reality by granting autonomy in specific high-need health care contexts while maintaining protections that recognize ongoing vulnerability—a balance particularly critical in substance use treatment.

LEGAL AND ETHICAL FRAMEWORK FOR ADOLESCENT CONFIDENTIALITY IN MEDICAL CARE

General Standards: Adults versus Minors

The legal and ethical frameworks governing consent and confidentiality in health care diverge significantly between adults and minors, reflecting presumptions about decisional capacity and autonomy. Adults (age 18 and older) are presumed competent to make independent health care decisions.[11,14] This presumption includes the capacity to understand risks, benefits, and reasonable alternatives required for informed consent.[11,14] Consequently, under the Health Insurance Portability and Accountability Act (HIPAA), adults retain the right to confidentiality and control over who can access their medical records.[22]

In contrast, minors (aged less than 18) are presumed to lack the legal capacity to provide informed consent for medical treatment, requiring parents or guardians to authorize care.[14,23] Minors may provide *assent*, an affirmative agreement to participate in care that acknowledges their developing autonomy without conferring full legal authority.[19,24] Under HIPAA, parents are designated as the minor's *personal representative* with access to the child's health information unless specific exceptions apply.[22] This default legal framework is grounded in constitutional principles, Supreme Court precedent, and longstanding Western cultural traditions that prioritize parental authority.[14]

Exceptions Granting Minors Control (Autonomy)

Despite this default presumption, significant legal exceptions exist to promote public health by removing parental barriers to care.[12,13] When these exceptions apply, minors gain legal authority to consent, and parents are no longer automatically entitled to access related medical records.[12,13,22] These exceptions fall into 2 major categories: status-based and service-based.[13,23]

Status-based exceptions grant adult-like decision-making authority to minors whose life circumstances justify greater autonomy.[23] For example, emancipated minors (e.g. married, military, financially independent) may gain authorization to consent to all aspects of their health care without parental permission.[12,23] Similarly, the 'mature minor' doctrine, recognized in some form in approximately 36 states, permits adolescents (typically age 14–15 and older) to consent if they demonstrate sufficient intelligence, maturity, and understanding of the intervention's nature, risks, benefits, and consequences.[23,25]

Service-based exceptions authorize minors to consent to specific 'sensitive services' without parental permission, based on the public health principle that adolescents may avoid essential or lifesaving care if confidentiality is not assured.[12,13] These services typically include testing and treatment of sexually transmitted infections (including HIV), reproductive and contraceptive services, mental health care, and SUD treatment, though specific minimum age thresholds, often between 12 and 16, and provisions vary by state.[12] When minors are legally authorized to consent to these sensitive services, they generally acquire corresponding confidentiality rights to control disclosure of information related to that care.[12,22] However, these protections are not absolute and may be limited in practice by insurance-related disclosures, safety exceptions, or institutional policies.[12,13]

Substance Use as an Axception to General Confidentiality Norms

In contrast to most medical care, the majority of US states permit minors to consent to SUD evaluation and treatment without parental permission, though the specific age thresholds, treatment modalities, and conditions vary by jurisdiction.[12] (**Table 1**)

These statutes are rooted in the ethical principles of beneficence and harm reduction, acknowledging that adolescents may forgo care if parental involvement is mandatory. Historically, minor consent provisions emerged in response to rising rates of adolescent alcohol and drug use and were later reinforced by the HIV and opioid epidemics, which highlighted the life-saving potential of confidential access to care.[13]

Table 1
Variation in state laws

General Policy	States
No Age Threshold Specified (Broad Authority)	Alabama, Colorado, Connecticut, Florida, Georgia[a], Hawaii[a], Idaho[a], Indiana, Iowa, Kansas, Kentucky[a], Louisiana[a], Maine[a], Maryland[a], Minnesota[a], Missouri[a], Montana[a], Nebraska, Nevada, New Jersey, New York[a], North Carolina, Ohio, Oklahoma[d], Pennsylvania[a], Rhode Island, South Dakota, Tennessee[a], Texas[a,b], Virginia[c], West Virginia
12 or Older	Arizona[c], California, Illinois, Massachusetts, New Hampshire, Vermont[c], Wisconsin[a], Wyoming[a]
13 or Older	Washington[c]
14 or Older	Delaware[c], Michigan, New Mexico[a], North Dakota, Oregon[c]
15 or Older	Mississippi
16 or Older	South Carolina
"Mature Minor" Standard (Capacity-Based)	Arkansas
No Explicit Policy	Alaska, Utah

Note: State laws vary in scope and may include additional restrictions based on age, treatment setting, or clinical circumstances.

[a] State law may permit or require parental notification.

[b] Parental consent may be required for inpatient treatment.

[c] Limited to outpatient services unless additional criteria are met.

[d] Includes restrictions based on clinical context (e.g., emergency status, emancipated, living circumstances, or treatment type).

Adapted from Sharko M, Jameson R, Ancker JS, Krams L, Webber EC, Rosenbloom ST. State-by-State Variability in Adolescent Privacy Laws. *Pediatrics*. 2022;149(6):e2021053458. https://doi.org/10.1542/peds.2021-053458

Although statutory details vary widely, minor consent laws in most jurisdictions authorize adolescents to independently consent to some or all components of SUD treatment, including screening, counseling, and, in some states, pharmacotherapy.[12] Given this variability, clinicians should consult their state-specific statutes and institutional policies to determine what services adolescents may consent to independently in their practice setting. Importantly, the ability to consent to treatment often confers corresponding confidentiality protections, limiting parental access to treatment records unless the adolescent authorizes disclosure or specific safety thresholds are met.[13] Federal regulations, including HIPAA and title 42 of the code of federal regulations (CFR) Part 2, further shape these protections by restricting disclosure of substance use treatment information.[17,22]

Importantly, these protections are neither uniform nor absolute. Some states permit minors to consent only to outpatient services but not inpatient care.[12,13] Others impose minimum age thresholds, restrict consent based on treatment modality, or perceived severity of substance use and/or differentiate between counseling and medication-based care.[12] Access to medications for substance use disorders, particularly opioid agonist therapies remains inconsistent, with some jurisdictions requiring parental consent despite allowing adolescents to consent to counseling services.[12]

Autonomy versus Parental Consent

Although minor consent laws are designed to promote access to care, they exist in ongoing tension with well-established benefits of family involvement in adolescent treatment.[13,26] Caregivers often provide logistical support, supervision, and emotional stability that enhance treatment adherence and outcomes.[26] At the same time, mandatory parental involvement can undermine trust, discourage disclosure, and deter adolescents from seeking care altogether.[6,13]

In clinical practice, this tension manifests as a need to balance legal autonomy with therapeutic alliance. Ethical practice does not equate independent consent with exclusion of caregivers. Rather, it calls for intentional efforts to engage families when safe and appropriate, while preserving the adolescent's right to confidential care. Encouraging adolescent assent to selective family involvement, such as participation in psychoeducation, safety planning, or family-based therapy, can help reconcile these competing imperatives.[24,26]

Importantly, parental involvement is not uniformly protective. In families affected by substance use, violence, or significant conflict, disclosure may expose adolescents to harm or destabilization.[13,23] Minor consent statutes implicitly recognize this reality by prioritizing adolescent access to care in circumstances where default parental control could function as a barrier rather than a safeguard.

CHALLENGES IN NAVIGATING CONSENT IN MANDATED TREATMENTS (EG, JUVENILE JUSTICE, SCHOOL REFERRALS)

Consent and confidentiality become especially complex in mandated treatment settings, including juvenile justice referrals, school-initiated evaluations, and court-ordered treatment.[13,26] In these contexts, adolescents may experience care as coercive, and disclosures may carry perceived or real legal consequences. Clinicians are often asked to share treatment information with probation officers, school administrators, or courts, creating tension between therapeutic confidentiality and external reporting requirements.[13]

From an ethical perspective, mandated treatment raises concerns about voluntariness, trust, and proportionality of disclosure. While some information sharing may be legally required, overly broad or nonspecific disclosures risk undermining the therapeutic relationship and discouraging meaningful engagement.[6,13] Best-practice profiling emphasizes clarity at the outset of care regarding what information will be shared, with whom, and for what purpose.[6] When disclosure is necessary, limiting shared information to disclosures of attendance, general progress, or safety-related concerns rather than detailed substance use histories can help preserve confidentiality while meeting external legal obligations.

School-based referrals present similar challenges, particularly when disciplinary frameworks intersect with health care. Adolescents may reasonably fear that disclosure of substance use will result in suspension, expulsion, or criminalization rather than support. Clinicians must remain vigilant to avoid inadvertently transforming clinical encounters into extensions of disciplinary systems.

Ethical Considerations and Dilemmas in Adolescent Confidentiality

Ethical decision-making around confidentiality in adolescent substance use treatment is rarely binary. Clinicians must continuously balance respect for emerging autonomy with obligations to protect safety, engage caregivers, and comply with legal mandates. These tensions are especially pronounced in substance use care, where disclosure may expose adolescents to punishment, family conflict, or disengagement, while nondisclosure may increase risk for overdose, self-harm, exploitation, or death.[5,6] Ethical practice, therefore, requires a principled, developmentally informed approach that distinguishes when confidentiality should be preserved, when disclosure is required, and how to navigate the space between these extremes.

Ethical Rationale for Maintaining Confidentiality

Maintaining confidentiality is ethically grounded in respect for autonomy, promotion of beneficence, and preservation of trust within the therapeutic relationship.[6,13] Adolescents are more likely to disclose substance use, overdose risk, suicidal ideation, and related behaviors when they believe their information will be handled with transparency and discretion.[6] Concerns about parental notification or punitive consequences consistently deter adolescents from seeking care or being forthcoming once engaged, particularly for stigmatized behaviors such as substance use.[6,13]

Confidentiality also serves a protective function in contexts where disclosure may itself cause harm. For some adolescents—particularly those in families affected by substance use, violence, or rigid disciplinary practices—disclosure can precipitate punitive responses, housing instability, or emotional or physical harm.[13,23] For youth involved in juvenile justice or child welfare systems, breaches of confidentiality may lead to legal consequences that exacerbate risk rather than mitigate it.[13,26] From an ethical standpoint, preserving confidentiality supports proportionality by reducing harm without introducing additional, foreseeable risks.

Importantly, confidentiality is not synonymous with secrecy. Ethical confidentiality involves deliberate, principled discretion that advances clinical goals while preserving the adolescent's dignity, agency, and engagement in care.

Ethical Justifications for Breaching Confidentiality

Despite its central importance, confidentiality is not absolute. Ethical and legal obligations require clinicians to breach confidentiality when there is a credible and imminent risk of serious harm to the adolescent or others.[17] In substance use care, this most commonly arises in situations involving imminent suicide risk, high likelihood of fatal overdose, severe impairment due to intoxication or withdrawal, or concerns related to coercion, trafficking, or abuse.[13,26]

In these circumstances, the principles of nonmaleficence and beneficence may override respect for autonomy, obligating clinicians to act to prevent serious injury or death. Legal mandates—including mandatory reporting statutes and duty-to-protect obligations—may further require disclosure irrespective of clinical preference.

Ethical justification for breaching confidentiality requires more than discomfort or uncertainty. Disclosures should be grounded in clearly articulated risk, proportional to the threat, and limited to the minimum necessary information required to address the safety concern.

Whenever feasible, clinicians should inform adolescents before breaching confidentiality, explaining the reasons for disclosure, what information will be shared, and with whom. This transparency helps preserve trust and supports continued engagement even when disclosure is unavoidable.

A PRAGMATIC *MIDDLE-GROUND* APPROACH

Between strict confidentiality and immediate disclosure lies a developmentally informed, pragmatic middle-ground approach. This framework emphasizes transparency, collaboration, and graduated disclosure rather than all-or-nothing decision-making.

Whenever possible, clinicians should preserve confidentiality while actively encouraging adolescents to involve caregivers in care. This may include framing caregiver involvement as a source of support rather than surveillance, identifying specific domains where family engagement enhances safety, and allowing adolescents some control over the timing and content of disclosure. For example, an adolescent may agree to caregiver involvement in treatment planning or medication management while retaining privacy around specific details of substance use.

Education and harm reduction are essential components of this middle-ground approach. Providing adolescents with overdose education, naloxone, guidance on avoiding solitary use, and information about fentanyl contamination can meaningfully reduce risk without necessitating immediate parental disclosure. In this way, harm reduction functions as an ethically sound strategy that respects autonomy while advancing beneficence and safety.

Clinical Vignette

James, a 15-year-old living in Baltimore, Maryland, presents with his father for his annual physical at a primary care pediatric clinic. His father expresses frustration regarding James's declining grades, frequent absences, and that he sometimes comes home smelling like weed. James appears guarded and avoids eye contact while his father remains in the room, but once his father reluctantly agrees to step out, James agrees to speak privately with the pediatrician.

Once alone, James eventually discloses daily cannabis use and intermittent vaping of THC cartridges. Upon further gentle probing, he reveals a significant recent stressor: he recently lost a close friend to an opioid overdose. While James denies using opioids himself, he admits he is struggling to cope with the loss. He denies current suicidal ideation but notes a history of superficial self-harm 6 months prior.

When the pediatrician suggests involving his parents to support treatment, James becomes visibly distressed, pleading, "You can't tell him. My dad is intense—he'll pull me out of all my activities and lock me down." He describes a home environment marked by rigid discipline and frequent high-conflict interactions, though he denies physical abuse.

At this juncture, the clinician faces a critical decision: whether the level of risk justifies breaching confidentiality or whether preserving privacy would better support engagement and reduce harm. Recognizing that immediate disclosure could fracture trust and escalate conflict, the pediatrician adopts a developmentally informed middle path. After determining that James has the capacity to consent to confidential care under Maryland law, the clinician prioritizes safety through harm-reduction strategies, including naloxone provision and a collaborative safety plan focused on minimizing overdose risk. The clinician validates James's privacy concerns while arranging close follow-up and working toward voluntary family involvement as the therapeutic relationship strengthens.

WHEN (AND HOW) TO BREACH CONFIDENTIALITY

When breaching confidentiality becomes necessary, *how* the breach occurs is ethically as important as *whether* it occurs. Best practice is to inform the adolescent in advance whenever feasible, explain the specific reasons for disclosure, and clarify what information will be shared and with whom.[13,23,25,26] This preserves transparency, mitigates feelings of betrayal, and supports continued engagement even after disclosure.

Risk to Self or Others

Imminent suicide risk, credible overdose risk, or behaviors that endanger others justify disclosure to caregivers or emergency services.[13,26] In substance use care, overdose risk may be more ambiguous than suicidality; clinicians should consider factors such as prior overdoses, fentanyl exposure, polysubstance use, tolerance changes, and access to naloxone when assessing imminence.

Legal Mandates

Mandatory reporting laws, duty-to-warn obligations, and child protection statutes may require disclosure irrespective of patient preference. Clinicians should be familiar with jurisdiction-specific requirements and limit disclosures to information necessary to meet the legal obligation.

Other Ethical Challenges

Family dynamics frequently complicate confidentiality decisions. Caregivers may have competing interests related to custody, legal exposure, or family conflict. Mandated treatment settings, such as juvenile justice or school-based referrals, introduce additional ethical tension, as adolescents may perceive care as coercive and disclosures as punitive. In these contexts, explicitly acknowledging limits of confidentiality at the outset is critical.

Balancing beneficence and respect for autonomy is further shaped by cultural considerations. Family structures, beliefs about authority, stigma surrounding substance use, and expectations of adolescent independence vary widely across cultures and should inform, but not override, ethical analysis. Culturally responsive care requires curiosity, humility, and avoidance of assumptions about family roles or adolescent preferences (**Table 2**).

PRACTICAL AND POLICY IMPLICATIONS AND IMPLICATIONS FOR TRAINING

Despite the centrality of consent and confidentiality to adolescent substance use care, formal training in these areas remains inconsistent across medical, nursing, and behavioral health disciplines. Many clinicians report uncertainty regarding minor consent laws, federal confidentiality regulations, and institutional policies, often relying on informal guidance or overly cautious practices that may inadvertently limit access to care. Standardized education that integrates legal principles with real-world clinical

Table 2
Summary of consent and confidentiality considerations in adolescent substance use

Domain	Key Legal Considerations	Common Clinical Pitfalls	Practical Implications for Clinicians
Minor consent to substance use treatment	Varies by state; many states allow adolescents to consent independently to substance use assessment and treatment	Assuming parental consent is always required; conflating consent to treatment with confidentiality of records	Verify state law; clarify what services adolescents can consent to independently and explain limits of confidentiality at the outset
Minor consent to mental health treatment	Often permitted at lower age thresholds than other medical care; scope may differ from substance use treatment	Applying mental health consent rules inconsistently to substance use care	Treat mental health and substance use consent as overlapping but distinct legal domains
Confidentiality of health information (HIPAA)	Parents generally personal representatives unless exceptions apply (eg, minor-consented care, best-interest determinations)	Over-disclosure of sensitive information via after-visit summaries, portals, or billing	Use developmentally appropriate confidentiality scripts; limit unnecessary documentation of sensitive disclosures
42 CFR Part 2	Provides heightened protection for substance use treatment records; recent updates allow some care coordination	Misunderstanding when Part 2 applies; assuming it fully prevents parental access	Know whether your setting/program is Part 2-covered; obtain consent when possible; consult compliance when uncertain
Naloxone distribution	Often legal without prescription; parental consent may not be required depending on jurisdiction and setting	Avoiding naloxone distribution due to fear of disclosure or documentation concerns	Treat naloxone as standard harm reduction; anticipate confidentiality implications in documentation and communication
Documentation in EHRs	Shared records increase risk of inadvertent disclosure	Detailed notes accessible to caregivers through portals	Use focused, clinically necessary documentation; understand institutional privacy controls
Emergency and inpatient settings	Safety concerns may justify broader disclosure; legal authority may be unclear	Inconsistent disclosure practices across teams	Default to transparency with adolescents about what will be shared and why
Parental requests for information	Rights vary based on consent authority and state law	Either blanket refusal or full disclosure without clinical judgment	Share themes and safety-relevant information while protecting specific disclosures when appropriate
High-risk situations (overdose, suicidality, and abuse)	Mandatory reporting and duty-to-protect obligations override confidentiality	Delayed disclosure due to uncertainty	Clearly explain limits of confidentiality early; document rationale for disclosure

scenarios—particularly those involving overdose risk and harm reduction—is essential to improving confidence and consistency in practice.

Health systems play a critical role in shaping how confidentiality is operationalized. Electronic health records, patient portals, billing systems, and after-visit summaries can unintentionally undermine confidentiality through default information-sharing practices that were not designed with adolescent substance use care in mind. Systems-level solutions, including configurable privacy controls, clear documentation standards, and workflows that anticipate harm reduction services such as naloxone distribution, are necessary to align institutional infrastructure with clinical and ethical goals.

Institutional policies must also evolve in response to the changing epidemiology of adolescent substance use. As overdose prevention becomes an expected component of pediatric and adolescent care, policies should explicitly address consent and confidentiality related to naloxone provision, toxicology testing, and follow-up care. Ambiguity in policy often results in inconsistent practice, with some clinicians withholding interventions due to perceived legal risk while others proceed without clear guidance.

At the policy level, ongoing variation in state minor consent laws creates inequities in access to confidential substance use care. Adolescents' ability to receive timely treatment or harm reduction services should not depend solely on geography. Greater harmonization of consent statutes, clearer guidance on the application of federal confidentiality regulations to adolescent care, and explicit inclusion of harm reduction within pediatric practice standards would support more equitable and effective care delivery.

Finally, consent and confidentiality should be recognized as core components of implementation science in adolescent substance use care. Interventions that fail to account for confidentiality concerns—particularly those requiring documentation, caregiver involvement, or system-level reporting—are unlikely to achieve sustained uptake. Incorporating adolescent and caregiver perspectives into policy development and quality improvement efforts can help ensure that evolving models of care remain both effective and acceptable.

SUMMARY

There is an urgent call for continued research, legal reform, and training in adolescent consent and confidentiality. In 2025, consent and confidentiality are no longer peripheral considerations in adolescent substance use care; they are central determinants of whether adolescents disclose risk, engage in treatment, and receive life-saving interventions. Rising rates of substance use disorders and overdose deaths among adolescents—particularly in the context of an increasingly unpredictable illicit drug supply—have elevated the stakes of clinical decision-making. As harm reduction strategies such as naloxone distribution become standard components of care, clinicians must navigate consent and confidentiality with greater intentionality, clarity, and consistency.

This article highlights that consent and confidentiality are not static legal hurdles, but dynamic clinical processes shaped by adolescent development, ethical principles, legal frameworks, and health system design. Thoughtful application of these principles can preserve trust, support family engagement, and promote safety, even in high-risk and acute care settings. Conversely, inconsistent or overly cautious practices risk undermining access to care and widening existing inequities.

Clinicians, institutions, and policymakers share responsibility for ensuring that consent and confidentiality frameworks evolve alongside the changing epidemiology of adolescent substance use. Investment in clinician training, alignment of health system infrastructure, and policy reform that centers adolescent safety and autonomy are essential to meeting this moment. By reframing consent and confidentiality as core clinical interventions, the field can better support adolescents and families while advancing equitable, effective, and compassionate substance use care.

CLINICS CARE POINTS

- Clarify consent and confidentiality early and explicitly. At the outset of care, clinicians should explain who can consent to treatment, what information is confidential, and the specific circumstances under which confidentiality may be breached. Transparent discussions support trust and reduce misunderstandings during high-risk situations.
- Distinguish consent to treatment from control over health information. Legal authority to consent does not automatically determine who may access medical records, and adolescent consent does not always guarantee full confidentiality from parents. Clinicians should clarify these distinctions when discussing care and anticipate real-world limitations, such as insurance disclosures and institutional policies.
- Use a developmentally informed approach to decisional capacity. Adolescents' ability to participate in consent and disclosure decisions is context-dependent. Decision-making may be intact in calm settings but impaired during emotionally charged or peer-influenced situations, which is particularly relevant in substance use care.
- Inform adolescents before breaching confidentiality whenever feasible. Explaining why disclosure is necessary, what information will be shared, and with whom helps preserve trust and supports continued engagement even when confidentiality cannot be fully maintained.

DISCLOSURE

There is nothing to disclose

REFERENCES

1. Friedman J, Godvin M, Shover CL, et al. Trends in drug overdose deaths among US adolescents, January 2010 to June 2021. JAMA 2022;327(14):1398–400.
2. Friedman J, Hadland SE. The overdose crisis among U.S. adolescents. N Engl J Med 2024;390(2):97–100.
3. Goldstick JE, Cunningham RM, Carter PM. Current causes of death in children and adolescents in the United States. N Engl J Med 2022;386(20):1955–6.
4. Tanz LJ, Dinwiddie AT, Mattson CL, et al. Drug overdose deaths among persons aged 10-19 years - united States, July 2019-December 2021. MMWR Morb Mortal Wkly Rep 2022;71(50):1576–82.
5. Simon KM, Levy SJ, Bukstein OG. Adolescent substance use disorders. NEJM Evid 2022;1(6):EVIDra2200051.
6. Agostino H, Toulany A. Considerations for privacy and confidentiality in adolescent health care service delivery. Paediatr Child Health 2023;28(3):172–83.
7. Diekema DS. Adolescent brain development and medical decision-making. Pediatrics 2020;146(Suppl 1):S18–24.
8. Carney T, Myers B. Effectiveness of early interventions for substance-using adolescents: findings from a systematic review and meta-analysis. Subst Abuse Treat Prev Policy 2012;7:25.
9. Panchal N, Zitter S. Teens, drugs, and overdose: contrasting pre-pandemic and current trends. KFF. 2024. Available at: https://www.kff.org/mental-health/teens-drugs-and-overdose-contrasting-pre-pandemic-and-current-trends/. Accessed January 5, 2026.

10. NCDAS. Substance abuse and addiction statistics [2025]. NCDAS. Available at: https://drugabusestatistics.org/. Accessed January 5, 2026.
11. Parmigiani G, Benevento M, Solarino B, et al. Decisional capacity to consent to treatment in children and adolescents: a systematic review. Psychiatry Res 2025;344:116343.
12. Sharko M, Jameson R, Ancker JS, et al. State-by-State variability in adolescent privacy laws. Pediatrics 2022;149(6):e2021053458.
13. Weddle M, Kokotailo PK. Confidentiality and consent in adolescent substance abuse: an update. AMA J Ethics 2005;7(3):239–43.
14. Shields JM, Johnson A. Collision between law and ethics: consent for treatment with adolescents. Bull Am Acad Psychiatry Law 1992;20(3):309–23.
15. Grootens-Wiegers P, Hein IM, van den Broek JM, et al. Medical decision-making in children and adolescents: developmental and neuroscientific aspects. BMC Pediatr 2017;17(1):120.
16. Icenogle G, Steinberg L, Duell N, et al. Adolescents' cognitive capacity reaches adult levels prior to their psychosocial maturity: evidence for a "maturity gap" in a multinational, cross-sectional sample. Law Hum Behav 2019;43(1):69–85.
17. 42 CFR § 2.14 - minor patients. LII/legal information institute. Available at: https://www.law.cornell.edu/cfr/text/42/2.14. Accessed January 8, 2026.
18. Hein IM, Troost PW, Lindeboom R, et al. Accuracy of the MacArthur competence assessment tool for clinical research (MacCAT-CR) for measuring children's competence to consent to clinical research. JAMA Pediatr 2014;168(12):1147–53.
19. Wendler DS. Assent in paediatric research: theoretical and practical considerations. J Med Ethics 2006;32(4):229–34.
20. Scott HK, Cogburn M. Piaget. In: StatPearls. StatPearls Publishing; 2025. Available at: http://www.ncbi.nlm.nih.gov/books/NBK448206/. Accessed January 9, 2026.
21. Hein IM, Troost PW, Broersma A, et al. Why is it hard to make progress in assessing children's decision-making competence? BMC Med Ethics 2015;16:1.
22. US Department of Health and Human Services. Health Insurance Portability and Accountability Act (HIPAA) Privacy Rule. Available at: https://www.hhs.gov/hipaa/for-professionals/privacy/index.html (Accessed 8 January 2026).
23. Sigman GS, O'Connor C. Exploration for physicians of the mature minor doctrine. J Pediatr 1991;119(4):520–5.
24. Navin MC, Wasserman JA. Capacity for preferences and pediatric assent implications for pediatric practice. Hastings Cent Rep 2019;49(1):43–51.
25. Brocato M. Growing pains? An overview of the mature minor doctrine and its patchwork criteria for application. Center for Children, Law & Ethics (CCLE) Online; 2025. Available at: https://www.cumberlandccleonline.com/post/growing-pains-an-overview-of-the-mature-minor-doctrine-and-its-patchwork-criteria-for-application. Accessed January 7, 2026.
26. Heward BJ, Yule AM, Jackson PR. How should harm reduction strategies differ for adolescents and adults? AMA J Ethics 2024;26(7):534–45.

Bullying and Substance Use

Jorge C. Srabstein, MD[a,b,*]

KEYWORDS

• Bullying • Substance use • PTSD • Impulsivity • Detection • Treatment

KEY POINTS

- There is research evidence documenting a significant link between bullying and substance use.
- The role of any trauma symptom as a moderator in this association needs further research.
- There is a need to prevent, detect, and treat substance use within the scope of health risks associated with bullying.

INTRODUCTION

In 2023, nearly one in 5 US high school students (19%) reported being bullied at school, and 16% experienced electronic bullying, according to the Centers for Disease Control and Prevention.[1]

The concept of bullying, initially explained by Olweus[2] in the 1990s, as "a student being exposed, repeatedly and over time, to negative actions on the part of one or more students," has gradually evolved to the present notion of being a multifaceted form of maltreatment that encompasses physical aggression, verbal harassment, and/or relational mistreatment (ignoring or excluding somebody). Furthermore, bullying is known to be prevalent across social settings, along the lifespan, and around the world, as well as occurring, concomitantly or at various times in the lifespan, with other forms of maltreatment (Srabstein J. 2024).[3] A substantial body of literature from the past 24 years documents the strong correlation between bullying involvement, as a victim, perpetrator, victim–perpetrator, or bystander, and adverse outcomes, including physical morbidity, emotional distress, and increased risk behaviors (Srabstein J. 2024).[3] Between 1996 and 2026, researchers focused heavily on the link between bullying and suicide, publishing twice as many articles on this connection as on the relationship between bullying and substance use.[4]

[a] Department of Psychiatry and Behavioral Sciences, Children's National Hospital; [b] Department of Psychiatry and Behavioral Sciences, Geoge Washington University, School of Medicine and Health Sciences

* Department of Psychiatry and Behavioral Sciences, Children's National Hospital, Montgomery County Regional Outpatient Center, 9850 Key West Avenue, Rockville, MD 20850.

E-mail address: jsrabste@childrensnational.org

Child Adolesc Psychiatric Clin N Am 35 (2026) 723–738
https://doi.org/10.1016/j.chc.2026.06.002 **childpsych.theclinics.com**

Abbreviations	
APA	American Psychiatric Association
EMDR	Eye Movement Desensitization and Reprocessing
HBSC	Health Behavior in School-aged Children
PTSD	Post-Traumatic Stress Disorder
SSRI	selective serotonin reuptake inhibitors
TF-CBT	Trauma-Focused Cognitive Behavioral Therapy

Objectives of this article:

1. *Synthesize* current evidence regarding the correlation between bullying involvement and substance use.
2. *Examine* the role of child and adolescent psychiatrists in detecting and treating bullying-related symptoms and risk behaviors, such as substance use.
3. *Propose* strategic directions for future research and clinical practice.

WHAT IS KNOWN?

Association Between Bullying and Substance Use: Cross-Sectional Studies

A literature review covering the years 2015 through early 2026 identified 12 cross-sectional studies[5–16] on adolescent bullying and substance use. These studies used large-scale, *non-clinical* samples from 50 countries, with participant groups ranging from 10,000 to 220,000 teenagers representing diverse national or regional populations. These surveys demonstrate a significant correlation between involvement in traditional bullying or cyberbullying and substance use. This heightened likelihood of drug and alcohol consumption applies to all roles within the bullying dynamic, including victims, perpetrators, bully-victims, and even those who witness the behavior as bystanders.

Of the existing research, just two reports (Perotte and colleagues, 2026[5]; Gaete and colleagues, 2017[16]) differentiated substance use risk levels across the full spectrum of bullying involvement (victims, perpetrators, and bully-victims). A closer examination of each of these two studies[5,16] shows that both were developed in South America (Brazil[5] and Chile[16]); based on analysis of national surveys (the 2019 Brazilian National School Health Survey[5] and the 2014 Chilean National Survey on Violence in School[16]) with total samples of more than 123,000 Brazilian adolescent students[5] and almost 38,000 Chilean teenagers,[16] respectively.

Both studies[5,16] indicate that the association with substance use is lower for only victims and also, both studies focused on the use of nicotine cigarettes, alcohol, and cannabis (**Table 1**), while Perotte and colleagues[5] have also concentrated on the use of hookah, E-cigarettes, illicit drugs, and crack (**Table 2**).

Given the cross-sectional nature of the studies, we can only infer the existence of a significant association without establishing cause and effect.

Association Between Bullying and Substance Use: Longitudinal Studies

Prospective studies across the United States,[17] Australia,[18] and the United Kingdom[19] show that peer[17,18] or sibling[19] bullying in early adolescence often leads to later substance use.

In 2004, Earnshaw and colleagues.[17] implemented a 3 wave longitudinal study, involving more than 4000, fifth-grade students from Alabama, Texas, and California, to ascertain whether peer victimization in fifth grade (at school or in other places,

Table 1
Degree of Association (OR) between distinct roles in bullying and use of cigarette nicotine, alcohol, and cannabis, in the previous month, data from Perrotte et al,[5] and Gaete et al[16]

Substance Used	Victims	Bully/Victims	Perpetrators
Cigarette Nicotine	OR: 1.14; 95% CI [1.00–1.29][a]	OR: 1.60;95%CI [1.40–1.83][a]	OR: 1.59;95% CI: [1.34–1.89][a]
	OR: 1.54; 95% CI [1.30–1.84] [b]	OR: 3.56; 95% CI: [3.06–4.13][b]	OR: 3.94;95% CI [3.21–4.84][b]
Alcohol	OR: 1.23; 95% CI [1.10–1.38][a]	OR: 1.72; 95% CI: [1.58–2.03][a]	OR: 1.81;95% CI: [1.55–2.13][a]
	OR: 1.35; 95% CI [1.26–1.44][b]	OR: 2.37;95%CI: [[2.17–2.59] [b]	OR 2.91; 95% CI [2.58–3.28] [b]
Cannabis	OR: 1.11;95% CI [0.95–1.29][a]	OR: 1.59;95% CI [1.35–1.87][a]	OR: 2.05; 95% [CI:1.69–2.48][a]
	OR: 1.47; 95% CI [1.29–1.67][b]	OR: 3.18; 95% CI: [2.68–3.78][b]	OR 4.22; 95% CI [3.52–5.04][b]

[a] Results from a survey of Chilean Adolescents Gaete, J., Tornero, B., Valenzuela, D., Rojas-Barahona, C. A., Salmivalli, C., Valenzuela, E., & Araya, R. (2017). Substance use among adolescents involved in bullying: a cross-sectional multilevel study. *Frontiers in psychology, 8*, 1056.
[b] Results from a survey of Brazilian Adolescents, Perrotte, G., Baruzzi, M. M., Torales, J., Ventriglio, A., & Castaldelli-Maia, J. M. (2026). Bullying and Psychoactive Substance Use Among Adolescents: Evidence from a Nationally Representative Survey in Brazil. *Substance Use & Misuse*, *61*(3), 385-393.

but not at home) was associated with alcohol, marijuana, and tobacco use in tenth grade, while exploring the role of depressive symptoms as experienced in seventh grade, within this association. Their results documented that peer victimization occurring in fifth grade was significantly associated with use of marijuana, alcohol, and tobacco in tenth grade, and that this association was mediated by depressive symptoms experienced in seventh grade.

In 2012, Kelly and colleagues.[18] tracked over 2000 Australian students over 2 years to examine the link between bullying and substance use. Their findings revealed that

Table 2
Degree of association (OR) between distinct roles in bullying and use hookah, e-cigarettes, illicit drugs and crack, Perrotte G et al 5[5]

Substance Used	Victims	Bully/Victims	Perpetrators
Hookah	OR:1.38; 95% CI [1.201.57]	OR:1.92;95% CI [1.59–2.32]	OR:1.38; 95% CI [1.20–1.57]
E-Cigarettes	OR:1.49; 95% CI [1.22–1.83]	OR:2.58; 95% CI [2.00–3.34]	OR: 3.08; 95% CI [2.35–4.02]
Illicit Drugs	OR:1.51; 95% CI [1.32–1.74]	OR:3.28; 95% CI [2.80–3.85]	OR: 4.20; 95% CI [3.55–4.98]
Crack	OR:2.7; 95% CI [1.67–4.37]	OR: 10.5; 95% CI [6.75–16.5]	OR:10.3; 95% CI [6.00–17.8]

Data from Perrotte G, Baruzzi MM, Torales J, et al. Bullying and psychoactive substance use among adolescents: evidence from a Nationally Representative Survey in Brazil. Subst Use Misuse 2026;61(3):385–393.

being a "bully-victim" at the age of 13 years predicted substance use at the age of 15 years, even when accounting for the students' bullying status at the time of the follow-up. There was evidence of increased odds of risky drinking (OR 3.8) and cannabis use (OR 7.4) among bully/victims as compared to students not involved.

A UK cohort prospective study, led by Dantchev and Wolke,[19] of nearly 7000 early adolescents found that those who were involved, at the age of 12 years, in sibling bullying both as perpetrators and victims, were 1.5 times at higher risk of nicotine dependence or cannabis use, in early adulthood, as compared to teenagers not involved in sibling bullying.

Current Evidence from Meta-Analyses

As of today, the latest meta-analysis on the prospective association between peer bullying perpetration in childhood and adolescence and later substance use was conducted by Vrijen and colleagues,[20] in 2019. This study[20] based on a review of 28 publications, reporting on 22 samples, which included more than 28, 000 participants, showed that bullying perpetration was positively associated with all types of substance use, while the results for those participants who were both perpetrators and victims were more mixed, with generally weaker effects.[20]

Psychiatric Symptoms as Moderators/Mediators in the Pathway from Bullying to Substance Use

A recent systematic review on the link between bullying and subtsance abuse[21] demonstrates that various psychiatric symptoms mediate or moderate the relationship between bullying involvement (both victimization and perpetration) and substance abuse. Key factors include

- Aggression[9]
- Anxiety[22]
- Depression/[6,17,23–28]
- Hopelessness[9]
- Impulsivity[22,29]
- Sadness[9]

Although research confirms that posttraumatic stress disorder (PTSD) is significantly associated with both bullying[30] and substance use,[31] this review[21] identified no studies investigating whether PTSD symptoms moderate the link between the two.

CLINICAL AND PUBLIC HEALTH IMPLICATIONS

The Role of Child and Adolescent Psychiatrists in Addressing Bullying and Other Risk Behaviors

Because bullying is a major public health issue[32] linked to significant morbidity and mortality, child and adolescent psychiatrists are uniquely positioned to prevent, detect, and treat its associated symptoms and risky behaviors.[33]

Prevention of Bullying-Related Health Problems

Pediatric practitioners, particularly child and adolescent psychiatrists, should utilize initial clinical encounters and school consultations to raise awareness of the toxicity of bullying. Beyond education, they must advocate for school programs that foster mutual respect and sensitivity, while highlighting the serious health risks associated with victimization and maltreatment, which impact victims, perpetrators, and bystanders alike.

As of 2024, published data indicate that current prevention strategies have yet to significantly reduce bullying-related morbidity or mortality. Even highly regarded primary prevention programs reduce incidents by only 50% to 60%. Given this gap, child and adolescent psychiatrists play a critical role in secondary and tertiary prevention—detecting bullying early to interrupt its cycle and treating victimization-related morbidity to prevent mortality.[33]

Detection

Clinical Identification of Bullying Involvement and Exposure Systematic screening for bullying exposure and participation during psychiatric evaluations is a vital public health instrument for the secondary prevention of ongoing victimization. Effective detection serves as a catalyst for interventions aimed at terminating bullying cycles and mitigating associated health risks.

One way to navigate this conversation is by informing patients and their families that, as a health professional, one is concerned about the significant health problems resulting from bullying and other forms of victimization. Consequently, routine inquiries should be made regarding whether patients are exposed to, or participating in, bullying within any environment or circumstance.

It is essential that the patient and the clinician reach a shared understanding of bullying, framed within the patient's specific cultural language and developmental stage. In this context, terminology may include being bothered, hurt, offended, teased, insulted, or harassed. Providing examples across distinct categories of mistreatment—including verbal, physical, emotional, and relational—further illustrates the multifaceted aspects of bullying.

If the patient identifies involvement in bullying, whether through exposure or participation, it must be determined if the victimization is current (within the last 2 months) or occurred in the past. This process further clarifies the specific type of bullying, its frequency, the social milieu or location, and what measures, if any, are being taken to intervene.

Detection of Bullying-Related Health Problems

Clinicians should routinely screen all new pediatric psychiatric patients for clinical manifestations of bullying exposure or involvement.[3] This evaluation must extend beyond the chief complaint to identify potential psychiatric symptoms, trauma, risk behaviors, and psychosocial stressors.

Detection of Symptoms

The approach uses a semi-structured interview to conduct a thorough anamnesis. The process begins by screening current, recent, or lifetime symptoms[34] as follows:

- *Mood and emotion* (depressed mood; anhedonia; irritability; hopelessness; worthlessness; grandiosity; emotional numbing; euphoria).
- *Cognitive and perception* (racing thoughts; inattention
  delusions; hallucinations; obsessions; suicidal or homicidal ideation; intrusion of thoughts; body preoccupation).
- *Anxiety and fears* (having multiple worries; worries about future events; feeling that something terrible is about to happen; hypervigilance; panic sensations; fear of being scrutinized or shamed by others).
- *Physical and somatic sensations* (headaches, abdominal pain, dizziness, nausea without organic cause; fatigue; appetite changes; hypersensitivity to sound, light, or touch; cravings for a specific substance).

- *Sleeping symptoms* (insomnia; hypersomnia, nightmares; decreased need for sleep).
- *Dissociation* (depersonalization [feeling like an outside observer of one's own body or mind]; derealization [a feeling that the world around is "foggy," "fake," or unreal]; flashbacks; feeling like multiple people).

For each symptom, clinicians should document the time of onset, frequency, duration, intensity (on a 1–10 scale), setting (eg, home, school), and potential triggers. Symptom anamnesis should be obtained directly from the patient using age-appropriate inquiry tailored to their intellectual and communicative abilities. However, parents may provide following essential collateral information, particularly regarding observed changes in emotion, behavior, cognition, perception, or sleep disturbance[34] :

- *Emotional and Behavioral Signs:* Frequent verbal or physical temper tantrums; loss of interest in play and/or meeting with friends; verbal or physical hostility toward others; flat affect or reduction in the expression of positive emotions; being constantly "on guard," jumpy or having an exaggerated startle response.
- *Cognitive and perceptual signs*: Difficulties in sustaining focus in school or play activities; hearing voices or seeing things that occurred without stimuli; loss of previously mastered skills, like toilet training or speech.
- *Sleep disturbance signs:* Difficulty in falling or staying asleep without parent intervention; frequent frightening dreams causing distress; difficulties in waking up or falling asleep at standard times.

Detection of Risks Behaviors

As part of the anamnesis gathered from the patient, parents, or other sources, there is a need to ascertain whether the patient has recently or in the past been involved in one or more of the following risk behaviors, including *bullying others*[3]:

- *Aggression: Verbally or physically bullying others*; threatening, using a weapon
- *Intentional property destruction*
- *Deceit and theft:* Lying for personal gain; breaking into homes or cars, stealing.
- *Rule violations:* Frequent school truancy; running away from home; staying away from home at night without permission.
- *Non-suicidal self-injury*
- *Suicidal or homicidal attempt*
- *Substance use*

Identifying Adverse Events and Victimization

The clinical assessment should encompass an evaluation of both direct and witnessed exposure to the following adverse, stressful, or traumatic events, whether current or historical.[34–37]

- *Bullying*: This includes physical aggression (eg, hitting, pushing), verbal harassment (eg, teasing, name-calling), and/or relational aggression (eg, social exclusion, rumors, peer pressure, discrimination) occurring in any social environment, such as schools, in cyberspace, at home between siblings, in the neighborhood, during sports activities, or in the workplace(for older adolescents).
- *Dating victimization*: Physical or sexual violence, stalking, or psychological aggression by a current or former boyfriend, girlfriend, dating, or sexual partners.[38]
- *Abuse:* Physical or sexual abuse of a child or adolescent by a parent or caregiver; or emotional abuse,[39] such as being rejected, degraded, or humiliated; isolated

from peers or adults; exploited or corrupted; denied emotional responsiveness; or neglected in their health, mental health, medical, or educational needs.
- *Medical trauma:* Experiencing a life-threatening illness, serious accident (eg, car crash), or painful medical procedures.
- *Academic stress:* Measured as "schoolwork pressure".[40,41] This is an item included in the Health Behavior in School-aged Children (HBSC)[42] survey. Responses are scored from 0 to 3, with higher scores indicating greater perceived pressure.
- *Loss of friendship*
- *Death and grief:* Sudden loss of a parent, caregiver, or closed loved one.
- *Domestic or intimate partner violence*
- *Living with a household member who has a substance use disorder or mental illness*
- *Parental separation or divorce*
- *Household member incarceration*
- *Community violence:* School shooting; mass violence; war; homicidal or suicidal death of a friend
- *Exposure to disasters:* Natural disasters like hurricanes, floods, or wildfires, as well as human-made disasters like terrorism or war,
- *Unmet health-related social needs:* Homelessness; extreme poverty; social isolation.

Intervention

Stopping ongoing bullying is a critical public health strategy to prevent recurrent victimization and persistent health complications. Clinicians who identify targeted patients must help them and their families report the abuse to school authorities and demand immediate action. If a patient is a perpetrator or a bully-victim, clinicians should provide targeted behavioral interventions aimed at terminating their aggressive behavior as a core component of their psychiatric treatment.

School Intervention

To prevent and mitigate bullying, schools have implemented various interventions,[42] including

- Disciplinary consequences for prohibited behavior (incorporated in many US statutes to prevent bullying).
- Restorative practices,[43] focusing on the perpetrator's recognition of harm and subsequent reparation to the victim.
- Victim empowerment,[44] specifically through assertive communication training
- Mediation[45] to resolve conflicts between the perpetrator and the victim.
- The Method of Shared Concern,[46] involving separate and eventual joint consultations to reach a solution.
- The Support Group Method,[47] a non-punitive intervention that engages perpetrators in a group setting (excluding the victim) to foster accountability for the harm caused and encourage proactive efforts to mitigate the impact of the maltreatment.

Limitations of current interventions

- *Psychosocial distress in victim-perpetrator interactions:* Direct confrontation with the perpetrator—a common component of mediation and the method of shared concern—can trigger avoidance behaviors and heightened anxiety in victims.

- *Victim responsibility in the intervention process:* Strategies centered on victim resilience place the onus on the injured party to endure maltreatment, failing to prioritize the cessation of the perpetrator's behavior.
- *Required to stop bullying:* Mandating participation in restorative practices or support groups can feel coercive. For emotionally vulnerable perpetrators, these methods may prove intimidating or even aggravate the situation rather than resolving it.

Brief health intervention to stop ongoing bullying

An established[48] framework outlines a recommended strategy for developing and validating a voluntary, 3 week health intervention targeting active bullying behavior. Designed for implementation by school health professionals with child psychiatric oversight, this program requires parental consent and rigorous emotional risk monitoring. The framework aligns directly with the Klomek and colleagues.[49] Bullying Prevention Plan, which is built upon the following core strategic objectives:

- *Environmental risk reduction:* Eliminating physical and digital spaces, as well as peer interactions, that prompt or facilitate bullying behavior.
- *Identifying prodromal signs of aggression:* Spotting early emotional markers, such as anger or behavioral urges, which precede active bullying.
- *Applying personal de-escalation strategies:* Using alternative behaviors and self-calming methods to suppress the urge to mistreat others.
- *Accessing interpersonal support for redirection:* Interacting with designated individuals to effectively neutralize and divert the urge to bully.
- *Addressing dual victimization and preventing retaliation:* Identifying if the perpetrator is concurrently a victim of bullying and mobilizing targeted clinical interventions to disrupt the cycle of mutual mistreatment.
- *Facilitating clinical escalation pathways:* Securing specialized child and adolescent psychiatric intervention when intense aggressive impulses resist standard self-regulation strategies.

This framework directly incorporates the core principles of Solution-Focused Brief Therapy.[50] It is designed for students with intact cognitive abilities, sound judgment, healthy empathy, and stable moods. However, practitioners must adapt the approach to align with the student's developmental stage and sociocultural background. Moving forward, this intervention model requires further standardization and formal efficacy testing.

Treatment

The diagnostic context for treatment

Treating the symptoms, risk behaviors, and psychosocial problems associated with past or present exposure to bullying falls under the diagnostic framework for stress and trauma-related disorders. Diagnoses within this framework include adjustment disorder, acute stress disorder, and PTSD.

- *Overlapping symptoms:* All 3 conditions can present with depressed mood, irritability, anxiety, sleep disturbances, nightmares, and intrusive memories.
- *Acute stress disorder and PTSD specifics:* Symptoms such as flashbacks, depersonalization, derealization, dissociation, inattention, hypervigilance, and nausea are primarily tied to acute stress disorder and PTSD.
- *Severe Complications:* Both adjustment disorder and PTSD are linked to suicidal ideation, hallucinations, headaches, backaches, and non-epileptic seizures.

- *Behavioral risks:* Substance abuse, self-injury, and suicide attempts represent critical behavioral risks experienced by individuals with PTSD and adjustment disorder.

These trauma-related and stress-related symptoms and behavioral risks are primarily experienced by youth with a history of past or current bullying victimization. However, they are also prevalent among "bully-victims" (perpetrators who are also victimized) and pure perpetrators, who frequently have histories of other forms of maltreatment or prior victimization.

Additionally, the symptoms of impulsivity and irritability leading to risky behaviors, including bullying, or mistreating others, may fall under several clinical diagnoses, such as

- Disruptive mood dysregulation disorder
- Conduct disorder
- Intermittent explosive disorder
- Attention deficit hyperactivity disorder (ADHD)
- Bipolar disorder (Mania)

And these need to be appropriately treated.

Treatment for bullying victims with stress and trauma symptoms

For victims of bullying who present with symptoms of an adjustment disorder, our practice recommends brief psychotherapy. Patients are typically treated with cognitive behavioral therapy (CBT) to mitigate stressors, facilitate adaptation, and modify maladaptive behavioral responses.[51] When pharmacotherapy is indicated, it is symptom-oriented and targets depressive mood, agitation, and anxiety using selective serotonin reuptake inhibitors (SSRIs), mood stabilizers, or antipsychotic medications.

For youth exposed to bullying who exhibit symptoms consistent with acute stress disorder or PTSD, our psychotherapy strategy has been guided by the findings of the network meta-analysis of evidence-based therapies by Mavranezouli and colleagues.[52] Based on this framework, we utilize:

- *First-line therapy:* Trauma-focused cognitive behavioral therapy (TF-CBT) as the primary intervention.
- *Alternative therapy:* Eye movement desensitization and reprocessing (EMDR) may be utilized as a secondary intervention.

While evidence-based psychotherapeutic interventions such as TF-CBT and EMDR have been studied in youth with trauma-related symptoms, evidence specific to pharmacologic treatment of bullying-related trauma remains limited. Our clinical observation indicates that standard American Psychiatric Association (APA)[53] guidelines recommending SSRIs as first-line therapy are often ineffective for bullying-induced PTSD. Specifically, SSRIs have frequently failed to resolve complex trauma symptoms, including mood instability, irritability, hyperarousal, impulsivity, flashbacks, and dissociation. The following recommendations reflect the author's clinical experience managing youth exposed to bullying and should be considered expert opinion rather than evidence-based treatment guidelines.

- *Primary pharmacotherapy:* Initiating treatment with an anticonvulsant medication like Lamotrigine.
- *Augmentation:* If necessary, augment this regimen with guanfacine or an atypical antipsychotic.

Treatment of mood dysregulation, impulsivity, and aggression

Treatment for youth who bully or victimize others may require strategies focused on mood regulation and impulse control. This process involves alleviating irritability, reducing intrusive thoughts that trigger negative urges, and correcting thought or perceptual distortions leading to delusions or hallucinations. Simultaneously, the treatment must enhance empathy, respect, and social sensitivity toward others.

These objectives can be seamlessly integrated into psychological frameworks such as cognitive-behavioral therapy for aggression and impulsivity.[54,55] Furthermore, these programs may incorporate elements of the Bullying Prevention Plan,[49] which was previously outlined in the subsection "Brief Health Intervention to Stop Ongoing Bullying."

In instances where the clinical severity of underlying symptoms drives aggressive or bullying behaviors, it may be necessary to initiate pharmacotherapy. Evidence supporting specific pharmacologic approaches for bullying-related aggression is limited, and medication selection should be guided by the underlying psychiatric diagnosis and symptom profile. In my clinical practice, starting with guanfacine and/or an anticonvulsant like lamotrigine has yielded effective outcomes. If a patient requires a more robust response, this baseline regimen can be successfully augmented by adding an atypical antipsychotic.

Addressing poly-victimization and revictimization in bullying treatment

When treating youth involved in bullying, whether as victims, perpetrators, or both, clinicians must recognize that bullying often co-occurs with other forms of victimization. Pivotal research by Finkelhor and colleagues.[56] demonstrates that among US children and adolescents who experienced one form of victimization in a single year, at least 60% experienced another form within that same year. Furthermore, 18% of youth in the US experience 4 or more distinct types of victimization within a single year, a phenomenon known as poly-victimization. Accounting for this concept is critical, as poly-victimization—as shown by Ford and colleagues[57] is significantly associated with PTSD diagnoses (OR = 11.77), severe aggressive behavior (OR = 5.93), and marked psychiatric impairment (OR = 4.57); consequently, it must be a core consideration in psychosocial treatment planning.

Furthermore, psychosocial interventions for both victims and perpetrators must account for the persistent threat of re-victimization. Longitudinal data from Finkelhor and colleagues.[56] demonstrate the severity of this cycle, showing that 66% of youth experiencing peer or sibling victimization in a given year suffer re-victimization the following year.

In this context, both psychosocial and psychopharmacological treatments must incorporate regular screening at every follow-up visit. Clinicians must actively assess whether exposure to bullying, other forms of victimization, or adverse life events remain ongoing or recurrent.

Integrating treatment for bullying and substance use

Research indicates that individuals exposed to trauma who exhibit PTSD symptoms display significantly higher levels of impulsivity and substance use than traumatized individuals without PTSD, suggesting that impulsivity acts as a mediator between PTSD and substance misuse.[58] Furthermore, the roles of emotion dysregulation and impulsivity have been heavily underscored in the association between PTSD and substance use.[59]

Consequently, treating individuals involved in bullying—as victims, perpetrators, or both—who present with co-occurring substance use requires a tailored approach. This involves integrating psychosocial and pharmacologic interventions targeted at

PTSD symptoms or focusing directly on impulsivity and mood dysregulation for patients who do not meet the full criteria for PTSD.

When treating youth with PTSD and substance use, clinicians should closely coordinate services with a child and adolescent psychiatrist who has training and clinical experience in addiction psychiatry. In this context, a comprehensive consultation should evaluate the following domains:

- *Diagnostic profile:* The specific classes of substances used, the quantity and frequency of consumption, and whether the youth meet criteria for a substance use disorder.[60,61]
- *Functional impact:* The direct and indirect consequences of substance use across different domains, including family, school, social, psychological, and medical.[60]
- *Contextual and behavioral factors:* The patient's view of substance use, their expectancies of use, the usual times and places of substance use, peer attitudes and use patterns, common behavioral or emotional antecedents, and the patient's overall social milieu.[60]
- *Diagnostic screening:* The clinical necessity for objective toxicologic screening.
- *Level of care:* The appropriate treatment setting, ranging from outpatient services to partial hospitalization or inpatient care.
- *Integrated psychosocial strategies:* The addition of family-based therapy, motivational interviewing, motivational enhancement therapy, or 12 step programs to supplement trauma-focused and aggression-focused modalities already planned, such as TF-CBT, EMDR, or cognitive-behavioral therapy for aggression and impulsivity.[54,55]
- *Pharmacologic management:* The optimization of medication regimens, evaluating the introduction of addiction-focused agents (eg, bupropion, naltrexone) alongside medications already planned, including guanfacine, sertraline, atypical antipsychotics, or antiepileptic medications such as lamotrigine, topiramate, or gabapentin.
- *Medication safety and efficacy*: How active substance use impacts the safety and efficacy of medications prescribed for bullying-related trauma.

FUTURE DIRECTIONS

There is a public health need to

- Conduct periodic national health surveys, such as the HBSC study,[51] to better understand how regional sociocultural determinants influence bullying prevalence and associated substance use patterns in non-clinical populations.
- Establish clinical studies across diverse health care settings to determine the prevalence of substance use among pediatric patients involved in bullying as victims, perpetrators, or both.
- Quantify the Global Burden of Disease[62] among populations affected by substance use tied to bullying involvement.
- Design longitudinal clinical trials to identify clusters of psychiatric symptoms (including trauma) and evaluate their roles as mediators or moderators in the relationship between bullying and substance use risk.
- Integrate bullying and substance use prevention efforts into a single, comprehensive school wellness strategy to protect at-risk students.
- Advocate for schools to consult with child and adolescent psychiatrists regarding students exposed to or participating in bullying to detect and mitigate associated health risks.

SUMMARY

Research evidence demonstrates a strong link between bullying and subsequent substance use. This association is especially pronounced among youth who are both perpetrators and victims—a dynamic driven by trauma symptoms, impulsivity, and irritability.

In this context, child and adolescent psychiatrists play a unique role in

- *Integrating prevention*: Advocating for the integration of bullying prevention strategies with substance use prevention programs.
- *Universal screening*: Evaluating all new psychiatric patients for both substance use and involvement in bullying.
- *School advocacy*: Campaigning for effective school interventions to halt ongoing bullying.
- *Targeted therapy*: Utilizing therapeutic strategies to address trauma, mood instability, and impulsivity, thereby treating bullying-related morbidity and curbing substance use.

CLINICS CARE POINTS

- Screen every new psychiatric patient for both substance use and bullying.
- Target underlying trauma, impulsivity, and iiritability to reduce substance use.
- Avoid separating substance use treatment from bullying and trauma history.
- Do not overlook bullies who are often victims themselves in need of trauma therapy.

ACKNOWLEDGMENTS

I acknowledge the use of Google Gemini (Google, May 8, 2026) to assist in organizing and tailoring, by categories, the list of psychiatric symptoms, signs and risk behaviors included in DSM V, for the detection/anamnesis section. I take full responsibility for the integrity and accuracy of the final content.

DISCLOSURES

The author of this article is also the published author of the book *Bullying, Impact on Health, and Beyond: Exploring the Spectrum of Maltreatment*. Oxford University Press; 2024.

REFERENCES

1. Centers for Disease Control and Prevention. Youth risk behavior survey data summary & trends report: 2013–2023. US Dept of Health and Human Services 2024;45–7. Available at: https://www.cdc.gov/yrbs/dstr/pdf/YRBS-2023-Data-Summary-Trend-Report.pdf. Accessed May 22, 2026.
2. Olweus D. Bullying at school: what we know and what we can do. MA: Blackwell; 1993.
3. Srabstein JC. Chapter four: morbidity associated with bullying and other forms of victimization and chapter 5: psychosocial problems and risk behaviors linked to bullying and other forms of victimization. In: Bullying, impact on health, and beyond: exploring the spectrum of maltreatment. New York (NY): Oxford University Press; 2024. p. 35–83.

4. Advanced PubMed Search with the terms "bullying" AND "suicide" as well as "bullying" AND "substance," respectively, appearing in the "Title/Abstract," from 1996 to 2026. Available at: https://pubmed.ncbi.nlm.nih.gov/advanced/. Accessed April 9, 2026.
5. Perrotte G, Baruzzi MM, Torales J, et al. Bullying and psychoactive substance use among adolescents: evidence from a Nationally Representative Survey in Brazil. Subst Use Misuse 2026;61(3):385–93.
6. Zhou H, Chen JK. Teacher–student relationship quality as a mediator in the Association of Parent–Child communication with adolescent bullying perpetration and substance use: evidence from the 2017/2018 HBSC study. Behav Sci Law 2026; 44(3):469–78.
7. Yang X, Yang Y. Adolescent polysubstance use: the intersection of social media use frequency and cyberbullying. Subst Use Misuse 2026;1–8.
8. Lehmann PS, Wingert AC, Jones MS. Bullying victimization, gender, and adolescent substance use: the moderating role of school connectedness. Crime Delinquen 2025;71(10):3269–98.
9. Azagba S, Ebling T, Korkmaz A. Mediators of bullying victimization and substance use among US high school students. Int J Ment Health Addiction 2025; 23(3):2402–14.
10. Boccio CM, Leal WE, Jackson DB. Bullying victimization and nicotine and marijuana vaping among Florida adolescents. Drug Alcohol Depend 2022;237: 109536.
11. Da Silva MA, Martins SS. Mutual influences on bullying perpetration and substance use among adolescents in the United States. J Adolesc Health 2020; 67(3):384–91.
12. Azagba S, Akofua Mensah N, Shan L, et al. Bullying victimization and e-cigarette use among middle and high school students. J Sch Health 2020;90(7):545–53.
13. Baiden P, Tadeo SK. Examining the association between bullying victimization and prescription drug misuse among adolescents in the United States. J Affect Disord 2019;259:317–24.
14. Turner S, Taillieu T, Fortier J, et al. Bullying victimization and illicit drug use among students in grades 7 to 12 in Manitoba, Canada: a cross-sectional analysis. Can J Public Health 2018;109(2):183–94.
15. Cénat JM, Blais M, Lavoie F, et al. Cyberbullying victimization and substance use among Quebec high schools students: the mediating role of psychological distress. Comput Hum Behav 2018;89:207–12.
16. Gaete J, Tornero B, Valenzuela D, et al. Substance use among adolescents involved in bullying: a cross-sectional multilevel study. Front Psychol 2017;8: 1056.
17. Earnshaw VA, Elliott MN, Reisner SL, et al. Peer victimization, depressive symptoms, and substance use: a longitudinal analysis. Pediatrics 2017;139(6): e20163426.
18. Kelly EV, Newton NC, Stapinski LA, et al. Concurrent and prospective associations between bullying victimization and substance use among Australian adolescents. Drug Alcohol Depend 2015;154:63–8.
19. Dantchev S, Wolke D. Sibling bullying at 12 years and high-risk behavior in early adulthood: a prospective cohort study. Aggress Behav 2019;45(1):18–32.
20. Vrijen C, Wiertsema M, Ackermans MA, et al. Childhood and adolescent bullying perpetration and later substance use: a meta-analysis. Pediatrics 2021;147(3): e2020034751.

21. Association of Bullying and Substance Use. Available at: https://pubmed.ncbi.nlm.nih.gov/advanced/ (Accessed 16 April 2026).
22. Laroque FM, Boers E, Afzali MH, et al. Personality-specific pathways from bullying victimization to adolescent alcohol use: a multilevel longitudinal moderated mediation analysis. Dev Psychopathol 2023;35(3):1454–67.
23. Vannucci A, Fagle TR, Simpson EG, et al. Perceived family and friend support moderate pathways from peer victimization to substance use in early-adolescent girls and boys: a moderated-mediation analysis. J Early Adolesc 2021;41(1):128–66.
24. Mei S, Hu Y, Sun M, et al. Association between bullying victimization and symptoms of depression among adolescents: a moderated mediation analysis. Int J Environ Res Publ Health 2021;18(6):3316.
25. Luk JW, Wang J, Simons-Morton BG. Bullying victimization and substance use among US adolescents: mediation by depression. Prev Sci 2010;11(4):355–9.
26. Richard J, Grande-Gosende A, Fletcher É, et al. Externalizing problems and mental health symptoms mediate the relationship between bullying victimization and addictive behaviors. Int J Ment Health Addiction 2020;18(4):1081–96.
27. Forster M, Dyal SR, Baezconde-Garbanati L, et al. Bullying victimization as a mediator of associations between cultural/familial variables, substance use, and depressive symptoms among Hispanic youth. Ethn Health 2013;18(4):415–32.
28. Lawrence TI, Hong JS, Espelage DL, et al. Antecedents of sibling aggression and bullying victimization: the parallel and serial contributions of depressive symptoms and substance use. J Affect Disord 2023;333:193–201.
29. Walters GD, Espelage DL. Exploring the victimization–early substance misuse relationship: in search of moderating and mediating effects. Child Abuse Negl 2018;81:354–65.
30. Idsoe T, Dyregrov A, Idsoe EC. Bullying and PTSD symptoms. J Abnorm Child Psychol 2012;40(6):901–11.
31. Brady KT, Back SE, Coffey SF. Substance abuse and posttraumatic stress disorder. Curr Dir Psychol Sci 2004;13(5):206–9.
32. Srabstein JC, Leventhal BL. Prevention of bullying-related morbidity and mortality: a call for public health policies. Bull World Health Organ 2010;88:403–4.
33. APA Official Actions. Joint AACAP and APA position statement on prevention of bullying-related morbidity and mortality, approved by the board. 2011. Available at: https://www.psychiatry.org/getattachment/b06fadeb-8b23-4c0e-922d-bda599cc370c/Position-2011-Bullying.pdf. Accessed April 30, 2026.
34. American Psychiatric Association. Diagnostic and statistical manual of mental disorders. 5th edition, text rev. Washington, DC: American Psychiatric Association; 2022.
35. Centers for Disease Control and Prevention. Preventing adverse childhood experiences: leveraging the best available evidence. Atlanta, GA: National Center for Injury Prevention and Control, Centers for Disease Control and Prevention, 40. 2019. Available at: https://stacks.cdc.gov/view/cdc/82316. Accessed August 5, 2026.
36. Idsoe T, Vaillancourt T, Dyregrov A, et al. Bullying victimization and trauma. Front Psychiatr 2021;11:480353.
37. Weathers FW, Blake DD, Schnurr PP, et al. The life events checklist for DSM-5 (LEC-5). Available at: https://www.ptsd.va.gov/professional/assessment/documents/LEC-5_Interview.pdf. Accessed May 8, 2026.

38. Breiding MJ, Chen J, Black MC. Intimate partner violence in the United States–20. 2014. Available at: https://stacks.cdc.gov/view/cdc/21961 (Accessed 8 May 2026).
39. Glaser D. Emotional abuse and neglect (psychological maltreatment): a conceptual framework. Child Abuse Negl 2002;26(6–7):697–714.
40. Cosma A, Stevens G, Martin G, et al. Cross-national time trends in adolescent mental well-being from 2002 to 2018 and the explanatory role of schoolwork pressure. J Adolesc Health 2020;66(6):S50–8.
41. Armitage JM, Lewis G, Page N, et al. Change over time in perceived schoolwork pressure and associations with emotional problems among 11–16-year-olds: a repeat cross-sectional study in Wales, UK. JCPP advances 2025;5(4):e70005.
42. Rigby K. How teachers address cases of bullying in schools: a comparison of five reactive approaches. Educ Psychol Pract 2014;30(4):409–19.
43. Morrison B. Restoring safe school communities. Federation Press; 2007, cited by Rigby42.
44. Savage R. Friendship and bullying patterns in children attending a language base in a mainstream school. Educ Psychol Pract 2005;21(1):23–36, cited by Rigby[42].
45. Johnson DW, Johnson RT, Dudley B. Effects of peer mediation training on elementary school students. Mediat Q 1992;10(1):89–99, cited by Rigby[42].
46. Pikas A. New developments of the shared concern method. Sch Psychol Int 2002; 23(3):307–26, cited by Rigby[42].
47. Robinson G, Bullying MB. A complete guide to the support group method. London, England: SAGE; 2008. cited by Rigby[42].
48. Srabstein JC. Chapter nine: intervention and treatment. In: Bullying, impact on health, and beyond: exploring the spectrum of maltreatment. Oxford University Press.; 2024. p. 144–6.
49. Klomek AB, Stanley B, Sourander A. Bullying prevention plan (BPP). Adolesc Psychiatry 2014;4:000.
50. Bond C, Woods K, Humphrey N, et al. Practitioner review: the effectiveness of solution focused brief therapy with children and families: a systematic and critical evaluation of the literature from 1990–2010. JCPP (J Child Psychol Psychiatry) 2013;54(7):707–23.
51. Casey P. Adjustment disorder: epidemiology, diagnosis, and treatment. CNS Drugs 2009;23(11):927–38.
52. Mavranezouli I, Megnin-Viggars O, Daly C, et al. Research review: psychological and psychosocial treatments for children and young people with post-traumatic stress disorder: a network meta-analysis. JCPP (J Child Psychol Psychiatry) 2020;61(1):18–29.
53. Ursano RJ, Bell C, Spencer E, et al. Practice guideline for the treatment of patients with acute stress disorder and posttraumatic stress disorder. Am J Psychiatry 2004;161(11 Suppl):3–31.
54. Soleimani-Rad H, Abolghasemi A, Shakerinia I, et al. Cognitive behavioural therapy for adolescents with impulsive aggressive behaviour: a randomised controlled trial. Early Intervention in Psychiatry 2026;20(3):e70146.
55. Zarei E, Mobbasser M, Karimpour S. Effectiveness of training anger management according to cognitive approach on the impulsivity in bully male students. Psychological Achievements 2024;31(2):49–70.
56. Finkelhor D, Ormrod RK, Turner HA. Polyvictimization and trauma in a national longitudinal cohort. Dev Psychopathol 2007;19(1):149–66.

57. Ford JD, Wasser T, Connor DF. Identifying and determining the symptom severity associated with polyvictimization among psychiatrically impaired children in the outpatient setting. Child Maltreat 2011;16(3):216–26.
58. Morris VL, Huffman LG, Naish KR, et al. Impulsivity as a mediating factor in the association between posttraumatic stress disorder symptoms and substance use. Psychol Trauma, Theory Res Pract Pol 2020;12(6):659.
59. Weiss NH, Tull MT, Anestis MD, et al. The relative and unique contributions of emotion dysregulation and impulsivity to posttraumatic stress disorder among substance dependent inpatients. Drug Alcohol Depend 2013;128(1–2):45–51.
60. Bukstein OG. Practice parameter for the assessment and treatment of children and adolescents with substance use disorders. J Am Acad Child Adolesc Psychiatr 2005;44(6):609–21.
61. About health behavior in school-aged children. Available at: https://www.hbsc.org/about/. Accessed April 19, 2026.
62. University of Washington, Institute for Health Metrics and Evaluation, Global burden of disease (GBD). Available at: https://www.healthdata.org/research-analysis/gbd. Accessed April 19, 2026.

Why Context Matters

Rethinking Minoritized Youth Substance Use Care and Outcomes

Lisa R. Fortuna, MD, MPH, MD[a,*], Michelle V. Porche, EdD[b], Mikaela Pulse, PhD[a]

KEYWORDS

- Substance use • Minoritized youth • Systems of care • Structural determinants
- School substance use care

KEY POINTS

- Minoritized youth experience distinct structural and sociocultural determinants of substance use, including racism-related stress, trauma, immigration stress, and inequitable access to care.
- Self-report and toxicology exhibit variable concordance across racial/ethnic groups, with implications for screening accuracy and disparities in identification.
- Family-based and motivational interventions, mindfulness-based therapies, and culturally grounded approaches demonstrate strong evidence for improving outcomes for minority youth.
- Religiosity, spirituality, and cultural identity may operate as protective factors against early alcohol use and progression to disorder, particularly among girls and certain ethnic-racial groups.
- Innovative, community-partnered models—including digital care, school-based, and trauma-focused substance use disorder interventions—can address gaps in access and retention among underserved youth.

INTRODUCTION

Substance use disorders (SUDs) in adolescence occur against a backdrop of dynamic neurodevelopment, shifting social contexts, and cumulative environmental stressors. Although national surveys show that Black, Latino, Asian American, multiracial, and some immigrant youth do not use substances at higher rates than White adolescents, minoritized youth experience *greater exposure to structural and sociopolitical risk*

[a] Department of Psychiatry & Neurosciences, University of California, Riverside, School of Medicine; [b] Department of Internal Medicine, University of California, Riverside, School of Medicine
* Corresponding author. Department of Psychiatry and Neuroscience, 900 University Avenue, Riverside, CA 92521.
E-mail address: lisa.fortuna@medsch.ucr.edu

Child Adolesc Psychiatric Clin N Am 35 (2026) 739–757
https://doi.org/10.1016/j.chc.2026.05.004 childpsych.theclinics.com

Abbreviations	
BSFT	brief strategic family therapy
CBT	cognitive behavioral therapy
CM	contingency management
EBP	evidence-based practice
MDFT	multidimensional family therapy
MI	motivational interviewing
MOUD	medication for opioid use disorder
PTSD	post-traumatic stress disorder
SUD	substance use disorder

factors, higher likelihood of punitive rather than therapeutic responses to substance use, and *significant disparities in access to evidence-based SUD treatment.*[1,2] These inequities are produced and perpetuated by structural racism, community disadvantage, trauma, discriminatory, or at minimum misinformed school and legal systems, and disparities in insurance and service availability.[3,4]

Further complicating equitable diagnosis and intervention are well-documented racial, ethnic, and gender-related differences in the validity, interpretation, and downstream consequences of substance use screening and identification. Studies demonstrate that concordance between adolescent self-report and objective toxicologic measures varies substantially across racial/ethnic subgroups and by gender, raising significant concerns about the reliability and fairness of commonly used screening tools in both clinical and research settings.[5] Gender norms, reproductive health issues, socialization patterns, and power dynamics shape both substance use behaviors and disclosure practices, contributing to systematic differences in who is identified, how risk is interpreted, and what interventions are offered.[6]

Evidence suggests that toxicologic methods used in research and clinical services, such as hair analysis and other longer-detection-window assays, may identify substance exposure that is frequently missed by self-report alone.[7] However, these approaches are not methodologically or socially neutral.[8] Hair-based testing, for example, shows differential sensitivity based on hair texture, cosmetic practices, melanin content, and hormonal influences—factors that intersect with race, ethnicity, and gender expression.[9] Gendered grooming practices (eg, hair treatments, braiding, shaving, or covering) and cultural norms around appearance may further affect assay reliability, raising concerns about differential false positives or negatives for girls, transgender youth, and gender-diverse adolescents. Without explicit attention to these dynamics, reliance on toxicology as a corrective to self-report risks reinforcing inequities rather than mitigating them.[10] In clinical settings, increased reliance on toxicology may have unintended consequences, including erosion of trust and perceptions of surveillance that negatively impact engagement in care, particularly among minoritized youth, and should be balanced with relationship-centered care through transparent, consent-based communication, attention to confidentiality, and shared decision-making.

SUBSTANCE USE DISORDER DISCLOSURE AND SCREENING

Regardless of whether toxicology methods are used, sociocultural and structural factors related to gender further influence disclosure and screening accuracy. Adolescent girls may under-report substance use due to heightened stigma, fear of moral judgment, or concern about reputational harm, particularly in primary care or school-linked settings, and patterns of use may vary by race.[11] Conversely, boys may over-report or normalize certain forms of substance use due to masculinity norms that valorize risk-taking or minimize perceived harm.[12] Transgender and gender-diverse youth may face additional barriers to accurate screening, including fear of misgendering, discrimination, or disclosure of substance use being used to invalidate their gender identity or access to gender-affirming care.[13,14] These concerns are compounded for youth who also experience racialization, immigration stress, or system involvement.

In primary care settings—where substance use screening is often brief, protocolized, and embedded within time-limited visits[15]—these biases may have significant implications. Universal screening tools that do not account for gendered patterns of use, disclosure, and risk interpretation may lead to underidentification of substance use among girls and gender-diverse youth, while disproportionately flagging boys or youth of color for further monitoring or referral.[16] Such misclassification can result in delayed intervention, inappropriate counseling, missed opportunities for early prevention, and/or escalation to punitive or stigmatizing pathways rather than supportive, developmentally appropriate care.

Clinical Example and Synthesis: In a school-based primary care clinic using a brief standardized screening tool, a minoritized adolescent who uses cannabis intermittently screens negative because they under-report use due to mistrust of confidentiality and concern about potential consequences (resulting in a false negative), while another adolescent who feels safer with the clinician discloses use and screens positive, prompting follow-up. Thus, differences in trust and perceived safety—rather than actual substance use—can drive misclassification, leading to missed intervention for some youth and greater surveillance for others. Addressing this requires trauma-informed, culturally and gender-affirming communication that emphasizes confidentiality, for example, asking about reasons for use such as sleep or coping with stress, patterns and settings of use, perceived benefits and harms, and barriers to honest disclosure including concerns about confidentiality or consequences.

Cultural and spiritual assets—including religiosity, spirituality, family cohesion, and ethnic identity—function as important protective factors that can delay alcohol use initiation and reduce risk for progression to alcohol use disorders.[17] These protective pathways vary by gender and ethnicity, with distinct patterns observed among Black, Latino, Asian American, and multiracial youth. At the same time, trauma and adversity—disproportionately experienced by minoritized adolescents—heighten SUD risk through effects on stress physiology, emotion regulation, and coping. This may vary by gender with elevated early life stress associated with increased risk of substance use initiation for girls and gender-specific patterns.[18,19] Trauma-integrated interventions show promise for racially diverse youth with co-occurring post-traumatic stress disorder (PTSD) and SUD, demonstrating feasibility and early efficacy.[20] Together, these findings inform a culturally grounded, equity-focused framework for identification of need, assessing and treating SUD in minoritized adolescents. The following vignette is illustrative rather than comprehensive, highlighting key considerations for youth navigating structural and contextual barriers to substance use care.

Clinical Vignette

Elena, a 16-year-old Mexican American girl, is referred to outpatient adolescent psychiatry after her school reports repeated absenteeism, episodes of tearfulness in class, declining academic performance, and suspected cannabis vaping on school grounds. The school counselor notes that Elena has become increasingly withdrawn and has been spending lunch periods alone. A recent disciplinary report described her as defiant when approached by staff, although the context suggests heightened anxiety and mistrust rather than oppositionality.

Elena lives with her mother and 9-year-old brother in a neighborhood that has experienced a sharp rise in community violence over the past year, in the context of aggressive immigration enforcement. Her mother recently lost her job following a reduction in hours at her workplace, leading to significant financial strain and periods of food and housing insecurity. Elena's family history includes multiple stressors: a previous immigration raid affecting her extended family, the deportation of an uncle who served as a key emotional support figure, and episodes of family separation during migration. Elena recalls these events vividly and describes them as formative moments of fear and instability.

During the clinical interview, Elena reports using cannabis nightly to sleep and stop my thoughts. She describes intrusive memories, hypervigilance, and panic attacks—particularly when hearing loud noises or sirens. She endorses occasional alcohol use at parties but denies other substances. Although a urine toxicology screen is negative, the clinician notes several factors that may account for underdetection: her pattern of use (primarily edibles/vaping), the timing of the test, and, importantly, Elena's guardedness around disclosure. Her hesitancy is shaped by previous experiences in school where substance use suspicion led to punitive measures rather than support. She fears that her words could be "used against her," reflecting a broader theme of mistrust toward institutional systems.

Elena's mother expresses deep worry about her daughter's withdrawal and panic symptoms. She describes her own spiritual distress and the sense that family members have become "disconnected from the traditions that once held us." She has sought guidance both from a local clinician and from their parish priest. Elena identifies her grandmother's spiritual rituals—lighting candles, prayer, and folk healing practices—as important but distant since her grandmother's death. She longs for a sense of connection but feels unsure of how to integrate these traditions into her current life.

In session, Elena responds positively to grounding and mindfulness exercises, noting that these practices help quiet her intrusive thoughts and "make my chest loosen." She expresses interest in learning additional skills to manage her trauma-related symptoms and stabilize her mood and is curious about combining these with spiritual elements that feel authentic to her cultural identity.

Clinical Pearls Illustrated by Elena's Case

- *Trauma exposure is cumulative and intersecting:* Immigration-related trauma, community violence, and chronic stress compound risk for early substance use.
- *Family separation and sociopolitical uncertainty matter clinically:* These experiences shape anxiety, mistrust, and engagement with care.
- *Structural instability drives risk:* Economic hardship and food or housing insecurity increases vulnerability and complicate treatment adherence.
- *School-based disciplinary responses can hinder care:* Punitive practices may reinforce silence and mistrust rather than facilitate early identification and support.
- *Screening requires clinical judgment:* Under-reporting is common, and standard toxicology testing may miss clinically meaningful use.
- *Substance use often serves a regulatory function:* Anxiety, trauma symptoms, and sleep disturbance frequently underlie use as a coping strategy.
- *Cultural and spiritual disruption is clinically relevant:* Loss of cultural or spiritual connection may exacerbate distress, while reconnection can be protective.
- *Early, culturally congruent, and family centered interventions are promising:* Culturally grounded approaches may enhance engagement and early response

Structural racism and social determinants of substance use disorder in minoritized youth

Minoritized adolescents from disadvantaged communities often navigate environments marked by discriminatory policing, inequitable school discipline, housing instability, community violence, and chronic poverty—each a potential driver of early substance use initiation and accelerated progression. Structural racism operates through restricted access to mental health services, under-resourced communities, and pathways that divert youth toward punitive justice systems rather than treatment. Research highlights how structural inequities—including socioeconomic disadvantage, cultural trauma, and racialized stress—shape risk exposure, limit access to care, and disrupt normative developmental trajectories, contributing to disparities in substance use, mental health, and educational outcomes.[3,21,22]

Carceral logics are embedded within the US K-12 education system, with the school-to-prison pipeline functioning as one component of a broader carceral continuum spanning major institutions of power.[23,24] Within schools, minoritized students are more likely than their White peers to experience overpolicing, exclusionary discipline practices (eg, zero-tolerance policies), and harsher punishment for comparable behaviors.[25] These practices erode trust, reduce access to supportive services, and increase contact with juvenile legal systems.

Disparities are further compounded for students with disabilities, and sex and gender minority youth, who face disproportionate disciplinary actions and heightened surveillance within educational settings.[26] Parallel racial and structural inequities persist within juvenile and criminal legal systems, reinforcing cycles of exclusion and criminalization.[24]

Collectively, this body of evidence underscores structural racism and bias as a fundamental determinant of health,[27] with schools serving as a critical site where inequities in discipline and access to support contribute directly to disparities in substance use, mental health, and life-course outcomes. While structural racism is often examined in relation to risk and outcomes, its effects on treatment engagement are equally consequential. For minoritized adolescents, engagement is shaped by prior experiences of institutional harm, perceived safety, and the relational quality of care environments. **Table 1** synthesizes these influences, highlighting clinical strategies for responding to structural, cultural, and developmental factors that affect engagement across screening, initiation, and retention in substance use care.

Childhood trauma, psychiatric disorders, and educational disengagement

Evidence from a nationally representative study demonstrated that childhood trauma and early-onset psychiatric disorders were strongly associated with school dropout among young adults, especially in the context of substance use, and independent of sociodemographic factors.[21] Trauma exposures—including family disruption, violence, and chronic adversity—were linked to elevated risk for mood, anxiety, and SUDs, which in turn increased the likelihood of educational disengagement. Recent studies support this association between trauma, adversity, and developmental outcomes such as disrupted education in Latinx youth.[28] These findings suggest that school dropout functions not merely as an educational outcome but as a downstream marker of cumulative adversity and unmet mental health and substance use needs. Educational disengagement reflects disruptions in developmental trajectories shaped by trauma, psychiatric symptoms, and structural stressors, limiting access to protective school-based supports and increasing vulnerability to substance use and justice-system involvement. This pathway is particularly salient for racially and ethnically minoritized youth, who are disproportionately exposed to both trauma and punitive institutional responses.

CLINICAL IMPLICATIONS

- *Reframe school disengagement as a clinical signal:* Absenteeism, disciplinary actions, or declining performance should prompt assessment for trauma exposure,

Table 1
Equity considerations shaping engagement in substance use care for minoritized adolescents

Engagement-Related Factor	How It Shapes Engagement	Risk to Engagement	Implications for Primary Care and School Settings	Engagement-Promoting Clinical Strategies
Privacy and Confidentiality	Concerns about information sharing with caregivers, schools, immigration, or child welfare systems reduce openness and follow-through	Limited disclosure; avoidance of screening or care	Low uptake of screening; delayed help-seeking; early dropout	Clearly explain confidentiality and limits; normalize screening; offer private time without caregivers; revisit consent across visits
Perceived Discrimination	Anticipated or prior bias undermines trust and willingness to engage	Selective disclosure; disengagement after initial contact	Differential referral patterns; lower retention for minoritized youth	Use trauma-informed, nonjudgmental language; validate experiences; reflect on implicit bias; engage in shared decision-making
Cultural Norms and Values	Family loyalty, stigma, gender roles, and respect for authority shape readiness to engage	Misalignment between clinical recommendations and youth priorities	Poor engagement with counseling or referrals	Use culturally responsive interviewing; explore meaning of use; engage family when appropriate and desired by the youth
Systemic Mistrust	Historical and ongoing institutional harms increase guardedness toward care systems	Avoidance of services; reluctance to accept referrals	Missed prevention opportunities; reliance on crisis-driven entry points	Acknowledge historical harms; prioritize transparency; build longitudinal relationships; partner with trusted community-based supports

Gender and Identity Safety	Fear of judgment, misgendering, or loss of gender-affirming care suppresses engagement	Underutilization of services by girls and gender-diverse youth	Missed early intervention and co-occurring needs	Ensure affirming environments; use inclusive language; tailor engagement strategies to lived experience
Assessment Approach	Single-method screening can feel impersonal or punitive	Early disengagement; mistrust of results	Inaccurate triage; disengagement after screening	Use relational, multimethod assessment; contextualize results; frame screening as supportive rather than evaluative

mental health symptoms, and substance use risk rather than assumptions of nonadherence or defiance.
- *Integrate educational context into assessment:* Routinely assess school experiences, including attendance patterns, sense of safety, disciplinary history, and connection to supportive adults.
- *Use brief, relational screening questions to deepen understanding.* Importantly, when asking these questions within a school setting, the school-based clinician (eg, school social worker) should be ready with appropriate resources and referrals. Proactively, school districts should develop a response protocol before using the following questions at their sites:
  - "How has school been feeling for you lately?"
  - "What makes it harder to go to school on some days?"
  - "Have there been times you didn't feel safe or supported at school?"
  - "Who at school do you feel you can trust or go to for help?"
  - "What helps you get through a difficult school day?"
- *Prioritize early, engagement-focused intervention:* Trauma-informed, culturally responsive approaches that emphasize trust, confidentiality, and collaboration can interrupt pathways toward disengagement and substance use.
- *Strengthen school–health care partnerships:* Coordinated, nonpunitive collaboration between schools and health care systems can reduce exclusionary discipline and improve continuity of care.

EVIDENCE-BASED TREATMENTS FOR MINORITIZED ADOLESCENTS WITH SUBSTANCE USE DISORDER

Effective treatment for minoritized adolescents requires both the use of *evidence-based practices (EBPs)* and *culturally responsive, structurally informed delivery*. Below, we synthesize core EBPs and highlight adaptations shown to improve engagement and effectiveness for youth with concerning substance use (eg, increasing use, use before school, use that is impacting functioning, or co-occurring with a mental health concern). To illustrate best approaches, we return to the vignette of *Elena* as an example of how these evidence-based approaches can be helpful.

Motivational Interviewing

In early sessions, Elena's clinician prioritizes trust-building and uses motivational interviewing (MI) to explore her cannabis use in the context of trauma symptoms and sleep disturbance. The clinician adopts a nonjudgmental, collaborative stance and uses open-ended, contextual probes rather than relying on initial screening alone, asking questions such as "Can you walk me through what nights are like when it's hardest to sleep?" "What do you notice cannabis helps with—and what doesn't it help with?" "What are some of the downsides you've noticed the next day?" and "How safe do you feel being open about this here?" Reflective listening and affirmations (eg, "It makes sense you're trying to find ways to quiet your thoughts") are used to validate her experience, while gently eliciting ambivalence (eg, "On the one hand it helps you fall asleep, and on the other hand it seems to make anxiety worse the next day."). This process supports disclosure, clarifies the coping function of use, and begins to align goals around improved sleep and emotional regulation.

MI is particularly well suited for adolescents who experience ambivalence about change, stigma, or fear of judgment[29]—common dynamics among youth. MI can also help align care with cultural values emphasizing respect, autonomy, relational connection, and collaborative decision-making, especially among youth who may have an elevated sense of mistrust.

Evidence supports MI can be helpful for exploring the following:

- The direct and indirect effects in reducing cannabis and alcohol use[30]
- Readiness to change
- Enhance engagement across diverse adolescent populations

Culturally responsive MI adaptations can include exploration of factors that may be part of substance use context, for example,:

- Racism-related and discrimination stress
- Immigration fears and legal vulnerability stress
- Family obligations, intergenerational expectations, and conflicts regarding identity (eg, LGBTQ youth)
- Cultural and spiritual beliefs shaping meaning and motivation[20,31]

Functional assessment and behavioral science approaches

A functional assessment (ABC framework) situates Elena's cannabis use within night-time hyperarousal and broader ecological stressors, including community violence and family strain. Using this framework, the clinician identifies antecedents such as lying in bed with intrusive memories, heightened vigilance to sounds (eg, sirens), and worry about family stressors; the behavior of vaping or using edibles to fall asleep; and consequences including rapid sleep onset and emotional numbing in the short term, but next-day fatigue, increased anxiety, and continued reliance on cannabis. This formulation guides targeted interventions: the clinician introduces a structured night-time routine (eg, limiting phone use, consistent sleep schedule), teaches grounding strategies for intrusive memories (eg, paced breathing, sensory-based exercises like the 5-4-3-2-1 technique), and develops a coping plan for high-arousal moments (eg, getting out of bed, using calming music, brief journaling). The clinician also collaborates with Elena to identify and reinforce replacement behaviors (eg, relaxation exercises, culturally meaningful rituals such as prayer or candle lighting) and to anticipate triggers (eg, nights following stressful school days), while gradually reducing reliance on cannabis through skills-building and supportive monitoring.

When paired with an *ecological assessment* (eg, Bronfenbrenner's ecological systems theory[32]), functional assessment helps clinicians understand how behavior is shaped across multiple contexts—family, school, peers, neighborhood, and systems involvement. This approach is particularly useful for minoritized youth whose substance use may function as coping in response to environmental stressors rather than individual pathology.

Cognitive behavioral therapy

Elena's clinician uses cognitive behavioral therapy (CBT)–informed interventions tailored to her trauma and sleep difficulties. Grounding skills are practiced in session (eg, paced breathing, 5-4-3-2-1 sensory exercises) and assigned for night-time use when intrusive memories arise. Sleep regulation strategies include establishing a consistent bedtime routine, reducing screen exposure, and developing a plan for periods of high arousal (eg, getting out of bed briefly, using calming music or journaling rather than remaining in distress). Trauma-related triggers (eg, sirens, night-time silence) are identified and linked to physiologic responses, with gradual practice of coping strategies in these moments. Cognitive strategies focus on labeling trauma-related thoughts (eg, "something bad is going to happen") and reframing them in ways that acknowledge real environmental stressors while reducing catastrophic interpretations (eg, "I feel unsafe right now, but I am in my home and can use my coping plan"). CBT effectively targets mechanisms central to adolescent substance use,33 including the following:

- Emotion dysregulation
- Negative or rigid thinking patterns
- Trauma-related cues that can trigger substance use and avoidance
- Peer influence and risk behaviors

CBT is highly adaptable across cultures when clinicians intentionally integrate *family context, cultural values, and structural stressors* into case formulation and skill selection.34

> *Clinical adaptation example:* A student experiences verbal conflict with his teacher and is sent to the principal's office for disrupting the classroom milieu. As a Black student, he often feels singled out and attributes this to bias and targeting by the adults in the school. After leaving school, the student engages in cannabis use to quell feelings of trepidation related to punitive discipline practices at school. While this behavior results in immediate emotional relief, other consequences include decreased academic participation and attendance issues. Applying an ecological perspective with an adolescent experiencing anxiety and cannabis use, the school-based clinician situates cognitive and behavioral patterns within caregiving responsibilities, financial strain, immigration-related stress, housing instability, and neighborhood violence. The ABC framework also provides a lens for understanding the student's cannabis use within the context of his day-to-day experience (eg, What is happening beforehand that leads to cannabis use? What is happening after that might be reinforcing the behavior? For example, when he is sent to the principal's office, he is able to escape the classroom where he feels targeted by the teacher. A skilled clinician will recognize this and work with the staff to appropriately address the student's concerns). Cognitive restructuring acknowledges realistic threats rather than pathologizing worry, while behavioral strategies emphasize problem-solving, communication with caregivers, and coping plans aligned with limited resources. This preserves core CBT mechanisms while enhancing relevance, engagement, and effectiveness.

Contingency management

Contingency management (CM) is a behavioral intervention grounded in operant conditioning, providing immediate, tangible reinforcement (eg, vouchers, privileges, and points) contingent on engagement or behavior change (eg, visit attendance and negative substance screens).35 CM has demonstrated robust efficacy for reducing cannabis and stimulant use in adolescents but remains underutilized among minoritized youth.36

To enhance feasibility in clinical practice, CM can be operationalized through a brief, collaborative process to identify culturally meaningful and nonstigmatizing incentives. Clinicians can incorporate structured questions such as the following:

- "What kinds of rewards or recognition would feel meaningful to you if you met your goals?"
- "Are there things your family values that could be part of celebrating your progress?"
- "What motivates you to keep going when things are hard?"

This approach allows incentives to emerge from the youth's and family's cultural context and preferences (eg, additional recreational time, family-approved activities, privileges, or opportunities for connection) rather than relying solely on standardized voucher systems. When appropriate, involving caregivers can help align incentives with family values and increase sustainability.

Additional strategies to support implementation include the following:

- *Reinforcement inventory:* Administer this assessment tool to understand what types of incentives the youth prefers.
- *Menu-based options:* Offer a flexible *menu* of incentive types (eg, social, activity-based, or recognition-based) that can be tailored collaboratively.
- *Low-cost, nonmonetary rewards:* Emphasize privileges (eg, later curfew and choice of family activity), roles (eg, leadership opportunities), or recognition (eg, verbal praise and certificates) to reduce stigma and increase feasibility.
- *Link incentives to function:* Align rewards with the youth's goals (eg, improved sleep, school attendance, and reduced use), reinforcing meaningful behavior change.
- *Iterative adjustment:* Revisit incentives over time to ensure they remain motivating and culturally congruent. Adjust rewards periodically to avoid satiation.
- *Transparency and autonomy:* Frame CM as a collaborative tool rather than a behavioral contract imposed by clinicians, reinforcing trust and shared decision-making.

> *Implementation considerations:* CM can be integrated into primary care and school-based health centers through billing, collaborative care models, or care coordination workflows. Low-cost incentives can be supported through clinic resources, community partnerships, or grants.

Family-based interventions (multidimensional family therapy, multisystemic therapy, brief strategic family therapy)

Family-based therapies remain the *strongest evidence-supported treatments* for adolescent SUD, consistently outperforming individual-only approaches.[37] Their effectiveness is especially pronounced for minoritized youth, for whom substance use is often embedded within family stress, intergenerational trauma, and school or justice-system involvement. Rather than locating risk solely within the adolescent, these models intervene at relational and ecological levels and align closely with developmental psychopathology, family dynamics/intergenerational processes, structural competency, and culturally responsive care.[38]

Multidimensional family therapy (MDFT)[39] is an evidence-based, family-centered treatment for adolescents with substance use and co-occurring conditions that targets multiple domains of functioning, including the individual, family, school, and broader social context. For Elena, whose cannabis use is closely tied to trauma-related sleep disturbance, family stress, and school disengagement, MDFT provides a structured framework to intervene across these domains. The clinician engages Elena and her mother in both individual and joint sessions: with Elena, focusing on coping with trauma symptoms and reducing cannabis use; with her mother, addressing stress, communication, and parenting under financial strain. In joint sessions, the clinician facilitates supportive communication, helping shift interactions from fear-based or reactive responses to understanding and collaboration around Elena's anxiety and sleep difficulties. The clinician also coordinates with the school counselor to address absenteeism through supportive planning rather than disciplinary responses. This multidimensional approach aligns family, school, and clinical goals, including improved sleep, school engagement, and reduced substance use.

Brief Strategic Family Therapy

In sessions where patterns of misunderstanding emerge (eg, mother interpreting withdrawal as defiance), the clinician uses in-session enactments to observe and gently restructure interactions. For example, the clinician may guide Elena to express her night-time anxiety directly while coaching her mother to respond with validation rather than criticism. Attention is also given to bicultural and intergenerational dynamics (eg, differing expectations around independence, coping, and expression of distress), helping the family develop more adaptive communication patterns that reduce the need for substance use as coping.

Brief strategic family therapy (BSFT) is an evidence-based, family-centered model designed for youth with substance use and behavioral problems, using a strategic and structural approach to treatment.[40]

- Research includes Latino and immigrant families[41]
- Focuses on restructuring maladaptive family and other interpersonal interaction patterns that can lead to substance use[41]
- Strong engagement and retention outcomes
- Addresses bicultural stress and intergenerational conflict

> *Clinical Synthesis:* Research suggests that effective SUD care for minoritized adolescents is not about selecting *different* treatments, but about delivering evidence-based models with cultural humility, structural awareness, and developmental sensitivity—and integrating them across family, school, health care, and community contexts.

Opioid use in minoritized adolescents: structural context, patterns, and clinical implications

Opioid use among adolescents has become increasingly lethal not only because of rising prevalence, but also due to the dramatically more toxic and unpredictable drug supply, particularly the proliferation of counterfeit pills containing fentanyl.[42] For minoritized adolescents—who consistently report lower or comparable levels of opioid misuse relative to White peers—this shift has produced a striking and troubling inversion: disproportionately higher overdose mortality despite lower self-reported use.[43] This paradox cannot be explained by individual behavior alone. Rather, it reflects the convergence of structural inequities—including differential exposure to illicit markets, limited access to harm-reduction resources, uneven surveillance and prevention infrastructure, criminalization, and barriers to timely medical care—that shape both patterns of exposure and outcomes among racially and ethnically marginalized youth.[44,45] Understanding adolescent opioid risk therefore requires situating substance use within these broader social, economic, and policy contexts, rather than attributing disparities to use prevalence alone. Clinically, this underscores the importance of maintaining a high index of suspicion for opioid exposure—even when adolescents report only nonopioid substance use—given the widespread presence of fentanyl in counterfeit pills and other substances, and the growing risk of unintentional opioid ingestion in the current drug supply.

Structural Drivers of Exposure and Risk

As outlined earlier in the chapter, structural racism, immigration stress, and chronic community disinvestment function as *fundamental determinants* of health disparities.[46,47] These forces shape opioid-related risk by influencing:

- *Availability and quality of substances*: Youth in segregated, under-resourced neighborhoods are more likely to encounter counterfeit pills and unpredictable drug compositions.
- *Access to prevention and treatment*: Minoritized youth consistently receive less screening, fewer brief interventions, and markedly lower rates of medication for opioid use disorder (MOUD).
- *Criminal-legal surveillance and fear of consequences*, which suppress disclosure and delay help-seeking for treatment or overdose situations.
- *Accumulated trauma and stress exposure*, which heighten vulnerability to experimenting with substances to manage affective or somatic distress.

Fear of deportation or family separation is associated with substance use mediated by depression,[48] and may intensify secrecy regarding use as a way of coping[49] among immigrant and minoritized youth, often even within families, complicating early identification and intervention. These dynamics are particularly consequential in opioid use, where even a single unrecognized exposure to fentanyl can be lethal. Many youth encounter opioids unintentionally—thinking they are taking *Percocet*, *M30*, or another prescription pill—highlighting that risk is not always linked to *misuse* in the intentional sense.[42]

Implications for Treatment and Equity

Treatment and prevention of opioid use in minoritized adolescents requires the same equity-centered principles discussed across this chapter:

- *Ensure access to MOUD*, especially buprenorphine, which remains dramatically underused among minoritized youth despite strong evidence for safety and efficacy.
- Provide psychoeducation that acknowledges cultural and familial values, addressing concerns about medication stigma or *substituting one drug for another*.
- Use trauma-informed and relational approaches that contextualize opioid use within the youth's developmental history, structural stress exposures, and family system.
- Integrate overdose prevention—including naloxone distribution—as part of routine care, recognizing that unintentional exposures are common.
- Reinforce continuity of care for co-occurring depression, anxiety, PTSD, or bipolar spectrum symptoms, which often interact with substance use in bidirectional ways.

> *Clinical Synthesis:* In minority adolescents, opioid-related harm cannot be understood through prevalence alone. Instead, it reflects the intersection of structural determinants, contextualized stress, racism, structural inequities, stigma and surveillance, and types of drug supply. As with other substances discussed in this chapter, clinical care must emphasize relational engagement, culturally attuned assessment, and equitable access to effective treatment, with the understanding that even small windows of experimentation can carry outsized risk for youth living in structurally marginalized contexts.

Systems of care approaches

While cross-system collaboration is essential, these partnerships are typically built through existing care pathways rather than individual clinician outreach. In routine practice, clinicians can leverage established referral networks (eg, school-based behavioral health programs, community mental health agencies, and faith- or community-based organizations), partner with community health workers or cultural navigators who bridge clinical and community settings, and engage in periodic case coordination with school counselors or multidisciplinary teams. These mechanisms translate systems-of-care principles into feasible clinical practice for clinicians with full patient panels. Clinicians can also play an important consultative role by supporting schools and community partners in implementing developmentally appropriate, trauma-informed approaches to substance use assessment and response—emphasizing engagement, confidentiality, and early intervention rather than punitive or exclusionary practices. Embedding collaboration within team-based care and existing institutional relationships enhances sustainability and impact. A systems-of-care approach prioritizes alignment across these settings so that schools and allied institutions function as gateways to supportive, culturally responsive, and trauma-informed care[50] rather than pathways to criminalization—particularly given that schools remain the primary access point for youth mental health services.[51]

Systems-level Implications

- Strengthen partnerships with faith-based and cultural organizations as engagement and re-engagement anchors
- Align school, legal, and foster-care systems with primary care and behavioral health through coordinated referral pathways by working within team-based care.
- Consult with schools to implement trauma-informed, culturally responsive systems design to reduce punitive escalation
- Use cultural brokers or navigators to support cross-system communication and family engagement
- Prioritize diversion and treatment-based responses over exclusionary or carceral practices

Integrating digital care into family-based substance use disorder treatment

Digital care can extend and strengthen family-based therapies for adolescent SUD when used as a *hybrid or adjunct*, rather than a replacement for relational work. Telehealth increases access for families facing transportation barriers, inflexible work schedules, immigration-related mobility concerns, or geographic isolation.[52] Asynchronous supports—such as secure messaging, brief skills videos, and parent coaching prompts—can reinforce therapeutic goals between sessions. For minoritized families, digital modalities may also reduce stigma and lower barriers to engagement when trust in care systems is fragile. When implemented with intention, digital components can enhance care coordination across settings (eg, schools, primary care, child welfare, probation), support treatment fidelity through structured check-ins and measurement-based care, and facilitate culturally tailored adaptations, including language options, flexible scheduling, and family-defined goals.[53–55] Equity-focused digital integration requires explicit attention to digital access, privacy, and caregiver burden, developed as co-design with platforms that are mobile-friendly, low-bandwidth, and aligned with reimbursement pathways in primary care and community-based settings.

CLINICS CARE POINTS

Actions within routine clinical encounters

- *Assess structural context:* Routinely evaluate the impact of racism, immigration-related stress, community violence, and economic instability on substance use risk and engagement.

- *Use multimethod assessment:* Combine self-report with clinical interviews and contextual information to reduce underestimation and misclassification.
- *Integrate trauma and SUD care:* Address co-occurring trauma using trauma-informed, evidence-based approaches, including mindfulness-based strategies when appropriate.
- *Leverage cultural and spiritual strengths:* Incorporate culturally and spiritually congruent practices that support identity, meaning-making, and resilience, aligned with youth preferences.
- *Practice cultural humility and antiracism:* Engage in reflective, developmentally attuned care that centers youth voice and acknowledges structural inequities.

Actions supported through consultation and cross-system teamwork:

- *Provide consultation to partner systems:* Offer guidance to schools, primary care, and community organizations on trauma-informed, developmentally appropriate substance use assessment and responses that emphasize engagement and confidentiality rather than punitive approaches.
- *Participate in team-based coordination:* Engage in periodic case consultation with school-based mental health professionals, primary care providers, and multidisciplinary teams to align care plans and improve continuity.
- *Leverage intermediaries:* Work with community health workers, peer navigators, or cultural brokers who can bridge clinical care with family, school, and community contexts.

Actions requiring broader systems-level or institutional support:

- *Prioritize family-based therapies:* Implement evidence-based family interventions (eg, MDFT, multisystemic therapy [MST], BSFT) that address relational and systemic drivers of substance use.
- *Partner beyond the clinic:* Integrate community, cultural, and faith-based supports to enhance engagement and continuity of care when desired by youth and families.

Ultimately, reducing disparities in adolescent SUD requires a coordinated clinical, public health, and community response that centers on responding to systemic barriers and bias, engages in cultural humility practice, and integrates the lived experiences of youth and families, supporting pathways toward resilience and recovery.

SUMMARY

SUDs among minoritized adolescents emerge within a complex interplay of structural inequities, trauma exposure, racism-related stress, and sociocultural pressures. Although minoritized youth do not use substances at higher rates than their non-Hispanic White peers, they experience disproportionate harm due to structural barriers and markedly lower access to evidence-based treatment. Effective care must therefore extend beyond symptom reduction to incorporate structural competency, trauma-informed practice, and culturally responsive intervention strategies. Evidence-based treatments are effective across diverse adolescent populations when delivered with cultural humility and attention to context. Family-based therapies remain the most strongly supported modalities and align with the relational values and structural realities of many minoritized families.

DISCLOSURES

There is nothing to disclose.

FUNDING

SAMHSA award 5H79TI087349 (PI–Fortuna).

REFERENCES

1. Lu W, Muñoz-Laboy M, Sohler N, et al. Trends and disparities in treatment for Co-occurring major depression and substance use disorders among US adolescents from 2011 to 2019. JAMA Netw Open 2021;4(10):e2130280.
2. Goings TC, Salas-Wright CP, Howard MO, et al. Substance use among bi/multi-racial youth in the United States: profiles of psychosocial risk and protection. Am J Drug Alcohol Abuse 2018;44(2):206–14.
3. Porche MV, Fortuna LR, Tolou-Shams M. Unpacking the layers: dismantling inequities in substance use services and outcomes for racially minoritized adolescents. Child Adolesc Psychiatr Clin N Am 2022;31(2):223–36.
4. Johnson ME, Lloyd SL, Bristol SC, et al. Black girls and referrals: racial and gender disparities in self-reported referral to substance use disorder assessment among justice-involved children. Subst Abuse Treat Prev Pol 2022;17(1):68.
5. Steinhoff A, Shanahan L, Bechtiger L, et al. When substance use is underreported: comparing self-reports and hair toxicology in an urban cohort of young adults. J Am Acad Child Adolesc Psychiatry 2023;62(7):791–804.
6. Oni HT, Buultjens M, Abdel-Latif ME, et al. Barriers to screening pregnant women for alcohol or other drugs: a narrative synthesis. Women Birth 2019;32(6):479–86.
7. Janousch C, Eggenberger L, Steinhoff A, et al. Words versus strands: reliability and stability of concordance rates of self-reported and hair-analyzed substance use of young adults over time. Eur Addctn Res 2025;31(1):60–74.
8. Folk JB, Hirschtritt ME, McCrary QD, et al. Agreement between youth self-report and biospecimen-confirmed substance use: a systematic review. Subst Use Misuse 2022;57(4):531–8.
9. Hubbard JA. Review on toxicology testing in hair. J Appl Lab Med 2025;10(4): 983–1000.
10. Fortuna LR, Bagot KS. Editorial: inconclusive (or "Elusive"): concordance between substance use self-report and toxicology for diverse youth populations. J Am Acad Child Adolesc Psychiatry 2023;62(7):721–3.
11. Sartor CE, Ye F, Simon P, et al. Cross-substance patterns of alcohol, cigarette, and cannabis use initiation in black and white adolescent girls. Prev Med 2022; 156:106979.
12. Reidy DE, Smith-Darden JP, Vivolo-Kantor AM, et al. Masculine discrepancy stress and psychosocial maladjustment: implications for behavioral and mental health of adolescent boys. Psychol Men Masc 2018;19(4):560–9.
13. Raynor PA, Nation A, Outlaw F. Exploring substance use and mental health for minority transgender youth: implications for advanced practice nurses. J Am Assoc Nurse Pract 2020;32(3):229–43.
14. Reisner SL, Poteat T, Keatley J, et al. Global health burden and needs of transgender populations: a review. Lancet 2016;388(10042):412–36.
15. Lai B, Good J, Singh G, et al. Adolescent substance use disorder in primary care: challenges in treatment referral beyond access availability. J Prim Care Community Health 2024;15:21501319241276817.
16. Kuhns LM, Carlino B, Greeley K, et al. A chart review of substance use screening and related documentation among adolescents in outpatient pediatric clinics: implications for practice. Subst Abuse Treat Prev Pol 2020;15(1):36.
17. Porche MV, Fortuna LR, Wachholtz A, et al. Distal and proximal religiosity as protective factors for adolescent and emerging adult alcohol use. Religions 2015; 6(2):365–84.

18. Bielas H, Barra S, Skrivanek C, et al. The associations of cumulative adverse childhood experiences and irritability with mental disorders in detained male adolescent offenders. Child Adolesc Psychiatr Ment Health 2016;10:34.
19. Donovan A, Assari S, Grella C, et al. Early life stress and pubertal predictors of subsequent substance use in a national diverse sample of adolescents: sex and substance type matter. Drug Alcohol Depend 2025;268:112551.
20. Fortuna LR, Porche MV, Padilla A. A treatment development study of a cognitive and mindfulness-based therapy for adolescents with co-occurring post-traumatic stress and substance use disorder. Psychol Psychother 2018;91(1):42–62.
21. Porche MV, Fortuna LR, Lin J, et al. Childhood trauma and psychiatric disorders as correlates of school dropout in a national sample of young adults. Child Dev 2011;82(3):982–98.
22. Bailey ZD, Feldman JM, Bassett MT. How structural racism works - racist policies as a root cause of U.S. racial health inequities. N Engl J Med 2021;384(8):768–73.
23.. Foucault M. Discipline and punish: the birth of the prison. New York (NY): Sheridan A. Vintage; 1979.
24. Tynan EK, Warren MR. Mass incarceration and the school-to-prison pipeline: the intergenerational transmission of criminalization. Int J Adolesc Youth 2025;30(1): 2435270.
25.. Nese RNT, Green AL. Best practices in equitable and culturally responsive behavioral strategies in the classroom. In: Harrison PL, Proctor SL, Thomas A, editors. Best practices in school psychology: students, systems, and family services. 7th edition. Bethesda (MD): National Association of School Psychologists; 2023. p. 147–58.
26. McCarter S. The school-to-prison pipeline: a primer for social workers. Soc Work 2017;62(1):53–61.
27. Gonçalves C, Ip KI, Stanton CA, et al. A review of the impact of structural racism on lived experiences of adolescents of African descent: implications for development, brain structure, and health. Neuropsychopharmacology 2026;51(1): 203–18.
28. Ai AL, Moore J, Petscher Y, et al. Pathways between childhood mistreatment/victimization, posttraumatic stress, and lifetime substance use disorders among Latinx nationwide. Psychol Trauma 2026;18(1):210–9.
29. Jensen CD, Cushing CC, Aylward BS, et al. Effectiveness of motivational interviewing interventions for adolescent substance use behavior change: a meta-analytic review. J Consult Clin Psychol 2011;79(4):433–40.
30. Feldstein Ewing S, Bryan AD, Dash GF, et al. Randomized controlled trial of motivational interviewing for alcohol and cannabis use within a predominantly Hispanic adolescent sample. Exp Clin Psychopharmacol 2022;30(3):287–99.
31. Fortuna LR, Martinez W, Porche MV. Integrating spirituality and religious beliefs in a mindfulness based cognitive behavioral therapy for PTSD with latinx unaccompanied immigrant children. J Child Adolesc Trauma 2023;16(3):481–94.
33.. Bronfenbrenner U. The ecology of human development: experiments by nature and design. Cambridge (MA): Harvard University Press; 1979.
34.. Steele DW, Becker SJ, Danko KJ, et al. AHRQ comparative effectiveness reviews. *Interventions for substance use disorders in adolescents: a systematic review.* Rockville (MD): Agency for Healthcare Research and Quality (US); 2020.
34. Burrow-Sánchez JJ, Minami T, Hops H. Cultural accommodation of group substance abuse treatment for Latino adolescents: results of an RCT. Cult Divers Ethnic Minor Psychol 2015;21(4):571–83.

35. Petry NM, Alessi SM, Olmstead TA, et al. Contingency management treatment for substance use disorders: how far has it come, and where does it need to go? Psychol Addict Behav 2017;31(8):897–906.
36. Stanger C, Budney AJ. Contingency management: using incentives to improve outcomes for adolescent substance use disorders. Pediatr Clin 2019;66(6): 1183–92.
37. Fadus MC, Squeglia LM, Valadez EA, et al. Adolescent substance use disorder treatment: an update on evidence-based strategies. Curr Psychiatry Rep 2019; 21(10):96.
38. Horigian VE, Anderson AR, Szapocznik J. Family-based treatments for adolescent substance use. Child Adolesc Psychiatr Clin N Am 2016;25(4):603–28.
39. Liddle HA, Dakof G, Rowe C, et al. Multidimensional family therapy for justice-involved young adults with substance use disorders. J Behav Health Serv Res 2024;51(2):250–63.
40. Szapocznik J, Muir JA, Duff JH, et al. Brief strategic family therapy: implementing evidence-based models in community settings. Psychother Res 2015;25(1): 121–33.
41. Horigian VE, Feaster DJ, Brincks A, et al. The effects of brief strategic family therapy (BSFT) on parent substance use and the association between parent and adolescent substance use. Addict Behav 2015;42:44–50.
42. Bell LA, Hadland SE. Unintentional overdoses: understanding the fentanyl landscape and reducing harm. Curr Opin Pediatr 2023;35(4):408–14.
43. Chen Y, Seiters H, Wang Z, et al. Trends in U.S. adolescent and young adult overdose fatalities, 1999-2023. J Adolesc Health 2025;77(5):997–1000.
44. Banks DE, Campbell KD, Paschke ME, et al. “Another one bite the dust-It happens so much in black neighborhoods”: structural barriers and grassroots resources among black men who use drugs facing fentanyl-era overdose and treatment disparities. J Subst Use Addict Treat 2026;181:209846.
45. Walls M, Hautala D, Sittner KJ, et al. A prospective longitudinal analysis of opioid and stimulant use in American Indian and first nations communities. Addict Behav 2025;171:108456.
46. Cotton NK, Shim RS. Social determinants of health, structural racism, and the impact on child and adolescent mental health. J Am Acad Child Adolesc Psychiatry 2022;61(11):1385–9.
47. Monroe P, Campbell JA, Harris M, et al. Racial/Ethnic differences in social determinants of health and health outcomes among adolescents and youth ages 10-24 years old: a scoping review. BMC Public Health 2023;23(1):410.
48. Herring J, Barnow B. Indirect effects of immigration enforcement on health care utilization among lawfully present older Hispanics. Soc Sci Med 2025;384: 118540.
49. Pinedo M, Montero-Zamora Z, Pasch K, et al. Immigration policies as political determinants of alcohol and drug misuse among US-born Latinos. Int J Drug Policy 2022;106:103754.
50. American Academy of Child and Adolescent Psychiatry (AACAP), American Academy of Child and Adolescent Psychiatry AACAP Committee on Community-Based Systems of Care and AACAP Committee on Quality Issues. Committee on community-based systems of care and AACAP Committee on quality issues. Clinical update: child and adolescent behavioral health care in community systems of care. J Am Acad Child Adolesc Psychiatr 2023;62(4): 367–84.

53. Carlson JS. Introduction to school psychopharmacology. In: Carlson JS, Barterian JA, editors. School psychopharmacology: translating research into practice. Cham, Switzerland: Springer; 2019. p. 1–11.
52. Vidal C, Kezar A, Platt R, et al. School-based screening and brief intervention for adolescent substance use with telehealth-delivered case consultation and education. Subst Use Addctn J 2024;45(4):598–609.
53. Fortuna LR, Porche MV, Shumway M, et al. Addressing youth mental health through schools and primary care clinics using the connected for wellness Mobile app: protocol for a stepped-wedge trial. JMIR Res Protoc 2025;14:e73721.
54. Folk JB, Gonzalez JC, Del Cid MV, et al. Lessons learned from Co-Designing a digital health app for foster youth: development and usability study. JMIR Form Res 2025;9:e73281.
55. Marsch LA, Borodovsky JT. Technology-based interventions for preventing and treating substance use among youth. Child Adolesc Psychiatr Clin N Am 2016;25(4):755–68.

Addressing Substance Use in Lesbian, Gay, Bisexual, Transgender, and Queer/ Questioning Youth

Jenny Shen, PhD[a,*], Skylar A. Jones, BA[b], Natalia Ramos, MD, MPH[a]

KEYWORDS

- LGBTQ+ • Minority stress • Substance use • Substance use disorder
- Family rejection

KEY POINTS

- LGBTQ+ youth face higher rates of substance use disorders compared to their cisgender, heterosexual counterparts.
- Structural and stigma-related risk factors increase the likelihood of substance use problems for LGBTQ+ youth, which often co-occurs with other mental health conditions among LGBTQ+ youth.
- Providers can engage with LGBTQ+ youth with substance use problems through health promotion, prevention, individual and family interventions, and harm reduction strategies.
- In addition to using individual-level interventions, providers can bolster the resilience of LGBTQ+ youth with substance use problems by increasing their social support networks through families and communities.
- A multimodal approach that addresses social determinants of health, leverages school and family systems, and tailors interventions to the individual's risk and severity of substance use is recommended in providing care for LGBTQ+ youth.

INTRODUCTION

Lesbian, gay, bisexual, transgender, and queer/questioning (LGBTQ+) youth experience disproportionately elevated rates of substance use and substance use disorders (SUDs)[1] compared to their non-LGBTQ+ counterparts. Approximately half of LGBTQ+ youth aged 13 to 17 report substance use, compared to one-fifth of non-LGBTQ+ youth.[1] Though national data on transgender and gender diverse (TGD)

[a] Department of Psychiatry and Biobehavioral Sciences, University of California, Los Angeles David Geffen School of Medicine, Los Angeles, CA, USA; [b] The Jane and Terry Semel Institute for Neuroscience and Biobehavioral Sciences, University of California, Los Angeles, Los Angeles, CA, USA
* Corresponding author. Department of Psychiatry and Biobehavioral Sciences, UCLA Semel Institute for Neuroscience and Human Behavior, 760 Westwood Plaza, A Floor Mailroom, Los Angeles, CA 90095.
E-mail address: jennyshen@mednet.ucla.edu

Child Adolesc Psychiatric Clin N Am 35 (2026) 759–779
https://doi.org/10.1016/j.chc.2026.05.005 childpsych.theclinics.com

Abbreviations	
ART	antiretroviral therapy
ASD	autism spectrum disorder
CBT	cognitive behavioral therapy
GSA	gay–straight alliance
LGBTQ+	lesbian, gay, bisexual, transgender, and queer/questioning
MI	motivational interviewing
SUD	substance use disorder
TGD	transgender and gender diverse

youth are lacking, regional studies consistently show that TGD adolescents are more than twice as likely as cisgender peers to use alcohol, marijuana, tobacco, and illicit drugs.[2–4] LGBTQ+ youth also initiate substance use *earlier* than their cisgender heterosexual peers,[3] a pattern that increases their risk of lifetime SUDs.[5]

Multiple complex factors contribute to observed substance use disparities impacting LGBTQ+ youth: chronic identity-related discrimination and social rejection; elevated rates of trauma and violence; and higher prevalence of co-occurring mental health conditions. LGBTQ+ youth face social stressors throughout critical (early) developmental stages, over prolonged periods of time, and across multiple social settings. In particular, LGBTQ+ youth face elevated rates of family rejection,[6] peer victimization,[7,8] school discipline and push-out,[9] and legal and welfare involvement compared to their cisgender or heterosexual peers.[10–12] Rejection and traumatic experiences compromise LGBTQ+ youths' self-esteem, school-engagement, and belonging,[13] and alienate youth from sources of potential social connection and support.[14]

The disparities in substance use among LGBTQ+ youth reflect the impacts of early childhood adversity, intersectional discrimination, and marginalization on neurodevelopmental processes; cognitive and emotional resilience; and health-promoting versus health risk behaviors. This chapter pairs the frameworks of minority stress and intersectionality, which explicate why SUD risk is elevated in this population, with the Behavioral Health Continuum of Care, which informs clinicians' practice. In the following sections, we will introduce these frameworks, describes the drivers they predict, map interventions onto the Behavioral Health Continuum of Care, and distill clinic care points and a summary on strategies providers can use to reduce use, bolster individual strengths and social connectedness, and promote healthy coping with stress.

CONCEPTUAL FRAMEWORKS

The disproportionately elevated rates of substance use observed among LGBTQ+ youth can best be understood through the frameworks of minority stress and intersectionality. These models explain how LGBTQ+ identity-related stressors adversely impact mental health outcomes and increase maladaptive coping mechanisms, especially for individuals who possess multiple minoritized identities.

Minority stress theory explains how both the expectation of rejection and stigma, in addition to actual experienced prejudiced events, impact psychological well-being and health behaviors in LGBTQ+ populations.[15,16] Brooks captured how vulnerable populations (specifically, sexual minority women) experience levels of stress related to discrimination, prejudice, and restricted access to economic opportunities that surpass *adaptive ranges* of coping abilities, while also lacking access to resources that mitigate the stressors. The duration, frequency, and intensity of the stressors ultimately determined the impact on the individual.[15,17]

Meyer further characterized minority stressors as unique, chronic, and socially based and emphasized that minoritized individuals experience identity-linked stressors in addition to general life stressors.[16,18] He differentiated between distal stressors, external events originating from people or institutions (eg, bullying, discrimination, family rejection), and proximal, or internal, stressors based on the individual's perceptions of experiences (eg, expectations of discrimination, internalized stigma, and concealment of identity). Proximal minority stress specifically predicts depression and anxiety among transgender youth.[19] Distal and proximal stressors both contribute to maladaptive coping and increase the risk of substance use.

Intersectionality, described by Crenshaw, explains how individuals who hold multiple marginalized social identities experience complex, compounding life stressors and social oppression.[20,21] LGBTQ+ youth of color, for example, experience discrimination on the basis of both gender and/or sexuality and race/ethnicity, which creates additive and/or multiplying forms of identity-based stressors.[22,23] Black trans girls, for example, are affected by transmisogynoir[24] (ie, transphobia,[25] misogyny, and racism) and face consistent threats of discrimination, police profiling,[26] and physical violence[26]; such heightened victimization pushes transgender girls of color into unsafe environments, increasing their exposure to carceral systems and substance use risk. Research has shown that racism is a stronger indicator of negative mental health outcomes and substance use than sexual minority status for LGBTQ+ individuals of color,[23] highlighting this as a potentially important risk factor for LGBTQ+ youth of color that merits further research.[27]

DRIVERS OF SUBSTANCE USE

Social Drivers of Substance Use

The development of SUDs is influenced by both genetically based vulnerabilities and environmental risk factors.[28] LGBTQ+ youth are uniquely at risk due to their experiences of minority stress.[29] Specifically, early exposure to trauma, family rejection, and chronic stressors can influence the onset of SUDs.[28] LGBTQ+ youth with both minoritized gender and sexual identities may experience more substance use.[30] Among LGBTQ+ young adults, those who disclosed sexual orientation and gender identity at different time points reported greater substance use at each stage.[30]

LGBTQ+ youth often experience marginalization across multiple settings (eg, school, home), amplifying their stress burden and vulnerability. Discrimination, family rejection, and school mistreatment are key social drivers for substance use for LGBTQ+ youth, with a lack of support in schools, health care settings, community spaces, and home environments contributing to minority stress and negatively impacting well-being. Factors such as socioeconomic disadvantage, low educational attainment, problems at school, and unsupportive social environments are associated with early substance use.[28]

Family

Family support plays a significant role in mental health outcomes for LGBTQ+ youth.[31,32] Family support and connectedness can bolster mental health outcomes,[33] while family rejection increases risk of maladaptive coping strategies and substance use.[34] Previous research has shown that lower family functioning (eg, less connectedness) predicts lower psychological function and more externalizing behavior.[35–37] Neglect and abuse in family settings may predict SUDs,[28] while rejection can influence the onset of depression and anxiety symptoms.[38]

LGBTQ+ youth who lack affirming home and/or school environments may also experience increased vulnerability to peer group environments that encourage substance use. They may seek out alternative social support in environments where substance use is normalized and/or experience peer pressure to fit in by using substances.[28]

School

Additional factors such as school push-out are also associated with higher risk of substance use. In addition to institutional discrimination, peer rejection, and victimization impact mental health outcomes for LGBTQ+ youth. Studies have found that bullying increases risk for substance use in TGD youth compared to their cisgender counterparts.[2] Peer victimization is associated with negative mental health outcomes such as depression, anxiety, suicidal ideation, and self-harm,[37,39] and can influence behavioral problems, leading to school suspension, and longer-term behavioral, disciplinary, and legal consequences.[40] Online harassment is also associated with lower functioning in school settings, in addition to greater reports of detention, suspension, and skipping school.[41] Among Black youth, perceived discrimination from teachers is associated with increased risk of substance use throughout high school among Black youth,[42] which may also be a risk factor for LGBTQ+ youth, particularly LGBTQ+ youth of color.

Welfare and carceral systems

Adverse school-based experiences like victimization, harassment, harsh discipline, and expulsion increase risk for criminal-legal system involvement for LGBTQ+ youth.[11] LGBTQ+ youth of color are over-represented within child welfare systems. Family history of substance use, early substance use exposure, mental health challenges, and economic and racial stressors—paired with a lack of family support—increase risk for child welfare systems involvement and to substance use.[12]

Community

Despite facing an elevated risk for mental health challenges and substance use, LGBTQ+ youth experience less access to mental health care than their cisgender heterosexual peers.[43] A US study examining availability of LGBTQ+-specific treatment programs found that only 12.6% of mental health and 17.6% of substance abuse facilities reported offering LGBTQ+-focused services, suggesting many programs are unable to meet the needs of LGBTQ+ clients.[44] Simultaneously, lack of access to mental health resources, affirming environments, and family support undermine their ability to seek support that would bolster resilience against negative health outcomes. TGD patients, in particular, report that there are not enough health care professionals trained to deliver high quality care.[45] Physicians also report feeling uncomfortable providing care to TGD patients due to a lack of adequate training, worries about using incorrect language, and missing side effects related to gender-affirming medications.[46]

Sociopolitical Climate

LGBTQ+ youth are experiencing historically high levels of LGBTQ+ visibility in media and culture while also facing severe stress from anti-LGBTQ+ initiatives and legislation in the United States. Current efforts aim to ban transgender people from sports and public spaces, ban gender-affirming care for youth, and weaken antidiscrimination protections.[47] Unsurprisingly, LGBTQ+ youth in the United States report negative impacts on their mental health from such legislation, including high anxiety, stress, and fear about their safety and access to services.[48]

Co-occurring Mental Health Conditions

The Centers for Disease Control and Prevention Youth Risk Behavior Surveillance System, a multisite survey of US students in grades 9 to 12, demonstrated that LGBTQ+ youth are more likely to use tobacco, alcohol, and drugs than heterosexual peers.[49,50] LGBTQ+ youth are also more likely to engage in early use (ie, before age 13) and to have used alcohol or drugs before their last sexual encounter.[49,50] Concurrently, LGBTQ+ youth also report greater rates of depressive symptoms, considering attempting suicide, making a suicide plan, and attempting suicide in the last 12 months. Interestingly, youth who identify as *unsure* of their sexual orientation also demonstrate markedly increased rates of suicidal ideation and attempts as well as substance use, compared to heterosexual youth.

TGD youth who presented to large general health care systems across multiple states experienced higher rates of mental health diagnoses than matched cisgender peers.[51] Among younger TGD youth (ages 3–9), prevalence rates were highest for attention-deficit/hyperactivity disorder and anxiety disorders. Meanwhile, TGD adolescents (aged 10–17) presented most frequently with depressive disorders, including 49% of transfeminine and 62% of transmasculine youth. Prevalence rates for suicidal ideation and nonsuicidal self-injury were also greatly elevated for both transfeminine and transmasculine adolescents. These data are congruent with prior smaller studies from specialized gender-focused clinics in Los Angeles,[52] Boston,[53,54] and London,[55] which showed varying but elevated rates of depression and suicidal thoughts among TGD adolescents presenting for care.

Depression, the most prevalent mental health condition among TGD youth,[51] is associated with an increased risk for substance use. Substance use is twice as common in adolescents with depression in the past year compared to those without depression.[56] Adolescent substance use and depression have reciprocal effects, wherein substance use worsens mood and lowers response to treatment, and depression itself increases risk for substance use.[56,57] Some psychological characteristics of depression—namely, low self-esteem, poor behavioral control, and low assertiveness—increase risk for substance use.[58] Early intervention for adolescent substance use is thus a key target for TGD youth, particularly those with co-occurring depression. Decreasing substance use is associated with improved response to depression treatment and reduces lifetime risk of SUDs.[56]

Of note, autism spectrum disorder (ASD) is over-represented among TGD youth in relation to cisgender youth, but the impacts of ASD on adolescent substance use are not well established.[59] Numerous studies have suggested that autistic adolescents may in fact use substances at *lower* rates than nonautistic counterparts.[60] Existing evidence to date does not suggest ASD traits or formal diagnosis as a risk factor for substance use for LGBTQ + youth.

CLINICAL INTERVENTIONS ACROSS THE CONTINUUM OF CARE

The Behavioral Health Continuum of Care, a public health framework from the Institute of Medicine, identifies 4 key areas of focus: *promotion*, *prevention*, *treatment*, and *recovery/maintenance*.[61] This model conceptualizes adolescent substance use risk and behaviors across a spectrum, wherein mental well-being anchors one end and severe SUD the other. Similarly, intervention strategies exist across the continuum.

Health Promotion

Promotion-focused interventions aim to decrease substance use among LGBTQ+ youth by improving overall mental well-being, promoting healthy and adaptive coping strategies for managing stress, and building resilience. Health promotion interventions should occur at individual, community, and population levels[62] and across all stages of substance use care.[61]

LGBTQ+ youth benefit from interventions that target individual, family, school, and community protective factors. At the individual level, cognitive therapeutic approaches can increase accurate knowledge about risks and clarify misperceptions about peer use (ie, that the majority of peers use substances, that substance use is normalized).[58] Emotional and behavioral interventions target emotional regulation (eg, coping without using substances), self-esteem, and self-agency. Adolescents are uniquely vulnerable to social influences when it comes to substance use initiation and escalation,[63] and thus the benefits of supportive, safe peers cannot be underestimated for vulnerable LGBTQ+ youth. Social engagement with peers and family members who do not engage in substance use lowers the risk of substance use initiation for adolescents.[64–66]

At the community level, social support from peers and schools mitigate internalized stigma experienced by LGBTQ+ youth.[67] Supportive school policies and practices are associated with improved mental health and fewer suicidal thoughts and behaviors in LGBTQ+ youth.[67] Specifically, the presence of a gay–straight alliance (GSA) or a similar LGBTQ+-affirming student organization on campus is associated with better mental well-being among students.[68] In addition to GSAs, LGBTQ+-inclusive curricula and antibullying/antiharassment policies with protections for LGBTQ+ students lower rates of victimization for TGD youth.[69] Extracurricular school-based activities that foster youth development also have significant positive impacts on mental health for LGBTQ+ youth,[70,71] as do school personnel who support healthy coping, provide social support, and connect families to local resources.[4] State-based education policies that ensure safety and support for LGBTQ+ students and LGBTQ+-affirming training for school personnel are key population-level initiatives to target.

Parents can benefit from education and support programs that teach protective parenting practices and identity-affirming practices. Specific parenting practices known to decrease risk for substance use include clear, consistent limit setting; supervision and monitoring; and nurturing, open communication patterns. Parental support and engagement have also been shown to lower the risk of alcohol and drug use in both general adolescent populations[72] and in LGBTQ+ adolescents.[32,73,74] In particular, parental trust, warmth, and involvement decrease tobacco, alcohol, and marijuana use.[75] Many caregivers lack the requisite information and skills to effectively affirm and guide LGBTQ+ youth despite their best intentions. Parents often assume that healthy development includes a heterosexual orientation and a gender identity aligned with one's assigned sex. Some parents may see diversity in sexual orientation and/or gender as *just a phase* or a reaction to outside influences. Others may view it as a willful rejection of important family or religious values. Fortunately, parents can gain new knowledge and learn concrete skills to better support their LGBTQ+ youth (eg, the Family Acceptance Project).[31,76]

Prevention

Prevention-focused interventions aim to stop negative consequences of substance use and prevent the development of an SUD. *Universal (primary)* prevention efforts target all youth, without consideration for specific substance use risk factors. They categorically aim to prevent initiation of substance use. Rates of youth substance use generally increase in early to late adolescence, then peak in early adulthood.[58] Among LGBTQ+ youth, the prevention of substance use initiation in early adolescence is key to lowering the risk of numerous health and psychological problems throughout the lifespan associated with early use.[58] Universal prevention initiatives typically include: school-based youth education initiatives; support and training for parents to help them speak with youth about substance use and effectively set boundaries and monitor use; mass media and public policy initiatives that provide accurate education and/or limit access to substances for youth.[58] As mentioned previously, data show that connecting youth with peers and adults who do not use substances decreases risk of use in adolescents.[63]

Selective (secondary) prevention strategies target subgroups at an elevated risk–such as LGBTQ+ youth, who inherently present with an increased risk of substance use, as compared to cisgender heterosexual peers, due to minority stressors. Effective interventions address risk and protective factors at the individual, family, and community levels.[77,78] Of note, so-called *abstinence-only* and *zero-tolerance* initiatives (eg, Project DARE) have been shown to be ineffective,[79–81] and we do not recommend them for use with LGBTQ+ youth. Educational initiatives aiming to reduce harmful consequences of use offer more effective alternatives.[82] Youth-facing selective prevention strategies should focus on the risks of substance use, safe levels of use, and strategies for managing use-related behaviors.[58]

Indicated (tertiary) prevention interventions target youth who are at high risk for SUDs, including those who already use substances (but have not yet developed an SUD). Tertiary interventions aim to prevent disease progression and harm. Data show that substance use during adolescence can progress to abuse and dependence rather quickly,[83] so intervention as close as possible to first use is warranted. An adolescent's risk of developing an SUD essentially increases as use becomes more regular and/or escalates to illicit substances.[58] Some studies have shown that school-based substance education and brief motivational interviewing (MI) can successfully reduce substance use and/or prevent escalation.[84,85] School interventions focused on managing peer pressure to use drugs also have demonstrated efficacy.[86]

Treatment

Treatment begins with case identification, a process in which an individual is screened for an SUD by a provider, who then determines whether pursuing treatment services would be beneficial.[87] SUD treatments for LGBTQ+ youth comprise multiple approaches, ranging from harm reduction and behavioral therapies to resilience-building strategies to support a youth's daily life. Family treatment approaches have become increasingly central to youth SUD treatment and are particularly critical for LGBTQ+ youth, for whom family acceptance is a robust protective factor against adverse mental health outcomes.[31] Conversely, pharmacologic treatments for youth SUDs remain largely limited. As such, prevention and behavioral strategies, particularly those that integrate family supports, are key clinical foci in minimizing risk and managing relapse among youth. Moving away from *one-size-fits-all* methodologies are also key, as effective treatment with LGBTQ+ youth must also be affirming, culturally responsive, trauma-informed, and adapted to address the unique minority stressors that frequently drive substance use behaviors in this population.[88]

Harm reduction

Given the increased risk-taking behaviors characteristic of adolescence and the specific minority stressors faced by LGBTQ+ populations, harm reduction approaches offer a vital pathway for youth for whom immediate cessation may not be desirable or feasible. Indeed, harm reduction provides a critical alternative to traditional abstinence-only models, which may inadvertently alienate LGBTQ+ youth who use substances as a coping mechanism for minority stress or gender dysphoria. Rather than demanding immediate cessation, harm reduction prioritizes the minimization of negative health and social consequences associated with use.[89] Harm reduction strategies often use MI to facilitate nonjudgmental, collaborative discussions that generate insight into the youth's perceived benefits and risks of substance use.[89] Such approaches use a public health prevention framework and increases LGBTQ+ youth's comfort with accurately reporting substance use. Further, this approach fosters an environment for providers and LGBTQ+ youth to explore underlying symptoms and stressors that substance use may be helping mitigate.

Providers can use MI prompts that explore the function, benefits, and disadvantages of substance use in the setting of specific social stressors or situations. For example, "I'm curious what cannabis does for you when you're hanging out with your friends. You mentioned before that you tend to feel nervous with new people. Help me understand this—what does it do that feels helpful? How does it affect you? What's less good, or even not good, about it"? Additionally, providers can use MI prompts adapted for minority stress when working with LGBTQ+ youth to evaluate for readiness for change and support decision-making. For example, "What do you think would change about your gender dysphoria/gender stress if you smoked less weed? What about if you used more?" Providers can also integrate psychoeducation on safer use while engaging in open discussions about use patterns (eg, encouraging LGBTQ+ youth to not use substances alone, keep naloxone accessible, arrange ride-shares, and use drug-checking test kits). Open communication increases youths' receptivity to discussing alternative coping strategies and interventions to manage these drivers, rather than focusing solely on the substance use itself,[89] which can be particularly effective for LGBTQ+ youth using substance use to manage identity-related stress.

Integrating cultural responsiveness in harm reduction strategies is important in working with LGBTQ+ youth. This includes providing education on safer drug use practices to prevent HIV and other sexually transmitted infections (STIs), providing fentanyl test strips and naloxone, and creating nonjudgmental clinical spaces where youth can discuss use without fear of losing access to other necessary care, such as gender-affirming hormone replacement therapy.[90,91] When working with TGD youth, clinicians can proactively acknowledge the harmful relationship the mental health field has historically held in gatekeeping access to gender-affirming care, and clarify that questions around substance use are not intended to jeopardize access to gender-affirming hormones or puberty suppressors, but rather to ensure TGD youth have access to appropriate supports and interventions while accessing care. Sample language may include "I know mental health providers have played the role of gatekeeper in accessing care, and my asking questions might feel really nerve-racking or frustrating. I am going to outline for you exactly what we will discuss. As a mental health professional, I will ask you a bit about symptoms of depression, anxiety, and other things like substance use. Many, many people experience these things. We know that by managing them you will likely have even better outcomes—so I might make referrals or suggestions for you, but this does not change your ability to access hormone replacement therapy or puberty suppressors." Providers can use this discussion to clarify that, unlike gender-affirming surgery, hormone replacement therapy and puberty suppressors do not require letters of readiness by a mental health professional, and that the provider's goal is to meet the LGBTQ+ youth where they are to support them in their goals (eg, "If substance use comes up, we can come up with a targeted plan around treatment to support you in your goals.") Research suggests that when providers adopt a harm reduction stance, it fosters a therapeutic alliance that can eventually bridge the gap toward reduced use or recovery, whereas rigid abstinence requirements often lead to treatment dropout among marginalized youth.[89,92]

Behavioral & parenting interventions. LGBTQ+ youth benefit from evidence-based behavioral treatments for SUDs, including 12-step programs, contingency management, cognitive behavioral therapy (CBT), and MI.[93] However, current literature on substance use in LGBTQ+ populations primarily focuses on adults, specifically those living with HIV.[94] Additionally, literature suggests that while evidence-based behavioral interventions may be sufficient for many LGBTQ+ youth, adaptations are often necessary, particularly for TGD youth and in treatment settings that lack culturally responsive training for providers.[93]

For instance, although 12-step interventions may be associated with abstinence-based outcomes, LGBTQ+ individuals have also reported experiences of prejudice and discrimination in these programs, which may contribute to higher relapse and attrition for LGBTQ+ youth.[95] As such, care must be taken when referring LGBTQ+ youth to such programs to ensure they obtain treatment in an affirming setting, given the role of minority stress in maintaining substance use behaviors. Increasing work suggests that more accessible interventions, like those in digital and messaging form, are effective with youth,[96] and may be particularly high-yield for LGBTQ+ youth, who frequently seek community and coping strategies online.[97] Further SUD treatment research is needed with TGD youth, LGBTQ+ girls, LGBTQ+ youth not living with HIV, and comorbid presentations with trauma-related and internalizing disorders that may benefit from transdiagnostic approaches integrating CBT and MI.[93,98]

Parenting interventions are a cornerstone in working with LGBTQ+ youth. Positive parenting practices that facilitate open communication and bolster attachment with youth are protective against increases in substance use and substance use in adulthood.[99,100] Providers can coach caregivers to move beyond punitive parenting practices and foster practices that include communication with youth about substance use early, frequently, and over time. This enables an open-dialog framework between caregiver and youth that validates difficult emotions with which the youth may be using substance use to cope, reduces shame, and positions the caregiver as a resource to the youth.

Resilience-building strategies and supports. The impact of resilience-building approaches and supports is integral in reducing the prevalence of SUDs among LGBTQ+ youth. Moving beyond symptom reduction, treatment must focus on buffering minority stress and bolstering resilience. Such approaches should involve a multisystemic approach targeting the family, community, and individual.

Family

Providing or offering referrals for family-based treatment is integral in treating substance use among LGBTQ+ youth, particularly as substance use has been linked to family rejection experienced in adolescence among LGBTQ+ youth.[32] A variety of family therapies have been demonstrated to be effective in treating youth substance use, including Brief Strategic Family Therapy,[101] Multidimensional Family Therapy,[102] Functional Family Therapy,[103] and Multisystemic Therapy.[104] Common factors across these family models can be flexibly applied to working with LGBTQ+ youth, including being prepared to facilitate family processing of the youth's LGBTQ+ identity; assist families in navigating anti-LGBTQ+ stigma; work toward increased acceptance around the youth's LGBTQ+ identity; and collaborate with the family to delineate the impact of cultural and familial beliefs around the youth's substance use.[88] Providers can collaborate with families to identify specific supportive behaviors, such as advocating for their youth at school or respecting chosen names and pronouns, which function as direct buffers against the psychological distress that leads to substance use behaviors. Given the high rates of comorbidity between trauma and substance use among youth, as well as the risk factors of bullying and harassment in increased substance use among TGD youth, the role of family members' behaviors in bolstering LGBTQ+ youth's resilience and self-esteem is critical.[2,105,106] The Family Acceptance Project has demonstrated that parental accepting behaviors of LGBTQ+ identity are associated with decreased substance use among LGBTQ+ youth, with greater rates of substance use in the past 5 years being associated with low familial acceptance.[31] Further, family acceptance of LGBTQ+ identity increases social support, self-esteem, and a positive relationship between parent and youth, leading to overall improved well-being with reduced rates of depression, suicide attempts, and suicidal thoughts, in addition to substance use.[31] Key accepting behaviors providers can encourage families to implement include expressing affection to their LGBTQ+ youth when learning about their identity, talking with their youth about their identity, supporting their youth's identity and gender expression, advocating for their youth when they are mistreated because of their LGBTQ + identity, connecting their youth with an LGBTQ+ role model to show them options for their future, bringing their youth to LGBTQ+ events, requiring other family members to treat their youth with respect, and welcoming their youth's LGBTQ+ friends into the home.[76]

Community

Connecting youth to affirming environments and events can also bolster resilience, provide positive peer modeling and mentorship, and reduce social isolation that often precipitates substance use. Providers can give resources to youth on LGBTQ+-affirming events in their communities, the proximity of which has been shown to be protective against substance use for LGBTQ+ youth.[107] Further, providers can also address social determinants of health that often disproportionately affect LGBTQ+ youth by equipping youth with appropriate resources and referrals, such as connecting youth to social workers or employment resources.

Additionally, the clinical environment itself serves as a critical touchpoint. Inclusive care environments facilitate rapport-building and increase comfort in disclosing risk behaviors among LGBTQ+ youth, including substance use.[88] Providers can demonstrate this by introducing themselves with pronouns; using intake forms with inclusive options for sexual orientation and gender; displaying LGBTQ+-affirming books or art in waiting rooms; and using the youth's chosen name and pronouns in communications and medical records.[108]

Individual

At the individual level, resilience-based interventions focus on fostering identity pride, distress tolerance, and emotion regulation.[109] Providers should aim to help youth develop coping mechanisms for general and minority stressors that do not rely on substances. Strengthening these coping skills also serves as a buffer against the psychological distress that often precipitates relapse.

Pharmacologic treatment. Pharmacologic treatment for LGBTQ+ youth with SUDs should adhere to typical pediatric standards of care. Notably, pharmacologic SUD treatment for youth is quite limited, with current literature primarily capturing studies conducted with adults.[96] To date, the only medication approved by the U.S. Food and Drug Administration for youth SUDs is buprenorphine, which is approved for opioid use disorder among youth aged 16 years and above.[110] Although there have been some clinical trials investigating pharmacologic treatment for youth

SUDs—including naltrexone for alcohol and *N*-acetylcysteine for cannabis use disorder—current findings are mixed for youth alcohol and stimulant use disorders.[96,110] For youth with tobacco use disorder, bupropion may have some beneficial effect, though it remains unclear whether it augments effectiveness of nicotine replacement therapy,[96] given that nicotine patch therapy combined with CBT has been shown to result in increased abstinence rates after 6 months.[111] Current guidelines for youth tobacco use disorders consist of behavioral interventions, with the potential addition of nicotine replacement therapy if youth demonstrate dependence.[110]

Notably, LGBTQ+ adolescents—in particular men of color who have sex with other men and transgender women of color[112,113]—face a higher burden of HIV infection as compared to cisgender heterosexual peers. Thus, consideration should be given to potential interactions between SUD medications and antiretroviral therapies (ARTs), medications used for both the prevention of HIV infection (eg, Pre-Exposure Prophylaxis [PrEP]) and for the treatment of HIV. PrEP, which is approved for at-risk adolescents over 77 lbs,[114] can and should be integrated into harm reduction conversations about substance use and sex. Multiple studies have established that PrEP can safely be administered with feminizing or masculinizing hormone therapies.[115,116]

Overall, substance use treatment, gender-affirming medications, and ART can be safely combined to serve at-risk LGBTQ+ adolescents. Furthermore, treating co-occurring psychiatric conditions is essential. Since LGBTQ+ youth exhibit higher rates of depression and anxiety due to chronic minority stress, the use of antidepressants can mitigate underlying drivers of substance use.[3] For TGD youth, access to gender-affirming medical care also acts as an important preventative and treatment intervention that can improve mental health outcomes,[117] thereby reducing reliance on substances for symptom management.[118]

SUD Medication	Gender Affirming Medication	Theoretic Interaction or Clinical Concern
Bupropion (sustained release formulation marketed as Zyban for smoking cessation)	Estradiol, often prescribed at 17β-estradiol (feminizing hormone therapy)	Both agents can lower seizure threshold. Estradiol increases glutaminergic (excitatory) neural transmission.[119–122]
	Testosterone (masculinizing hormone therapy)	Both agents can lower seizure threshold. Testosterone has multiple metabolites, one of which is 17β-estradiol. *Tip*: Limit bupropion dose (no more than 300 mg daily for extended release formulation) as seizure risk is dose dependent.[123,124]
Methadone	Spironolactone (androgen blocker, also a diuretic)	Increased risk of electrolyte disturbance, for example, hypokalemia, hypomagnesemia[125]

SUD Medication	Sexual Health Medication	Theoretic Interaction or Clinical Concern
Bupropion	Emtricitabine/tenofovir disoproxil fumarate (brand name Truvada)	CYP2B6 inducers may lower the concentration and efficacy of bupropion.[126–128]
Methadone	Emtricitabine/tenofovir disoproxil fumarate (brand name Truvada)	CYP2B6 inducers may lower exposure to methadone (and may cause withdrawal).[129]

Several other potentially relevant drug interactions may occur that are not directly related to gender-affirming or sexual health care, including the following:

- Buprenorphine or buprenorphine/naloxone (brand name Suboxone) combined with bupropion increases risk of seizure as both medications lower seizure threshold.
- Opioids, including buprenorphine and methadone, should generally not be coadministered with other central nervous system depressants like clonidine, gabapentin, and benzodiazepines due to a potential risk of sedation and respiratory depression.
- Disulfiram is a CYP2B6 inhibitor and thus increases exposure to methadone and/or bupropion (CYP2B6 substrates) if coadministered.
- Bupropion and methadone have complex interactions, wherein bupropion may increase concentration of methadone due to its CYP2D6 inhibition.[130]

MAINTENANCE, RECOVERY, AND RELAPSE PREVENTION

As the final stage of the care continuum, compliance with long-term treatment and continuing care is essential for cementing positive outcomes. For LGBTQ+ youth, effective relapse prevention requires moving beyond generic maintenance models to a framework that specifically addresses the unique interplay of identity, minority stress, and general stressors contributing to substance use risk.[131] Addressing both tonic (stable) and phasic (situational) variables contributing to relapse is integral as part of the Dynamic Model of Relapse,[132] and tailoring this for LGBTQ+ youth is essential for sustained recovery.[131] See **Table 1** for tonic SUD risk factors providers can inventory at intake, and phasic SUD triggers for which providers can support LGBTQ+ youth in planning around and developing coping strategies. Providers can address these by gathering information on LGBTQ+ youth's experiences in these areas, and integrating coping strategies for stigma, safety planning, and trauma-related treatment referrals when collaborating with youth on their relapse prevention plans.[131] Identifying strategies early on to avoid engaging in behavioral patterns that may lead to relapse is important, and may include the need to assess potential connections between dating/sexual networking applications and substance use, which have been shown to have a significant association among sexual minority men.[131,133] Similarly, providers can address the impact of gender dysphoria and coming out experiences on relapse by integrating skills-training for youth with psychoeducation for families. Such psychoeducation can comprise options to support youth around age-appropriate medical interventions, social transitions, and coming out processes.[131]

Notably, minimizing relapse also hinges on stabilizing key social determinants of health impacting recovery, including increasing family support; improving social connectedness, particularly with peers who support abstinence; administering trauma interventions as needed; decreasing the impact of stressors through emotion regulation strategies; and facilitating access to quality care.[63] Participating in recovery group

Table 1
Tonic and phasic factors contributing to relapse for LGBTQ+ youth

Tonic Factors	Phasic Factors
• Familial substance use • Anti-LGBTQ+ stigma exposure • Adverse LGBTQ+ childhood experiences	• Coming-out events • Gender dysphoria flares • Anti-LGBTQ+ incidents • Dating-app and chemsex contexts

work, being used, having social support from family and friends, developing new habits and coping skills, and creating a sober, LGBTQ+ identity all predict better recovery outcomes.[63,134]

SUMMARY

LGBTQ+ youth face heightened risk for SUDs compared to their cisgender, heterosexual peers. Nonetheless, literature demonstrates that prevention and intervention can reduce the risk, severity, and recurrence of SUDs among LGBTQ+ youth. Prevention models that mitigate the effects of minority stress on LGBTQ+ youth, as well as intervention approaches that focus on community-building and integrating social support, are particularly important for this population. Growing work indicates that an integrative model using prevention, behavioral intervention, as well as familial and community supports are imperative to mitigating substance use risk, severity, and relapse among LGBTQ+ youth.

CLINICS CARE POINTS

Universal Prevention

- Initiatives should target youth in *early* adolescence to reduce and/or delay substance initiation
- Support school-based education initiatives focused on reduction of harmful consequences
- Support parents/caregivers in implementing clear, consistent limit setting; supervision and monitoring; and open communication with their youth
- Help youth identify peers and adults who are trustworthy and do not use substances themselves

Targeted Prevention and Identification of Early Substance Use

- Conduct ongoing assessment of substance use behaviors among lesbian, gay, bisexual, transgender, and queer/questioning (LGBTQ+) youth
- Provide psychoeducation of effects of substance use for LGBTQ+ youth, particularly as related to potential adverse health consequences
- Engage in advocacy to increase awareness and psychoeducation of substance use among LGBTQ+ youth, as well as increase use of preventive measures
- Assist schools with educational initiatives to discuss substance use
- Consider collaborating with community LGBTQ+ youth groups to provide education and mentorship

Interventions for Mild to Moderate Substance Use

- Use cognitive behavioral therapies, including harm reduction approaches and behavioral interventions, to help youth manage stressors more effectively and engage in values-based behaviors consistent with their goals
- Use evidence-based family-based modalities to increase support and improve prognoses for LGBTQ+ youth
- Help caregivers understand drivers of their youth's substance use behaviors and nonjudgmentally support their youth in practicing more effective stress management strategies

Interventions & Management for Substance Use Disorders

- Monitor substance use disorder symptoms and effectiveness of treatment approaches, and collaborate with LGBTQ+ youth and families to tailor treatment approaches as needed
- Stay updated on current guidelines on administering pharmacologic support, ensuring risks are mitigated while effective dosages are used
- Collaborate with social workers and case managers to support LGBTQ+ youth and families around barriers to treatment, including helping them obtain socioeconomic support, implement daily routines, and keep up with structured follow-up appointments and treatment plans

FUNDING

Dr N. Ramos receives research support from the National Institute on Drug Abuse of the National Institutes of Health under the AACAP NIDA K12 program (K12 DA000357).

DISCLOSURE

The authors have no relevant financial disclosures or conflicts of interest to declare.

REFERENCES

1. Human rights campaign. Growing up LGBT in America: at home, at school, and in the community. Human rights campaign. 2012. Available at: https://assets2.hrc.org/files/assets/resources/Growing-Up-LGBT-in-America_Report.pdf.
2. Reisner SL, Greytak EA, Parsons JT, et al. Gender minority social stress in adolescence: disparities in adolescent bullying and substance use by gender identity. J Sex Res 2015;52(3):243–56.
3. Day JK, Fish JN, Perez-Brumer A, et al. Transgender youth substance use disparities: results from a population-based sample. J Adolesc Health 2017;61(6):729–35.
4. De Pedro KT, Gilreath TD, Jackson C, et al. Substance use among transgender students in California public middle and high schools. J Sch Health 2017;87(5):303–9.
5. Adolescent substance use: America's #1 public health problem. National Center on addiction and substance abuse at Columbia university. 2011. Available at: https://eric.ed.gov/?id=ED521379. Accessed January 12, 2026.
6. Sterzing PR, Ratliff GA, Gartner RE, et al. Social ecological correlates of polyvictimization among a national sample of transgender, genderqueer, and cisgender sexual minority adolescents. Child Abuse Negl 2017;67:1–12.
7. Earnshaw VA, Bogart LM, Poteat VP, et al. Bullying among Lesbian, Gay, Bisexual, and transgender youth. Pediatr Clin 2016;63(6):999–1010.
8. Kosciw JG, Greytak EA, Bartkiewicz MJ, et al. The 2011 national school climate survey: the experiences of lesbian, gay, bisexual and transgender youth in our nation's schools. Gay, lesbian and straight education network (GLSEN). 2012. Available at: https://eric.ed.gov/?id=ED535177. Accessed January 12, 2026.
9. Himmelstein KEW, Brückner H. Criminal-justice and school sanctions against nonheterosexual youth: a national longitudinal study. Pediatrics 2011;127(1):49–57.
10. Irvine A, Canfield A. The overrepresentation of lesbian, gay, bisexual, questioning, gender nonconforming and transgender youth within the child welfare to juvenile justice crossover population. Soc Pol 2015;24.
11. Rosentel K, López-Martínez I, Crosby RA, et al. Black transgender women and the school-to-prison pipeline: exploring the relationship between anti-trans experiences in school and adverse criminal-legal system outcomes. Sex Res Soc Pol 2021;18(3):481–94.
12. Mountz S, Capous-Desyllas M. Exploring the families of origin of LGBTQ former foster youth and their trajectories throughout care. Child Youth Serv Rev 2020;109:104622. https://doi.org/10.1016/j.childyouth.2019.104622.
13. Galliher RV, Rostosky SS, Hughes HK. School belonging, self-esteem, and depressive symptoms in adolescents: an examination of sex, sexual attraction status, and urbanicity. J Youth Adolesc 2004;33(3):235–45.

14. Heck NC, Poteat VP, Goodenow CS. Advances in research with LGBTQ youth in schools. Psychol Sex Orientat Gend Divers 2016;3(4):381–5.
15. Brooks VR. Minority stress and Lesbian women. Lexington (MA): Lexington Books; 1981.
16. Meyer IH. Minority stress and mental health in gay men. J Health Soc Behav 1995;36(1):38–56.
17. Rich AJ, Salway T, Scheim A, et al. Sexual minority stress theory: remembering and honoring the work of Virginia brooks | LGBT health. LGBT Health 2020;7(3): 124–7.
18. Meyer IH. Prejudice, social stress, and mental health in lesbian, gay, and bisexual populations: conceptual issues and research evidence. Psychol Bull 2003;129(5):674–97.
19. Chodzen G, Hidalgo MA, Chen D, et al. Minority stress factors associated with depression and anxiety among transgender and gender-nonconforming youth. J Adolesc Health 2019;64(4):467–71.
20. Crenshaw K. Demarginalizing the intersection of race and sex: a black feminist critique of antidiscrimination doctrine. Feminist Theory and Antiracist Politics Univ Chic Leg Forum 1989;1989:139.
21. Crenshaw K. Mapping the margins: intersectionality, identity politics, and violence against women of color. Stanf Law Rev 1991;43(6):1241–99.
22. Mallory AB, Russell ST. Intersections of racial discrimination and LGB victimization for mental health: a prospective study of sexual minority youth of color. J Youth Adolesc 2021;50(7):1353–68.
23. Thoma BC, Huebner DM. Health consequences of racist and antigay discrimination for multiple minority adolescents. Cult Divers Ethnic Minor Psychol 2013;19(4):404–13.
24. LaMartine S, García JJ, Nakamura N. "scars on your heart and PTSD in your mind": Transmisogynoir and the well-being of black transgender women in Los Angeles. J Prev Health Promot 2024;5(2–3):235–63.
25. Krell EC. Is transmisogyny killing trans women of color?: black trans feminisms and the exigencies of white femininity. TSQ Transgender Stud Q 2017;4(2): 226–42.
26. Carpenter L, Marshall R. Walking while trans: profiling of transgender women by law enforcement, and the problem of proof. William Mary J Race Gend Soc Justice 2017;24(1):5.
27. Hughes D, Del Toro J, Harding JF, et al. Trajectories of discrimination across adolescence: associations with academic, psychological, and behavioral outcomes. Child Dev 2016;87(5):1337–51.
28. Thomasius R, Paschke K, Arnaud N. Substance-use disorders in children and adolescents. Dtsch Ärztebl Int 2022;119(25):440–50.
29. Hatzenbuehler ML, Nolen-Hoeksema S, Dovidio J. How does stigma "get under the skin"?: the mediating role of emotion regulation. Psychol Sci 2009;20(10): 1282–9.
30. Felner JK, Wisdom JP, Williams T, et al. Stress, coping, and context: examining substance use among LGBTQ young adults with probable substance use disorders. Psychiatr Serv 2020;71(2):112–20.
31. Ryan C, Russell ST, Huebner D, et al. Family acceptance in adolescence and the health of LGBT young adults. J Child Adolesc Psychiatr Nurs 2010;23(4): 205–13.

32. Ryan C, Huebner D, Diaz RM, et al. Family rejection as a predictor of negative health outcomes in white and Latino Lesbian, Gay, and bisexual young adults. Pediatrics 2009;123(1):346–52.
33. Gower AL, Rider GN, Brown C, et al. Supporting transgender and gender diverse youth: protection against emotional distress and substance use. Am J Prev Med 2018;55(6):787–94.
34. Katz-Wise SL, Rosario M, Tsappis M. LGBT youth and family acceptance. Pediatr Clin 2016;63(6):1011–25.
35. Levitan N, Barkmann C, Richter-Appelt H, et al. Risk factors for psychological functioning in German adolescents with gender dysphoria: poor peer relations and general family functioning. Eur Child Adolesc Psychiatry 2019;28(11):1487–98.
36. Sievert ED, Schweizer K, Barkmann C, et al. Not social transition status, but peer relations and family functioning predict psychological functioning in a German clinical sample of children with Gender dysphoria. Clin Child Psychol Psychiatr 2021;26(1):79–95.
37. Wittlin NM, Kuper LE, Olson KR. Mental health of transgender and gender diverse youth. Annu Rev Clin Psychol 2023;19:207–32.
38. Pariseau EM, Chevalier L, Long KA, et al. The relationship between family acceptance-rejection and transgender youth psychosocial functioning. Clin Pract Pediatr Psychol 2019;7(3):267–77.
39. Hatchel T, Valido A, De Pedro KT, et al. Minority stress among transgender adolescents: the role of peer victimization, school belonging, and ethnicity. J Child Fam Stud 2019;28(9):2467–76.
40. Talaugon AR, Turanovic JJ, Siennick SE. The consequences of peer victimization for suspension: specifying a pathway through school problem behaviors in early adolescence. J Sch Violence 2026;25(1):104–18.
41. Ybarra ML, Diener-West M, Leaf PJ. Examining the overlap in internet harassment and school bullying: implications for school intervention. J Adolesc Health 2007;41(6, Supplement):S42–50.
42. Fuller-Rowell TE, Cogburn CD, Brodish AB, et al. Racial discrimination and substance use: longitudinal associations and identity moderators. J Behav Med 2012;35(6):581–90.
43. Bränström R, Pachankis JE. Sexual orientation disparities in the co-occurrence of substance use and psychological distress: a national population-based study (2008–2015). Soc Psychiatr Psychiatr Epidemiol 2018;53(4):403–12.
44. Williams ND, Fish JN. The availability of LGBT-specific mental health and substance abuse treatment in the United States. Health Serv Res 2020;55(6):932–43.
45. Grant JM, Motter LA, Tanis J. Injustice at every turn: a report of the national transgender discrimination survey. Washington: National Center for Transgender Equality and National Gay and Lesbian Task Force; 2011.
46. McPhail D, Rountree-James M, Whetter I. Addressing gaps in physician knowledge regarding transgender health and healthcare through medical education. Can Med Educ J 2016;7(2):e70–8.
47. Mapping attacks on LGBTQ rights in U.S. State legislatures in 2023. American civil liberties union. Available at: https://www.aclu.org/legislative-attacks-on-lgbtq-rights-2023. Accessed January 6, 2026.
48. Issues impacting LGBTQ youth. The Trevor Project; 2023.
49. Kann L, Olsen EOM, McManus T, et al. Sexual Identity, Sex of Sexual Contacts, and Health-Risk Behaviors Among Students in Grades 9-12: Youth Risk Behavior Surveillance, Selected Sites, United States, 2001-2009. Morbidity and Mortality

Weekly Report. Early Release. Volume 60. Vol 60. ERIC Clearinghouse; 2011. Available at: https://www.cdc.gov/mmwr/preview/mmwrhtml/ss6007a1.htm?s_. Accessed January 11, 2026.
50. Kann L, Olsen EO, McManus T, et al. Sexual identity, sex of sexual contacts, and health-related behaviors among students in grades 9–12 — united States and selected sites, 2015. MMWR Surveill Summ 2016;65. https://doi.org/10.15585/mmwr.ss6509a1.
51. Becerra-Culqui TA, Liu Y, Nash R, et al. Mental health of transgender and gender nonconforming youth compared with their peers. Pediatrics 2018; 141(5):e20173845. https://doi.org/10.1542/peds.2017-3845.
52. Olson J, Schrager SM, Belzer M, et al. Baseline physiologic and psychosocial characteristics of transgender youth seeking care for gender dysphoria. J Adolesc Health 2015;57(4):374–80.
53. Reisner SL, Vetters R, Leclerc M, et al. Mental health of transgender youth in care at an adolescent urban community health center: a matched retrospective cohort study. J Adolesc Health 2015;56(3):274–9.
54. Spack NP, Edwards-Leeper L, Feldman HA, et al. Children and adolescents with gender identity disorder referred to a pediatric medical center. Pediatrics 2012; 129(3):418–25.
55. Holt V, Skagerberg E, Dunsford M. Young people with features of gender dysphoria: demographics and associated difficulties. Clin Child Psychol Psychiatr 2016;21(1):108–18.
56. Goldstein BI, Shamseddeen W, Spirito A, et al. Substance use and the treatment of resistant depression in adolescents. J Am Acad Child Adolesc Psychiatry 2009;48(12):1182–92.
57. Substance Abuse and Mental Health Services Administration. Key substance use and mental health indicators in the United States: results from the 2018 National Survey on drug use and health. Center for behavioral health statistics and quality, substance abuse and mental health services administration. 2019. Available at: https://www.samhsa.gov/data/.
58. Griffin KW, Botvin GJ. Evidence-based interventions for preventing substance use disorders in adolescents. Child Adolesc Psychiatr Clin 2010;19(3):505–26.
59. de Vries ALC, Noens ILJ, Cohen-Kettenis PT, et al. Autism spectrum disorders in gender dysphoric children and adolescents. J Autism Dev Disord 2010;40(8): 930–6.
60. McLeod JD, Hawbaker A, Meanwell E. The health of college students on the autism spectrum as compared to their neurotypical peers. Autism 2021;25(3): 719–30.
61. National Research Council and Institute of Medicine. Preventing mental, emotional, and behavioral disorders among young people: progress and possibilities. Washington, DC: National Academies Press; 2009.
62. World Health Organization. Well-being and health promotion. 2022. Available at: https://apps.who.int/gb/ebwha/pdf_files/WHA75/A75_R19-en.pdf. Accessed December 30, 2025.
63. Lin C, Cousins SJ, Zhu Y, et al. A scoping review of social determinants of health's impact on substance use disorders over the life course. J Subst Use Addict Treat 2024;166:209484. https://doi.org/10.1016/j.josat.2024.209484.
64. Davis JP, Merrin GJ, Berry DJ, et al. Examining within-person and between-person effects of victimization and social risk on cannabis use among emerging adults in substance-use treatment. Psychol Addict Behav 2016;30(1):52–63.

65. Brook JS, Lee JY, Rubenstone E, et al. Longitudinal determinants of substance use disorders. J Urban Health 2013;90(6):1130–50.
66. Atherton OE, Conger RD, Ferrer E, et al. Risk and protective factors for early substance use initiation: a longitudinal study of mexican-origin youth. J Res Adolesc 2016;26(4):864–79.
67. Durwood L, Eisner L, Fladeboe K, et al. Social support and internalizing psychopathology in transgender youth. J Youth Adolesc 2021;50(5):841–54.
68. Toomey RB, Ryan C, Diaz RM, et al. High school gay–straight alliances (GSAs) and young adult well-being: an examination of GSA presence, participation, and perceived effectiveness. Appl Dev Sci 2011;15(4):175–85.
69. Greytak EA, Kosciw JG, Boesen MJ. Putting the "T" in "Resource": the benefits of LGBT-related school resources for transgender youth. J LGBT Youth 2013;10-(1–2):45–63.
70. Eccles JS, Barber BL, Stone M, et al. Extracurricular activities and adolescent development. J Soc Issues 2003;59(4):865–89.
71. Zaff JF, Moore KA, Papillo AR, et al. Implications of extracurricular activity participation during adolescence on positive outcomes. J Adolesc Res 2003;18(6): 599–630.
72. Resnick MD, Bearman PS, Blum RWM, et al. Protecting adolescents from harm: findings from the National longitudinal study on adolescent health. JAMA 1997; 278(10):823–32.
73. Needham BL, Austin EL. Sexual orientation, parental support, and health during the transition to young adulthood. J Youth Adolesc 2010;39(10):1189–98.
74. Eisenberg ME, Resnick MD. Suicidality among gay, lesbian and bisexual youth: the role of protective factors. J Adolesc Health 2006;39(5):662–8.
75. Hundleby JD, Mercer GW. Family and friends as social environments and their relationship to young adolescents' use of alcohol, tobacco, and marijuana. J Marriage Fam 1987;49(1):151–64.
76. Ryan C. Supportive families, healthy children: helping families with lesbian, gay, bisexual & transgender children. San Francisco (CA): Family Acceptance Project, San Francisco State University; 2009.
77. Hawkins JD, Catalano RF, Miller JY. Risk and protective factors for alcohol and other drug problems in adolescence and early adulthood: implications for substance abuse prevention. Psychol Bull 1992;112(1):64–105.
78. Petraitis J, Flay BR, Miller TQ. Reviewing theories of adolescent substance use: organizing pieces in the puzzle. Psychol Bull 1995;117(1):67–86.
79. Moskowitz JM. The primary prevention of alcohol problems: a critical review of the research literature. J Stud Alcohol 2015;50(1):54–88.
80. Lynam DR, Milich R, Zimmerman R, et al. Project DARE: no effects at 10-Year Follow-Up. Washington, DC: American Psychological Association; 2009. p. 196. https://doi.org/10.1037/11855-008.
81. Beck J. 100 years of "Just Say No" Versus "Just say know": reevaluating drug education goals for the coming century. Eval Rev 1998;22(1):15–45.
82. Marlatt GA. Harm reduction: come as you are. Addict Behav 1996;21(6):779–88.
83. Wittchen HU, Behrendt S, Höfler M, et al. What are the high risk periods for incident substance use and transitions to abuse and dependence? Implications for early intervention and prevention. Int J Methods Psychiatr Res 2008;17(S1): S16–29.
84. Barnett E, Spruijt-Metz D, Unger JB, et al. Boosting a teen substance use prevention program with motivational interviewing. Subst Use Misuse 2012;47(4): 418–28.

85. Stewart DG, Siebert EC, Arlt VK, et al. READY or not: findings from a school-based MI intervention for adolescent substance use. J Subst Abuse Treat 2016;71:23–9.
86. Riggs NR, Chou CP, Pentz MA. Preventing growth in amphetamine use: long-term effects of the midwestern prevention project (MPP) from early adolescence to early adulthood. Addiction 2009;104(10):1691–9.
87. Miller T, Lauer A, Mihok B, et al. A continuum of care approach: western pennsylvania's response to the opioid epidemic. University of Pittsburgh. 2016. Available at: https://dscholarship.pitt.edu/29950/1/IOPOpioidReport2016.pdf.
88. Simpson SKJ, Hawkins JM, Bean RA. Family therapy for substance use among sexual minority youth: a review of treatment options. Am J Fam Ther 2020;48(5):431–45.
89. Winer JM, Yule AM, Hadland SE, et al. Addressing adolescent substance use with a public health prevention framework: the case for harm reduction. Ann Med 2022;54(1):2123–36.
90. Kimmel SD, Gaeta JM, Hadland SE, et al. Principles of harm reduction for young people who use drugs. Pediatrics 2021;147(Supplement 2):S240–8.
91. Krieger MS, Goedel WC, Buxton JA, et al. Use of rapid fentanyl test strips among young adults who use drugs. Int J Drug Policy 2018;61:52–8.
92. Bagot KS, Kaminer Y. Harm reduction for youth in treatment for substance use disorders: one size does not fit all. Curr Addict Rep 2018;5(3):379–85.
93. Wallace BC, Santacruz E. Addictions and substance abuse in the LGBT community: new approaches. In: LGBT psychology and mental health: emerging research and advances. Bloomsbury Publishing USA; 2017. p. 153–75.
94. Copenhaver MM, Johnson BT, Lee IC, et al. Behavioral HIV risk reduction among people who inject drugs: meta-analytic evidence of efficacy. J Subst Abuse Treat 2006;31(2):163–71.
95. McGeough BL, Paceley MS, Zemore SE, et al. Understanding the social and community support experiences of sexual and gender minority individuals in 12-Step programs. J Gay Lesb Soc Serv 2023;35(4):398–419.
96. Van Amsterdam J, Van Den Brink W. Pharmacological perspectives and clinical applications in substance use disorders in adolescents. Expert Opin Pharmacother 2025;26(7):787–90.
97. Liu Y, Wu YC, Fu H, et al. Digital intervention in improving the outcomes of mental health among LGBTQ+ youth: a systematic review. Front Psychol 2023;14. https://doi.org/10.3389/fpsyg.2023.1242928.
98. Harkness A, Rogers BG, Puccinelli M, et al. Engaging, retaining, and providing transdiagnostic integrated cognitive–behavioral therapy and motivational interviewing for underserved people with HIV. Psychotherapy 2020;57(1):15–22.
99. Simons-Morton B. Social influences on adolescent substance use. Am J Health Behav 2007;31(6):672–84.
100. Boden JM, Crossin R, Cook S, et al. Parenting and home environment in childhood and adolescence and alcohol use disorder in adulthood. J Adolesc Health Off Publ Soc Adolesc Med 2021;69(2):329–34.
101. Robbins MS, Feaster DJ, Horigian VE, et al. Brief strategic family therapy versus treatment as usual: results of a multisite randomized trial for substance using adolescents. J Consult Clin Psychol 2011;79(6):713–27.
102. Liddle HA, Dakof GA, Rowe CL, et al. Multidimensional family therapy as a community-based alternative to residential treatment for adolescents with substance use and co-occurring mental health disorders. J Subst Abuse Treat 2018;90:47–56.

103. Slesnick N, Prestopnik JL. Comparison of family therapy outcome with alcohol-abusing, runaway adolescents. J Marital Fam Ther 2009;35(3):255–77.
104. Baldwin SA, Christian S, Berkeljon A, et al. The effects of family therapies for adolescent delinquency and substance abuse: a meta-analysis. J Marital Fam Ther 2012;38(1):281–304.
105. Ryan C, Barba A, Cohen JA. Family-based psychosocial care for transgender and gender-diverse children and youth. Child Adolesc Psychiatr Clin N Am 2023;32(4):775–88.
106. Simmons S, Suárez L. Substance abuse and trauma. Child Adolesc Psychiatr Clin N Am 2016;25(4):723–34.
107. Watson RJ, Park M, Taylor AB, et al. Associations between community-level LGBTQ-supportive factors and substance use among sexual minority adolescents. LGBT Health 2020;7(2):82–9.
108. Shen J, Seager van Dyk I, Cohen JM. Talking with youth about sexual orientation and gender identity. Pediatr Rev 2024;45(12):721–5.
109. Rogers AH, Seager I, Haines N, et al. The indirect effect of emotion regulation on minority stress and problematic substance use in lesbian, gay, and bisexual individuals. Front Psychol 2017;8. https://doi.org/10.3389/fpsyg.2017.01881.
110. Squeglia LM, Fadus MC, McClure EA, et al. Pharmacological treatment of youth substance use disorders. J Child Adolesc Psychopharmacol 2019;29(7):559–72.
111. Bailey SR, Hagen SA, Jeffery CJ, et al. A randomized clinical trial of the efficacy of extended smoking cessation treatment for adolescent smokers. Nicotine Tob Res 2013;15(10):1655–62.
112. Clark H, Babu AS, Wiewel EW, et al. Diagnosed HIV infection in transgender adults and adolescents: results from the national HIV surveillance system, 2009–2014. AIDS Behav 2017;21(9):2774–83.
113. Becasen JS, Denard CL, Mullins MM, et al. Estimating the prevalence of HIV and sexual behaviors among the US transgender population: a systematic review and meta-analysis, 2006–2017. Am J Publ Health 2019;109(1):e1–8.
114. Martin EG, Avila Acosta M, Pepin DA, et al. HIV preexposure prophylaxis prescriptions, consent laws, and uptake barriers among adolescents. Pediatrics 2025;156(4):e2024069808. https://doi.org/10.1542/peds.2024-069808.
115. Yager JL, Anderson PL. Pharmacology and drug interactions with HIV PrEP in transgender persons receiving gender affirming hormone therapy. Expert Opin Drug Metab Toxicol 2020;16(6):463–74.
116. Senneker T. Drug–drug interactions between gender-affirming hormone therapy and antiretrovirals for treatment/prevention of HIV. Br J Clin Pharmacol 2024;90-(10):2366–82.
117. Connolly MD, Zervos MJ, Barone CJ, et al. The mental health of transgender youth: advances in understanding. J Adolesc Health 2016;59(5):489–95.
118. Girouard MP, Goldhammer H, Keuroghlian AS. Article commentary: understanding and treating opioid use disorders in Lesbian, Gay, Bisexual, transgender, and queer populations. Subst Abuse 2019;40(3):335–9.
119. Reddy DS. Testosterone modulation of seizure susceptibility is mediated by neurosteroids 3α-androstanediol and 17β-estradiol. Neuroscience 2004;129(1):195–207.
120. Foy MR, Xu J, Xie X, et al. 17β-Estradiol enhances NMDA receptor-mediated EPSPs and long-term potentiation. J Neurophysiol 1999;81(2):925–9.
121. Lange SC, Julien RM. Re-evaluation of estrogen-induced cortical and thalamic paroxysmal EEG activity in the cat. Electroencephalogr Clin Neurophysiol 1978;44(1):94–103.

122. Pottoo FH, Javed MN, Barkat MA, et al. Estrogen and serotonin: complexity of interactions and implications for epileptic seizures and epileptogenesis. Curr Neuropharmacol 2019;17(3):214–31.
123. ZYBAN(R) sustained-release oral tablets, bupropion hcl sustained-release oral tablets. Prescribing information. Research Triangle Park (NC): GlaxoSmithKline; 2007.
124. Merative. *Bupropion Hydrochloride*. Micromedex solutions. 2026. Available at: https://www.micromedexsolutions.com/. Accessed May 14, 2026.
125. Merative. *Methadone Hydrochloride-Spironolactone*. Micromedex solutions. 2026. Available at: https://www.micromedexsolutions.com/. Accessed May 14, 2026.
126. Robertson SM, Maldarelli F, Natarajan V, et al. Efavirenz induces CYP2B6-mediated hydroxylation of bupropion in healthy subjects. J Acquir Immune Defic Syndr 2008;49(5):513–9.
127. Hogeland GW, Swindells S, McNabb JC, et al. Lopinavir/ritonavir reduces bupropion plasma concentrations in healthy subjects. Clin Pharmacol Ther 2007; 81(1):69–75.
128. Hesse LM, Greenblatt DJ, von Moltke LL, et al. Ritonavir has minimal impact on the pharmacokinetic disposition of a single dose of bupropion administered to human volunteers. J Clin Pharmacol 2006;46(5):567–76.
129. Merative. Methadone hydrochloride - emtricitabine/tenofovir disoproxil fumarate. Micromedex Solutions 2026. Available at: https://www.micromedexsolutions.com/. Accessed May 14, 2026.
130. APLENZIN(R) oral extended-release tablets, Bupropion hydrobromide oral extended-release tablets. Prescribing Information. Bridgewater (NJ): Bausch Health US LLC; 2021.
131. Chaney MP, Mason N. Queering recovery: a proposed model for LGBTQ+-affirmative relapse prevention. J Addict Offender Couns 2024;45(1):98–110.
132. Witkiewitz K, Marlatt GA. Relapse prevention for alcohol and drug problems: that was zen, this is Tao. Am Psychol 2004;59(4):224–35.
133. Goedel WC, Duncan DT. Contextual factors in geosocial-networking smartphone application use and engagement in condomless anal intercourse among gay, bisexual, and other men who have sex with men who use Grindr. Sex Health 2016;13(6):549–54.
134. Nieder A, Schachter J, Ajayi AA. Minority stress, substance use, and resilience: examining long-term sobriety in the LGBTQ community. Alcohol Treat Q 2025; 43(2):290–305.

Substance Use Disorders in Adolescents with Bipolar Disorder

A Developmental Approach to Assessment and Treatment

Lisa R. Fortuna, MD, MPH*, Suren Najaryan, MD,
Edder Duarte, MD, PhD, Omar Abbas, MD

KEYWORDS

- Adolescent bipolar disorder • Substance use disorders • Co-occurring disorders
- Integrated care

KEY POINTS

- Substance use disorders are associated with earlier onset of substance use, mood instability, increased suicidality, and poorer functional outcomes.
- Differentiating BD from substance-induced mood symptoms requires longitudinal assessment tracking across periods of abstinence, collateral information, and careful attention to developmental context.
- Evidence-based pharmacologic treatments for pediatric BD are needed to safely control symptoms, even in the presence of active substance use.
- Family-based treatments, cognitive-behavioral approaches, and motivational interviewing constitute the strongest evidence-supported psychosocial interventions.
- Integrated, family-centered approaches that address mood symptoms, substance use, and contextual stressors concurrently are recommended to improve care and outcomes.

INTRODUCTION

Substance use disorders (SUDs) are common and clinically consequential among adolescents with bipolar disorder (BD).[1,2] Epidemiologic studies consistently demonstrate youth with bipolar spectrum disorders are at substantially elevated risk for early initiation of substance use, rapid escalation to problematic use, and development of SUDs compared with peers without mood disorders.[3,4] The presence of comorbid substance

Department of Psychiatry and Neuroscience, School of Medicine, University of California Riverside, 900 University Avenue, Riverside, CA 92521, USA
* Corresponding author.
E-mail address: Lisa.fortuna@medsch.ucr.edu

Child Adolesc Psychiatric Clin N Am 35 (2026) 781–796
https://doi.org/10.1016/j.chc.2026.05.007 childpsych.theclinics.com

Abbreviations	
ADHD	attention-deficit/hyperactivity disorder
BD	bipolar disorder
CBT	cognitive behavioral therapy
FFT	family-focused treatment
IPSRT-A	interpersonal and social rhythm therapy for adolescents
MDFT	multidimensional family therapy
SGA	second-generation antipsychotic
SUD	substance use disorder

use complicates diagnosis, worsens illness course, increases suicide risk, and contributes to significant family, academic, and social impairment.[3]

Adolescence represents a particularly vulnerable developmental period in which ongoing brain maturation, heightened reward sensitivity, and evolving autonomy intersect with the onset of serious mood disorders and exposure to substances.[5] For youth with BD, substance use may emerge as an attempt to regulate mood symptoms, sleep disturbance, or emotional dysregulation.[3] Cannabis use during adolescence is associated with mood dysregulation and increased psychiatric vulnerability, with effects that vary by developmental timing and individual risk.[6] The association between cannabis use and mood outcomes is likely bidirectional and may reflect shared underlying vulnerabilities, rather than a primarily unidirectional causal relationship. However, longitudinal evidence indicates that cannabis use is associated with subsequent depressive symptoms and affective morbidity across populations, supporting its role as a risk factor for worse mood outcomes, though causal pathways appear heterogeneous.[7]

Despite the high prevalence and clinical impact of co-occurring BD and SUDs, adolescents with comorbidity are frequently underrepresented in clinical trials.[8] Clinicians must therefore integrate evidence from pediatric BD trials, adolescent substance use treatment studies, and family-based intervention models to guide care.[9]

DEVELOPMENTAL EPIDEMIOLOGY AND CLINICAL DECISION MAKING

BD affects approximately 1% to 3% of adolescents, with broader bipolar spectrum presentations occurring at higher rates.[10] Among adolescents with BD, 30% to 60% develop a lifetime SUD, with risk increasing with age and illness severity.[3] Youth with BD are at significantly elevated risk for SUDs compared with peers, and this vulnerability often emerges early in the illness course.[4] However, given the current state of the evidence, clinicians are often required to make developmentally informed, individualized treatment decisions in the absence of directly applicable clinical trial and other research data.

Cannabis and alcohol are the most commonly used substances by adolescents and these are associated with greater clinical complexity,[4] including earlier illness onset, increased symptom burden, more frequent mood episodes, poorer treatment adherence, and worse psychosocial functioning.[11,12] Adolescents with co-occurring BD and SUDs are also at substantially increased risk for suicidal ideation and attempts, underscoring the severity of this comorbidity.[13]

From a developmental perspective, adolescence is characterized by a maturational imbalance between heightened reactivity of limbic and reward-related neural systems and still-developing top-down cognitive control, resulting in increased sensitivity to incentives and socioemotional contexts.[5] In adolescents with BD—who often exhibit heightened emotional reactivity and impulsivity—this neurodevelopmental profile may further amplify vulnerability to substance use and risk-taking during periods of mood instability. Together, these epidemiologic, clinical, and developmental findings highlight early identification and timely, comprehensive intervention as a critical opportunity to reduce illness severity, limit secondary morbidity, and improve long-term functioning among adolescents with BD.

SHARED RISK FACTORS AND INTEGRATED CARE

BD and SUDs reflect both genetic and environmental liabilities that shape risk, symptom burden, and longitudinal course.[14,15] Converging mechanistic work—from patient-derived cellular models to preclinical paradigms—supports disruptions in neuronal excitability, reward/stress responsiveness, and regulatory control processes that are plausibly relevant to both mood dysregulation and addiction vulnerability.[16–19] Human neuroimaging consortia demonstrate reproducible structural differences in BD, including subcortical volumetric alterations and widespread white matter microstructural abnormalities, consistent with involvement of distributed frontolimbic circuitry.[20,21]

Clinical Synthesis

Adolescence represents a critical developmental window in which shared genetic vulnerability, ongoing maturation of frontolimbic and reward circuits, and heightened sensitivity to environmental stressors converge to increase risk for both BD and SUDs. Understanding this comorbidity as a developmentally dynamic process underscores the importance of early, integrated interventions that address mood symptoms, substance use risk, and contextual factors simultaneously.

From a developmental perspective, adolescence is a period when manic/hypomanic symptoms can amplify approach behavior and reward-driven decision-making, potentially increasing susceptibility to experimentation and escalation in substance use among vulnerable youth.[22] At the same time, early adversity is associated with later risk behaviors and mental health problems, underscoring how stress exposures can compound developmental risk.[23] In a small study, youth with depression associated with BD demonstrated disruptions in family environment across domains of cohesion, independence, achievement orientation, and organization.[24] Consistent with this, other studies have found prognosis is shaped by social context, history of abuse and stressed family environments,[25] underscoring the importance of addressing environmental factors and parent psychopathology alongside symptom treatment.[24]

Clinical Presentation and Differential Diagnosis

Differentiating BD from substance-induced symptoms in adolescents is challenging, as intoxication and withdrawal may closely resemble manic, hypomanic, or depressive episodes, while ongoing substance use can obscure the episodic course required for diagnosis under Diagnostic and Statistical Manual of Mental Disorders, Fifth Edition, Text Revision (DSM-5-TR) criteria. With increasing adolescent cannabis use nationally, careful assessment of its temporal relationship to mood and psychotic symptoms is essential for diagnostic accuracy, prognosis, and treatment planning.[26] Key considerations include symptom onset relative to substance exposure, persistence of mood symptoms during sustained abstinence, family history of BD, and the presence of cardinal manic features such as decreased need for sleep, grandiosity, and episodic increases in goal-directed activity.[27] Longitudinal assessment and collateral information from caregivers and schools are therefore critical.

Comprehensive Assessment

Assessment of adolescents with suspected BD and comorbid substance use should be multimethod, developmentally informed, and culturally responsive. Screening tools such as the Mood Disorder Questionnaire-Adolescent Version and Child Bipolar Questionnaire may help identify youth requiring further evaluation; although positive predictive value is low, high negative predictive value supports their use in ruling out BD in lower-risk populations.[28] Diagnosis remains clinical and requires evaluation across multiple time points and settings.

Structured interviews such as the Kiddie Schedule for Affective Disorders and Schizophrenia (K-SADS) remain the diagnostic standard and allow systematic assessment of manic symptoms alongside alcohol, tobacco, and other SUDs.[29] Given informant discrepancies and stigma-related under-reporting, particularly around substance use, multi-informant assessment incorporating youth, caregivers, and school sources improves diagnostic accuracy.[30–32]

Ongoing evaluation should include standardized symptom monitoring (eg, Young Mania Rating Scale [YMRS] and Children's Depression Rating Scale [CDRS]) and assessment of trauma exposure, family functioning and parental psychopathology, sleep and circadian regulation, academic functioning, and social determinants of health, all of which influence relapse and recovery trajectories.[33–36] Systematic substance use screening with youth-validated tools such as the CRAFFT or ASSIST is recommended.[37,38] Comorbid substance use and BD requires an approach of integrated assessment and care planning.[3,39]

Although it is important to remember that youth can also have more than one psychiatric diagnosis, an integrated and longitudinal approach is important for differential diagnosis.

Differential Diagnosis

Attention-deficit/hyperactivity disorder

Chronic, nonepisodic inattention and impulsivity across contexts; symptoms are not confined to discrete mood episodes, and mood reactivity lacks sustained elation or grandiosity.

Disruptive mood dysregulation disorder

Persistent, nonepisodic irritability with frequent temper outbursts across settings; absence of distinct mood episodes and no periods of elevated or expansive mood.

Trauma-related disorders (eg, posttraumatic stress disorder [PTSD])

Mood lability and irritability linked to trauma reminders, with re-experiencing, avoidance, and hyperarousal rather than episodic mania.

Substance-induced mood disorder

Mood symptoms emerge during or shortly after intoxication or withdrawal and improve with sustained abstinence; persistence beyond expected substance effects raises concern for a primary mood disorder.

An integrated approach is also applicable across care settings. Clinicians should tailor assessment, diagnosis, and care planning to the clinical setting, using strategies appropriate to time, acuity, and available information, and emphasizing evaluation across multiple time points and settings.

Emergency settings: Prioritize rapid safety and risk assessment (eg, suicidality, mania, and psychosis), brief screening for substance use, and focused history from available caregivers or records. Use structured tools when feasible, clarify immediate disposition, and arrange close follow-up to enable reassessment over time, particularly after periods of stabilization or abstinence.

Outpatient settings: Conduct longitudinal, developmentally informed assessments across multiple visits, incorporating detailed history, standardized rating scales, and collateral information from caregivers, schools, and prior providers. Monitor symptom trajectories, include periods of abstinence when relevant, and use follow-up intervals to refine diagnosis as patterns emerge.

Inpatient settings: Use extended observation and a multidisciplinary approach (eg, psychiatry, psychology, nursing, and social work) to clarify diagnosis, assess family and environmental factors, and evaluate treatment response. Integrate daily behavioral observations, family meetings, and collateral data, and use the duration of admission and postdischarge follow-up to support diagnostic clarity across settings.

PHARMACOLOGIC TREATMENT

In psychopharmacologic management of co-occurring mood and substance use conditions, clinicians should prioritize acute mood stabilization while generally initiating concurrent treatment for substance use, with ongoing reassessment at defined time points—particularly following periods of abstinence—to refine diagnosis and adjust treatment as needed.[9] Pharmacologic treatment target mood symptoms in adolescents with BD who have co-occurring substance use, as effective medication management of manic and mixed states reduces behavioral disinhibition, impulsivity, and dysphoria often contribute to substance initiation and persistence. Second-generation antipsychotics (SGAs), lithium, and anticonvulsants constitute the primary evidence-based treatments for adolescent mania, with SGAs demonstrating the strongest antimanic effects and lower discontinuation rates compared to traditional mood stabilizers.[40]

Lithium remains an effective agent for mania and for relapse prevention, with evidence supporting its utility in reducing symptom severity, improving global functioning, and suicidality.[40,41] Early work also demonstrated that lithium may reduce both mood- and substance-related impairment in adolescents with BD and secondary substance dependence,[42] suggesting that stabilization of affective symptoms may indirectly attenuate substance-related morbidity.

Treatment guidelines for bipolar depression in adolescents remain more limited. Lurasidone and the olanzapine–fluoxetine combination has demonstrated short-term improvements in depressive symptoms in randomized trials, though the latter carries substantial risk of increased appetite, with concomitant weight gain and metabolic disturbance.[40] Lamotrigine shows potential benefit for bipolar depression and maintenance treatment in youth, though rare and sometimes life-threatening dermatologic complications can restrict its widespread use in younger patients.[40] Depressive symptoms, when insufficiently treated, may contribute to self-medication patterns observed in youth with BD, reinforcing the importance of optimized mood treatment in reducing SUD vulnerability and relapse.

High rates of comorbidity with attention-deficit/hyperactivity disorder (ADHD), anxiety disorders, and externalizing behavior further influence pharmacologic decision-making in bipolar youth with substance use. Stimulants may be used to treat co-occurring ADHD only following adequate mood stabilization, as stimulant monotherapy has been associated with treatment-emergent mania.[40] Antidepressants are generally avoided or deferred for anxiety or depressive symptoms in bipolar youth due to the risk of mood switching and mixed states,[40] a consideration that is relevant for youth using substances for anxiolysis or affect regulation. However, in practice they may be cautiously used in select cases—typically with concurrent mood stabilizer coverage and close monitoring—when depressive symptoms are severe, persistent, or impairing.[9]

SGAs carry significant metabolic adverse effects in pediatric populations, necessitating structured monitoring of body mass index, glucose, lipids, and blood pressure due to increased risk for metabolic syndrome.[40] These metabolic risks may interact with substance-related caloric excess, appetite dysregulation, or metabolic load, particularly with heavy alcohol or cannabis use. Novel metabolic supports such as glucagon-like peptide-1 receptor agonists may mitigate these effects, though pediatric evidence is limited.[40] Finally, the narrow therapeutic index and teratogenic risks associated with some anticonvulsants—including valproate—underscore the need for reproductive counseling in adolescents of reproductive potential.[43]

Despite the significant potential drawbacks of the medications discussed above, it is important to balance these effects against the substantial risks associated with untreated BD during adolescence and young adulthood, when manic states and substance use can lead to life-threatening behaviors, disruption of normative developmental trajectories, and long-lasting impairments in educational, social, and vocational functioning. During this developmental period, ongoing maturation of cognitive control, emotion regulation, and reward processing systems may heighten vulnerability to both mood dysregulation and substance use, increasing the potential consequences of delayed or inadequate treatment.

Although pharmacotherapy is essential for mood stabilization and may indirectly reduce substance-related harm by improving affect regulation and behavioral containment, medication alone is rarely sufficient to address the developmentally salient cognitive, motivational, interpersonal, and environmental processes that sustain substance use in adolescents. These include emerging autonomy, heightened sensitivity to peer influence, evolving identity formation, family dynamics, and exposure to stressors within school and community contexts. Integrated treatment models that combine mood-stabilizing pharmacotherapy with developmentally tailored psychosocial and family-based interventions for SUDs are therefore most appropriate for adolescents and young adults, supporting both symptom control and healthy progression through critical developmental milestones.

Medication selection for adolescents with bipolar disorder + substance use disorder is further influenced by:

Adherence variability and real-world barriers: Consider factors such as chaotic environments, caregiver inconsistency, and system transitions (eg, foster care, juvenile justice), and favor simpler regimens or long-acting formulations when adherence is uncertain.

Withdrawal and intoxication effects: Account for acute substance-related symptoms (eg, alcohol withdrawal agitation and cannabis withdrawal irritability/insomnia) when selecting agents and timing adjustments.

Drug–drug and physiologic interactions: Consider factors such as dehydration affecting lithium levels or alcohol increasing valproate-related hepatotoxicity.

Reproductive and sexual health considerations: Incorporate risk–benefit discussions, particularly with agents such as valproate.

Continuity across systems: Select treatments that are feasible and sustainable across care settings (eg, school, foster care, and juvenile justice).

Risks of nontreatment or discontinuation: Weigh the increased risk of relapse, hospitalization, disease progression, and mortality when medications are deferred or stopped.

PSYCHOSOCIAL AND INTEGRATED TREATMENTS

In routine outpatient care, clinicians can implement core elements of integrated and family-informed treatment, including psychoeducation, brief family sessions, care coordination, and monitoring of symptoms and substance use. More intensive approaches—such as structured family therapy models (eg, family-focused treatment [FFT], multidimensional family therapy [MDFT]), multidisciplinary team-based care, or programs requiring frequent contact and cross-system coordination—typically require specialized, resource-intensive settings. Even when full evidence-based models are not feasible, key components of these interventions can still be incorporated into community-based treatment settings to enhance care. Though frequently underutilized, recommendations for management of BD include incorporation of both psychotherapy and psychopharmacological treatment.[9,44] First-line psychotherapeutic treatment also includes cognitive behavioral therapy (CBT) and motivational enhancement therapy combined with CBT, which can be particularly effective in group formats.[45]

Given family-based interventions represent the strongest evidence-supported treatments for adolescent SUDs, they are quintessential in approaching adolescents with comorbid bipolar and SUDs. MDFT incorporates parents/families along with community partners for a more wrap around approach and has demonstrated efficacy across multiple randomized trials.[46,47] Research has demonstrated decreases in substance use frequency and delinquent behaviors that are comparable to residential treatment, with sustained results 18 months postbaseline.[47]

Additional considerations include multisystemic therapy–substance abuse which has likewise shown significant reductions in substance use and delinquent behavior, particularly among justice-involved youth[48,49] and FFT which has demonstrated efficacy as an adjunct to pharmacotherapy for adolescents with BD, improving time to recovery, symptom severity, and family functioning.[50] Interpersonal and social rhythm therapy for adolescents (IPSRT-A) has established efficacy in small studies for adolescents.[50–52] IPSRT-A focuses on interpersonal stress, circadian rhythm dysregulation, and medications nonadherence. Components that can be integrated across systems of care include psychoeducation about BD, psychotropics, assessing for interpersonal issues and addressing them, and stabilizing sleep, building structure, and social routines.

Table 1 summarizes the core elements of these intervention modalities, supporting the rationale for integrated dual-diagnosis care in adolescents, in which mood stabilization, substance use reduction, and family functioning.

Clinical Care Pathways Bipolar Disorder and Co-occurring Substance Use

Table 2 describes how these considerations can inform clinical care pathways and can integrate care for adolescents with co-occurring bipolar and SUD, using the evidence-based approaches, and tailored to current symptom phenotype. Treatment integration emphasizes family systems, motivational processes, sleep and circadian regulation, school functioning, and social determinants of health, with deliberate attention to transitions across levels of care and the high-risk youth-to-adult system transfer period.[53,54] This framework aligns with emerging evidence from dual-diagnosis youth literature describing the clinical, functional, and developmental interdependencies of bipolar and substance use trajectories, including elevated risk of SUD among adolescents with BD and the impact of comorbidity on course and outcomes.[4,39,55,56]

Table 1
Psychotherapy modalities for adolescent bipolar disorder + substance use disorder

Modality	Core Elements
MDFT	• *Youth domain:* Build motivation for change, mood awareness, emotion regulation, and coping skills; strengthen decision-making during mood fluctuations; challenge substance-related beliefs tied to mood management; and promote alternative, prosocial activities that support routine, sleep stability, and mood regulation. • *Parent domain:* Strengthen parental commitment, monitoring, and consistent limit-setting; enhance teamwork and communication around early mood warning signs and substance use; and when indicated, support parents in accessing their own mental health or substance use treatment to improve the family recovery environment.
Multisystemic therapy–substance abuse	• Intensive, home- and community-based intervention targeting multiple systems (family, peers, school, and neighborhood) • Integration of contingency management: caregivers are coached to implement a structured reward and consequence system tied to objective evidence of use/nonuse • Systematic drug testing protocol • Drug refusal skills training using extensive role-plays with youth and family • Self-management planning and cognitive-behavioral strategies to help youth anticipate risk, cope with cravings, and structure time toward prosocial, sober activities
Cognitive behavioral therapy (CBT)	• Psychoeducation about BD, substance use, and mood–behavior links • Cognitive restructuring to address maladaptive thoughts driving mood instability and substance use • Behavioral regulation (routine, sleep, and activity pacing) to reduce relapse risk • Emotion regulation and problem-solving skills for stress, irritability, and impulsivity • Relapse prevention planning for mood episodes and substance use • Caregiver involvement to support skill generalization
Motivational enhancement therapy combined with CBT	• Motivational interviewing stance that accounts for fluctuating insight across mood states • Exploration of ambivalence about substance use in relation to mood stability and functioning • Goal alignment linking change to stability, autonomy, and developmental milestones • CBT skills training timed to euthymic or stabilized periods when possible • Coping strategies for substance urges during mood episodes • Relapse prevention addressing both mood recurrence and substance use
FFT	Psychoeducation: • Patient is expert on their illness • Family contribution on what they are seeing • Discussion of suicide and risk factors • Develop relapse prevention plan

(*continued on next page*)

Table 1
(*continued*)

Modality	Core Elements
	Communication enhancement training: • Interrupting negative interaction patterns • Increased active listening and statements of empathy • Rebalancing praise vs criticism • Clear agenda when speaking • Improve skills and designating speaker and listener. Problem-solving: • Identify specific conflicts • Brainstorm solutions as a group • Assess pros and cons of each • Choose solutions • Develop implementation plans
IPSRT-A	• Psychoeducation • Addressing interpersonal problems • Sleep stabilization • Building social routine and structure

SYSTEMS OF CARE AND TREATMENT INTENSITY CONSIDERATIONS

Using the American Society of Addiction Medicine (ASAM) framework, clinicians should generally prioritize the highest indicated level of care across conditions, particularly when safety risks are present.[57] When BD and SUD severity suggest different levels, placement should be guided by the domain with the greatest acute risk and instability (eg, suicidality, mania, severe withdrawal), while ensuring capacity to address both conditions. In practice, this often means selecting a level of care that can safely manage the more severe condition and integrate treatment for both BD and SUD, with ongoing reassessment and step-down or step-up as clinical status evolves. Attention to transitions across services—including the youth-to-adult period—remains essential, as discontinuities in care during this time are common and associated with increased clinical risk.[58] Level-of-care determination for adolescents with SUDs should be guided by the American Society of Addiction Medicine (ASAM) Criteria. **Table 3** incorporates developmentally informed assessment across six dimensions, including biomedical risk, emotional and behavioral conditions, readiness to change, relapse potential, and recovery environment, with specific considerations for adolescents and co-occurring psychiatric disorders.[57]

Gender and Culturally Specific Considerations

Gender and cultural factors influence the clinical presentation, risk pathways, and treatment engagement of adolescents with co-occurring BD and SUDs and should be explicitly incorporated into assessment and care planning. Epidemiologic studies suggest that girls with BD are more likely to present with depressive and mixed features with higher rates of anxiety and self-harm, whereas boys more commonly exhibit earlier onset, externalizing symptoms, and behavioral dysregulation.[10] Gender differences in substance use pathways also emerge during adolescence, with girls more likely to use substances in the context of affect regulation and interpersonal stress and boys more influenced by externalizing, sensation-seeking, and peer dynamics.[59] However, these descriptions of gender differences reflects population-level patterns

Table 2
Clinical care pathways for adolescents with bipolar disorder and co-occurring substance use

Pathway	Profile/Entry Phenotype	Core Treatment Focus	Primary Goals
A. BD-dominant with emerging SUD	Early bipolar presentations; episodic or experimental substance use; limited functional impairment	Mood stabilization prioritized; early MI and psychoeducation for SUD; sleep/circadian and school coordination; trauma-informed monitoring	Prevent SUD escalation and stabilize bipolar trajectory
B. SUD-Dominant with bipolar vulnerability	Heavy cannabis/alcohol/nicotine use; mood lability, irritability, and sleep disruption; often identified in schools or primary care	MI + SUD treatment; BD screening; family engagement; SDOH and school interventions	Prevent conversion to full mood disorder and reduce substance-related harms
C. Fully co-occurring BD + SUD	Diagnosed BD + sustained SUD; high functional impairment; increased suicide risk and hospitalizations	Concurrent BD + SUD treatment; family-focused therapy; contingency management; medication + CBT/MET/DBT-SUD combinations; care coordination	Reduce relapse in both disorders and improve functional recovery
D. Crisis/safety pathway	Acute suicidality; intoxication/withdrawal; severe mania/mixed states	ED/inpatient stabilization; withdrawal management; lethal-means counseling; structured discharge + step-down	Stabilize acute risk and prevent recurrent ED/inpatient cycling
E. Transition to adult systems	Persistent BD + SUD into late adolescence; discontinuity between pediatric and adult services	Transition planning (ages 16–18); bridge visits; warm handoffs; navigation; legal/autonomy considerations	Minimize discontinuity during the high-risk transition period

Abbreviations: DBT, dialectic behavioral therapy; ED, emergency department; MI, motivational interviewing.

on average, and individual presentations may vary considerably, underscoring the importance of individualized assessment.

Transgender and gender-diverse adolescents often experience elevated rates of mood concerns, substance use, and trauma exposure, as well as barriers to care, frequently related to minority stress and limited access to affirming services.[60] Missed or delayed diagnosis can occur when youth avoid clinical settings due to anticipated stigma or when providers lack experience with gender-affirming care,

Table 3
Application of ASAM criteria for level-of care decisions

ASAM Dimension	Core Focus	Clinical Considerations in Adolescents with BD	Implications for Level-of-Care Decisions
Dimension 1: Acute intoxication and/or withdrawal potential	Risk of acute substance effects or withdrawal	Withdrawal syndromes are less common in adolescents, but intoxication may exacerbate mood instability, impulsivity, or suicidality	Acute risk may necessitate brief medical stabilization, but does not alone determine long-term level of care
Dimension 2: Biomedical conditions and complications	Co-occurring medical conditions	Consider medication effects (eg, lithium monitoring and antipsychotic metabolic risk), sleep disruption, and substance-related medical issues	Requires coordination with medical providers; rarely primary driver of residential placement
Dimension 3: Emotional, behavioral, or cognitive conditions	Psychiatric comorbidity	BD symptoms (mania, depression, suicidality, and psychosis) may drive risk independent of substance use severity	Mood instability and suicide risk may justify higher intensity psychiatric services even when SUD severity is moderate
Dimension 4: Readiness to change	Motivation and engagement	Adolescents may have limited insight; readiness often fluctuates with mood state and family dynamics	Motivational approaches (MI) are indicated; low readiness alone should not exclude outpatient care
Dimension 5: Relapse, continued use, or continued problem potential	Risk of ongoing substance use	Mood episodes, peer influences, and poor impulse control increase relapse risk	Supports need for integrated relapse prevention within mental health treatment
Dimension 6: Recovery/living environment	Family, school, and community supports	Family conflict, trauma exposure, and school disruption are common; caregiver involvement is critical	Strong rationale for family-based and community-based interventions (eg, MDFT and multisystemic therapy) over isolated residential SUD care

resulting in crisis-driven help-seeking and fragmented treatment access. These disparities parallel patterns observed among racial and ethnic minority youth, who also face structural and cultural barriers that reduce access to specialty care and contribute to higher unmet need.[61] Taken together, these patterns highlight the importance of integrated and affirming care models that combine psychiatric treatment with reproductive health counseling, family support, and identity-affirming services and move toward a precision approach aligned with developmental context, identity, and clinical risk.

CLINICS CARE POINTS

- *Screen early and repeatedly:* Use validated tools (eg, CRAFFT) at initial and follow-up visits.
- *Diagnose longitudinally:* Reassess over time and across settings; evaluate persistence of symptoms during *periods of abstinence* and incorporate collateral information (caregivers, school).
- *Timing and reassessment:* Observe across *multiple time points* (eg, early follow-up and postabstinence); no single duration defines diagnosis—clinical patterns over time are key.
- *Stabilize mood:* Initiate evidence-based treatment for bipolar disorder even with ongoing substance use; do not delay stabilization.
- *Treat concurrently:* Use integrated approaches to address both bipolar disorder and substance use together.
- *Level of care:* Apply and revisit ASAM Criteria, prioritizing safety and reassessing as clinical status evolves.
- *Engage families and evidence-based care:* Incorporate family involvement and use developmentally appropriate psychosocial treatments.
- *Monitor risk:* Continuously assess suicide risk and adjust care accordingly.
- *Coordinate across systems and plan for transitions:* Collaborate with primary care, schools, juvenile legal, and community services, particularly during key transitions (eg, school changes or aging out of pediatric care), which are periods of heightened risk.

Together, these considerations underscore that effective care for adolescents with co-occurring bipolar disorder and substance use disorders must be developmentally grounded, family-centered, and guided by structured level-of-care framework.

ACKNOWLEDGMENTS

This work was supported by the Susbatnce Use and Mental Health Administration (SAMHSA) under grant #5H79TI1087349 PI Lisa Fortuna. The content is the sole responsibility of the authors and does not represent the views of SAMHSA and the U.S. Department of Health and Human Services.

DISCLOSURE

None of the authors report any commercial or financial relationships that can be construed as potential conflicts of interest related to the subject or content of this article.

REFERENCES

1. Cerullo MA, Strakowski SM. The prevalence and significance of substance use disorders in bipolar type I and II disorder. Subst Abuse Treat Prev Pol 2007;2:29.

2. Grant BF, Stinson FS, Hasin DS, et al. Prevalence, correlates, and comorbidity of bipolar I disorder and axis I and II disorders: results from the National Epidemiologic Survey on Alcohol and Related Conditions. J Clin Psychiatry 2005;66(10): 1205–15.
3. Goldstein BI, Strober MA, Birmaher B, et al. Substance use disorders among adolescents with bipolar spectrum disorders. Bipolar Disord 2008;10(4):469–78.
4. Wilens TE, Biederman J, Kwon A, et al. Risk of substance use disorders in adolescents with bipolar disorder. J Am Acad Child Adolesc Psychiatry 2004;43(11): 1380–6.
5. Casey BJ, Jones RM, Hare TA. The adolescent brain. Ann N Y Acad Sci 2008; 1124:111–26.
6. Levine A, Clemenza K, Rynn M, et al. Evidence for the risks and consequences of adolescent cannabis exposure. J Am Acad Child Adolesc Psychiatry 2017;56(3): 214–25.
7. Lev-Ran S, Roerecke M, Le Foll B, et al. The association between cannabis use and depression: a systematic review and meta-analysis of longitudinal studies. Psychol Med 2014;44(4):797–810.
8. Wong JJ, Jones N, Timko C, et al. Exclusion criteria and generalizability in bipolar disorder treatment trials. Contemp Clin Trials Commun 2018;9:130–4.
9. McClellan J, Kowatch R, Findling RL, et al. Practice parameter for the assessment and treatment of children and adolescents with bipolar disorder. J Am Acad Child Adolesc Psychiatry 2007;46(1):107–25.
10. Van Meter A, Moreira ALR, Youngstrom E. Updated meta-analysis of epidemiologic studies of pediatric bipolar disorder. J Clin Psychiatry 2019;80(3). https://doi.org/10.4088/JCP.18r12180.
11. Goldstein BI, Levitt AJ. The specific burden of comorbid anxiety disorders and of substance use disorders in bipolar I disorder. Bipolar Disord 2008;10(1):67–78.
12. Cardoso TA, Jansen K, Zeni CP, et al. Clinical outcomes in children and adolescents with bipolar disorder and substance use disorder comorbidity. J Clin Psychiatry 2017;78(3):e230–3.
13. Carrà G, Bartoli F, Crocamo C, et al. Attempted suicide in people with co-occurring bipolar and substance use disorders: systematic review and meta-analysis. J Affect Disord 2014;167:125–35.
14. Stahl EA, Breen G, Forstner AJ, et al. Genome-wide association study identifies 30 loci associated with bipolar disorder. Nat Genet 2019;51(5):793–803.
15. Hatoum AS, Colbert SMC, Johnson EC, et al. Multivariate genome-wide association meta-analysis of over 1 million subjects identifies loci underlying multiple substance use disorders. Nat Ment Health 2023;1(3):210–23.
16. Arban R, Maraia G, Brackenborough K, et al. Evaluation of the effects of lamotrigine, valproate and carbamazepine in a rodent model of mania. Behav Brain Res 2005;158(1):123–32.
17. Koob GF, Volkow ND. Neurobiology of addiction: a neurocircuitry analysis. Lancet Psychiatry 2016;3(8):760–73.
18. Logan RW, McClung CA. Animal models of bipolar mania: the past, present and future. Neuroscience 2016;321:163–88.
19. Mertens J, Wang QW, Kim Y, et al. Differential responses to lithium in hyperexcitable neurons from patients with bipolar disorder. Nature 2015;527(7576):95–9.
20. Favre P, Pauling M, Stout J, et al. Widespread white matter microstructural abnormalities in bipolar disorder: evidence from mega- and meta-analyses across 3033 individuals. Neuropsychopharmacology 2019;44(13):2285–93.

21. Hibar DP, Westlye LT, van Erp TG, et al. Subcortical volumetric abnormalities in bipolar disorder. Mol Psychiatr 2016;21(12):1710–6.
22. Leibenluft E, Charney DS, Towbin KE, et al. Defining clinical phenotypes of juvenile mania. Am J Psychiatry 2003;160(3):430–7.
23. Felitti VJ, Anda RF, Nordenberg D, et al. Relationship of childhood abuse and household dysfunction to many of the leading causes of death in adults. The adverse childhood experiences (ACE) study. Am J Prev Med 1998;14(4):245–58.
24. Danielyan A, Patino LR, Benanzer T, et al. Cognitive, family, and quality-of-life characteristics of youth with depression associated with bipolar disorder. J Child Adolesc Psychopharmacol 2023;33(6):225–31.
25. Shalev A, Merranko J, Gill MK, et al. Longitudinal course and risk factors associated with psychosis in bipolar youths. Bipolar Disord 2020;22(2):139–54.
26. Schaefer JD, Nelson KM, Wilson S. The effects of adolescent cannabis use on psychosocial functioning: a critical review of the evidence. Psychiatr Clin 2023; 46(4):677–89.
27. Geller B, Zimerman B, Williams M, et al. Bipolar disorder at prospective follow-up of adults who had prepubertal major depressive disorder. Am J Psychiatry 2001; 158(1):125–7.
28. Miguez M, Weber B, Debbané M, et al. Screening for bipolar disorder in adolescents with the mood disorder questionnaire-adolescent version (MDQ-A) and the child bipolar questionnaire (CBQ). Early Interv Psychiatry 2013;7(3):270–7.
29. Kaufman J, Birmaher B, Brent D, et al. Schedule for affective disorders and schizophrenia for school-age children-present and lifetime version (K-SADS-PL): initial reliability and validity data. J Am Acad Child Adolesc Psychiatry 1997;36(7):980–8.
30. De Los Reyes A, Kazdin AE. Informant discrepancies in the assessment of childhood psychopathology: a critical review, theoretical framework, and recommendations for further study. Psychol Bull 2005;131(4):483–509.
31. Hadland SE, Levy S. Objective testing: urine and other drug tests. Child Adolesc Psychiatr Clin N Am 2016;25(3):549–65.
32. Kelly TM, Daley DC. Integrated treatment of substance use and psychiatric disorders. Soc Work Publ Health 2013;28(3–4):388–406.
33. Alloy LB, Urošević S, Abramson LY, et al. Progression along the bipolar spectrum: a longitudinal study of predictors of conversion from bipolar spectrum conditions to bipolar I and II disorders. J Abnorm Psychol 2012;121(1):16–27.
34. Hafeman DM, Merranko J, Axelson D, et al. Toward the definition of a bipolar prodrome: dimensional predictors of bipolar spectrum disorders in at-risk youths. Am J Psychiatry 2016;173(7):695–704.
35. Miklowitz DJ, Chang KD. Prevention of bipolar disorder in at-risk children: theoretical assumptions and empirical foundations. Dev Psychopathol 2008;20(3): 881–97. Summer.
36. Fazel M, Hoagwood K, Stephan S, et al. Mental health interventions in schools 1: mental health interventions in schools in high-income countries. Lancet Psychiatry 2014;1(5):377–87.
37. Humeniuk R, Ali R, Babor TF, et al. Validation of the alcohol, smoking and substance involvement screening test (ASSIST). Addiction 2008;103(6):1039–47.
38. Knight JR, Sherritt L, Shrier LA, et al. Validity of the CRAFFT substance abuse screening test among adolescent clinic patients. Arch Pediatr Adolesc Med 2002;156(6):607–14.
39. Goldstein BI, Goldstein TR, Collinger KA, et al. Treatment development and feasibility study of family-focused treatment for adolescents with bipolar disorder and comorbid substance use disorders. J Psychiatr Pract 2014;20(3):237–48.

40. Wozniak J, O'Connor H, Iorini M, et al. Pediatric bipolar disorder: challenges in diagnosis and treatment. Paediatr Drugs 2025;27(2):125–42.
41. Hafeman DM, Rooks B, Merranko J, et al. Lithium versus other mood-stabilizing medications in a longitudinal study of youth diagnosed with bipolar disorder. J Am Acad Child Adolesc Psychiatry 2020;59(10):1146–55.
42. Geller B, Cooper TB, Sun K, et al. Double-blind and placebo-controlled study of lithium for adolescent bipolar disorders with secondary substance dependency. J Am Acad Child Adolesc Psychiatry 1998;37(2):171–8.
43. Tomson T, Battino D, Perucca E. Teratogenicity of antiepileptic drugs. Curr Opin Neurol 2019;32(2):246–52.
44. National Institute for Health and Care Excellence (NICE). Bipolar disorder: assessment and management: clinical guideline CG185. 2014. Available at: https://www.nice.org.uk/guidance/cg185.
45. Dennis M, Godley SH, Diamond G, et al. The cannabis youth treatment (CYT) study: main findings from two randomized trials. J Subst Abuse Treat 2004;27(3):197–213.
46. Liddle HA, Dakof GA, Turner RM, et al. Treating adolescent drug abuse: a randomized trial comparing multidimensional family therapy and cognitive behavior therapy. Addiction 2008;103(10):1660–70.
47. Liddle HA, Dakof GA, Rowe CL, et al. Multidimensional family therapy as a community-based alternative to residential treatment for adolescents with substance use and co-occurring mental health disorders. J Subst Abuse Treat 2018;90:47–56.
48. Multisystemic therapy for antisocial behavior in children and adolescents, 2nd ed. New York, NY, US.
49. van der Stouwe T, Asscher JJ, Stams GJ, et al. The effectiveness of multisystemic therapy (MST): a meta-analysis. Clin Psychol Rev 2014;34(6):468–81.
50. Miklowitz DJ, Chung B. Family-focused therapy for bipolar disorder: reflections on 30 years of research. Fam Process 2016;55(3):483–99.
51. Goldstein TR, Merranko J, Krantz M, et al. Early intervention for adolescents at-risk for bipolar disorder: a pilot randomized trial of Interpersonal and Social Rhythm Therapy (IPSRT). J Affect Disord 2018;235:348–56.
52. Hlastala SA, Kotler JS, McClellan JM, et al. Interpersonal and social rhythm therapy for adolescents with bipolar disorder: treatment development and results from an open trial. Depress Anxiety 2010;27(5):457–64.
53. Carini-Graves F. Treatment of youth with bipolar disorder and substance use: the youth ACT care model and self determination theory. Journal of Mental Health & Clinical Psychology 2025;9(2):12–7.
54. Sesso G, Brancati GE, Masi G. Comorbidities in youth with bipolar disorder: clinical features and pharmacological management. Curr Neuropharmacol 2023;21(4):911–34.
55. Merikangas KR, Herrell R, Swendsen J, et al. Specificity of bipolar spectrum conditions in the comorbidity of mood and substance use disorders: results from the Zurich cohort study. Arch Gen Psychiatry 2008;65(1):47–52.
56. Bonner-Reid FT, Dar A, Zerin A, et al. Comprehensive review on association of bipolar disorder and substance abuse: dual diagnosis and treatment approaches. Cureus 2025;17(6):e86363. https://doi.org/10.7759/cureus.86363.
57. American Society of Addiction Medicine. The ASAM criteria®: treatment criteria for addictive, substance-related, and Co-Occurring conditions. 4th ed. American Society of Addiction Medicine; 2023.

58. Singh SP, Paul M, Ford T, et al. Process, outcome and experience of transition from child to adult mental healthcare: multiperspective study. Br J Psychiatry 2010;197(4):305–12.
59. Keyes KM, Platt JM. Annual research review: sex, gender, and internalizing conditions among adolescents in the 21st century - trends, causes, consequences. JCPP (J Child Psychol Psychiatry) 2024;65(4):384–407.
60. Toomey RB, Syvertsen AK, Shramko M. Transgender adolescent suicide behavior. Pediatrics 2018;142(4). https://doi.org/10.1542/peds.2017-4218.
61. Hoffmann JA, Alegría M, Alvarez K, et al. Disparities in pediatric mental and behavioral health conditions. Pediatrics 2022;(4):150. https://doi.org/10.1542/peds.2022-058227.

Gambling and Gaming Disorders, Problematic Pornography Use, and Other Addictive Behaviors (Use of Social Media and Artificial Intelligence Chatbots) in Youth

Jennifer J. Park, PhD[a], Marc N. Potenza, MD, PhD[b,c,d,e,f,*]

KEYWORDS

• Gaming disorder • Gambling disorder • Problematic pornography use
• Problematic use of social media • Problematic use of AI chatbots • Diagnosis
• Treatment • Youth

KEY POINTS

- Diagnosis and screening practices may benefit from greater attention to functional impairment and harm in youth. High engagement does not necessarily indicate a disorder.
- Behavioral addictions require assessment beyond symptom counts alone. Subthreshold problems may still be clinically meaningful and warrant support depending on severity, distress, and impairment.
- Emerging problematic online behaviors require nuanced clinical considerations (eg, moral incongruence for problematic pornography use and maladaptive reassurance-seeking for problematic AI chatbot use).
- CBT appears to be the most frequently studied and supported psychotherapeutic approach, and its effectiveness for youth may be strengthened through developmentally tailored adaptations.
- Treatment models should be flexible, accessible, and responsive to severity and need. Online interventions may reduce treatment barriers, but sustained participation would require engagement strategies.

[a] Department of Psychiatry, Yale University School of Medicine, New Haven, CT, USA; [b] Child Study Center, Yale University School of Medicine, New Haven, CT, USA; [c] Department of Neuroscience, Yale University School of Medicine, New Haven, CT, USA; [d] Connecticut Council on Problem Gambling, Wethersfield, CT, USA; [e] Connecticut Mental Health Center, New Haven, CT, USA; [f] Wu Tsai Institute, Yale University, New Haven, CT, USA
* Corresponding author. Wu Tsai Institute, Yale University, New Haven, CT.
E-mail address: marc.potenza@yale.edu

Child Adolesc Psychiatric Clin N Am 35 (2026) 797–811
https://doi.org/10.1016/j.chc.2026.06.001 **childpsych.theclinics.com**

Abbreviations	
ADHD	attention deficit hyperactivity disorder
AI	artificial intelligence
CSBD	compulsive sexual behavior disorder
DSM-5	*Diagnostic and Statistical Manual of Mental Disorders*, fifth edition
ICD-11	11th revision of the *International Classification of Diseases*

INTRODUCTION

In recent decades, the concept of "addiction" has undergone a meaningful and necessary expansion. Once confined to substance use, addiction now encompasses nonsubstance-related behaviors, including gaming/gambling disorders and emerging problematic online behaviors, such as problematic use of pornography, social media, and artificial intelligence (AI) chatbots. Most addictive behaviors occur in digital environments that are highly accessible and appealing to youth, who are in a critical period of development during which emotion-regulation, inhibitory control, and reward sensitivity are still maturing.[1–3] This may partially explain why behavioral addictions appear to disproportionately impact youth, who may require greater clinical attention in screening and treatment.[4–10] In youth, addictive behaviors have been frequently associated with impaired academic and social functioning, sleep difficulties, substance use (including excessive energy drink consumption), and other co-occurring psychiatric concerns (eg, attention deficit hyperactivity disorder [ADHD], depression, and anxiety), which further highlights the need for effective and developmentally responsive interventions in this vulnerable population.[11–16] This clinical complexity has raised questions regarding the order of treatment provision (ie, whether clinicians should prioritize the addictive behavior, the co-occurring psychiatric condition, or both concurrently). Although the evidence base is limited, a concurrent/integrated approach may be recommended, with early attention to co-occurring concerns (eg, ADHD) that may impede treatment engagement.[17] At the same time, it is important to recognize that behavioral addictions are distinct clinical conditions that can arise independently, rather than as manifestations or consequences of other disorders.[18,19]

Although youth behavioral addictions are evolving rapidly (eg, the relatively recent emergence of problematic use of social media and AI chatbots), diagnostic frameworks and treatment studies remain comparatively underdeveloped.[17,20] Although gambling and gaming disorders are formally recognized in diagnostic nomenclature and studied more extensively than emerging addictive behaviors, there remain limitations with diagnostic tools and gaps in knowledge regarding evidence-based treatment that should be addressed to improve the well-being of youth. The present review synthesizes current evidence on diagnosis, screening, and treatment of addictive behaviors in youth, including gaming/gambling disorders and problematic use of pornography, social media, and AI chatbots. The review also explicitly discusses gaps in evidence and provides specific recommendations for future research and clinical practice regarding diagnosis, screening, and treatment. To note, this article focuses on youth aged 10 to 24 years, consistent with United Nations guidance. Given the relatively wide age range of youth, clinicians should consider that behavioral addictions may present differently across preadolescence, adolescence, and emerging adulthood. Currently, the treatment literature for behavioral addictions in youth does not appear sufficiently developed to support robust age-stratified recommendations,[17] but screening and treatment planning in clinical contexts should be developmentally calibrated and consider parental involvement, school-based support systems, and considerations around consent.

OVERVIEW AND DISCUSSION

Clinical Characteristics and Important Considerations for Diagnosis/Screening

Gaming disorder, gambling disorder, and problematic pornography use

Gambling disorder and gaming disorder are currently the only behavioral addictions explicitly recognized in the 11th revision of the *International Classification of Diseases* (ICD-11).[21] Although compulsive sexual behavior disorder (CSBD) is not classified as a behavioral addiction in the ICD-11, the addictive behavior of problematic pornography use may be clinically represented within, and fall under, the CSBD diagnosis (as reflected under the "Additional Clinical Features" section). In the ICD-11, gambling and gaming disorders are characterized by the following core triad of symptoms, which are typically evident over at least 12 months prior to diagnosis, although this duration may be shorter when symptoms are severe and clinical judgment supports diagnosis: (1) impaired control over gambling/gaming, (2) prioritization of gambling/gaming over other activities and interests in life, and (3) continuation or escalation of gambling/gaming despite negative consequences; there must also be impairments to social, family, academic, occupational, and other life domains or severe psychological distress.[21] For gaming disorder, experts have identified gaming-related health consequences (eg, sleep deprivation, wrist pain, and significant weight changes related to eating irregularities and sedentary behaviors) as a potential additional indicator with diagnostic validity, which may be considered in clinical contexts.[22] Furthermore, although gaming duration is frequently discussed in research/clinical practice and may indicate the extent to which gaming occupies a young person's daily life, it is important to recognize that it may have limited diagnostic value on its own.[23] High gaming engagement does not necessarily indicate problematic use and thus should be interpreted alongside gaming-related harms and other contextual factors among youth.[23]

The diagnostic features of CSBD overlap with those of gambling and gaming disorders, while also introducing distinct nuances (eg, continuation of repetitive sexual activities despite *little or no satisfaction*) and an additional core symptom (ie, numerous unsuccessful attempts to significantly reduce the behavior, which is presented as an "additional clinical feature" for gambling and gaming disorders). Notably, CSBD is distinguished by an important diagnostic caveat, where distress arising solely from moral disapproval of sexual urges or behaviors is described as insufficient for diagnosis. This distinction may be clinically and conceptually meaningful, particularly for pornography-related concerns, where self-perceived problematic use may reflect moral incongruence (ie, misalignment between moral beliefs and behaviors) rather than a behavioral dysregulation or addiction.[24,25] Moral incongruence has also been reported to play a statistically significant moderating role in the relationship between frequency of pornography use and problematic pornography use or self-perceived pornography addiction,[26] suggesting the importance of considering this factor when screening youth.

For context, gambling disorder is formally recognized in the *Diagnostic and Statistical Manual of Mental Disorders*, fifth edition (DSM-5), and remains the only clinical condition listed under the "Non-Substance-Related Disorders" section. By contrast, Internet gaming disorder is placed in the "Condition for Further Study" section, while problematic pornography use, problematic use of social media, and other emerging addictive behaviors (eg, problematic use of AI chatbots) are not formally recognized in the DSM-5. In this section, we have focused on the ICD-11 diagnostic criteria rather than the DSM-5, considering recent expert-consensus study suggesting that the ICD-11 criteria for gaming disorder may be better positioned to distinguish a clinically significant disorder from characteristics of normative or intensive gaming engagement.[22] Several DSM-5 criteria for Internet gaming disorder (eg, tolerance, deceiving others about gaming, and gaming to escape negative mood) have been discussed to potentially have limited clinical relevance or risk pathologizing nonproblematic gaming.[22] This aligns with research with youth and young adults, which reported that escape and deception had poor diagnostic accuracy, while continuation of gaming despite problems and negative consequences due to gaming showed superior diagnostic accuracy.[27] Additionally, escapism and preoccupation were the most frequently endorsed DSM-5 Internet gaming disorder criteria by middle school students, but the criteria that contributed most strongly to a diagnosis were continued gaming despite problems, loss of interest in other hobbies due to gaming, and negative consequences.[28] Given debates regarding the equal weighting of the 9 DSM-5 items,[29] clinicians who wish to use the DSM-5 to screen youth for Internet gaming disorder may place greater emphasis on these more diagnostically informative symptoms, which appear to largely overlap with the ICD-11 criteria. Similar concerns have been raised in the field of gambling disorder regarding the 9 DSM-5 items.[29] For example, a study suggested that weighting more severe criteria may improve diagnostic accuracy, with chasing losses and preoccupation being the least severe, and relying on others for financial assistance due to situations caused by gambling, jeopardizing or losing relationships and opportunities, and withdrawal (ie, feeling irritable or restless when reducing or stopping gambling) showing the greatest severity and discriminatory power.[30] A summary of relevant "clinical pearls" has been provided in **Table 1**.

Another important consideration is that the support for gaming/gambling-related problems should not be restricted to individuals who meet formal diagnostic thresholds. Although existing treatment approaches typically target more severe presentations, evidence that many treatment-seeking individuals do not meet diagnostic criteria suggests gaming/gambling-related harms occur along a broader continuum,

Table 1
If you only have time for a few questions: *Diagnostic and Statistical Manual of Mental Disorders*, fifth edition and 11th revision of the *International Classification of Diseases* criteria to assess for gaming and gambling disorders

Concern	DSM-5 and ICD-11 Criteria that May Carry More Diagnostic Weight
Gaming disorder	*DSM-5*[a]: • Negative consequences due to gaming • Continuation of gaming despite problems • Loss of interest in other hobbies and entertainment due to gaming *ICD-11:* • Continuation or escalation of gaming despite negative consequences
Gambling disorder	*DSM-5:* • Negative consequences due to gambling • Reliance on others for financial assistance due to situations caused by gambling • Withdrawal (ie, feeling irritable or restless when reducing or stopping gambling) *ICD-11:* • Continuation or escalation of gambling despite negative consequences

[a] Gaming disorder is included in the "Conditions for Further Study" section in the DSM-5.

and that available treatment options should be responsive to this clinical reality.[23,31–34] For example, a study of treatment-seeking individuals from adolescent and adult outpatient psychiatric care and hospital-based gaming units found that only 36% met the gaming disorder (ICD-11) diagnostic criteria and 61% met the internet gaming disorder (DSM-5) criteria.[31] Another study, which was a prepost feasibility trial for a brief online intervention for youth and adults, found that 92% were in the problematic range, inclusive of only 40% who met the cutoff for gaming disorder using a tool based on the DSM-5.[32] Although categorical diagnosis is valuable for helping clinicians and patients understand concerns/symptoms, guide clinical communication, and identify more severe forms of disorder, a public health lens also requires attention to the broader spectrum of gaming-related and gambling-related harm among youth. A stepped-care approach that prioritizes health equity may, therefore, be more responsive and appropriate, where the type, intensity, and modality of treatment can be flexibly matched to the severity, needs, and preferences of each treatment-seeking individual.[34,35] Although this stepped-care approach may depend on the availability of resources and service infrastructure within a given health system, clinicians may consider: (1) providing individuals with subthreshold problematic gaming symptoms with psychoeducation, brief motivational interviewing, and online self-help resources,[36] (2) providing or referring individuals with moderate gaming-disorder severity for cognitive behavioral therapy (CBT),[17] and (3) referring individuals with severe gaming disorder and substantial functional impairment to specialized hospital-based gaming disorder or addiction medicine services.[37]

Problematic use of social media and artificial intelligence chatbots

Problematic use of social media and problematic use of AI chatbots are not officially recognized in diagnostic nomenclature. However, there have been important advancements in the development of valid and reliable screening tools over the last decade. For assessing severity of problematic use of social media in youth, clinicians and researchers may consider the use of the self-reported 6 item Bergen Social Media Addiction Scale[38] or the self-reported 6 item Social Media Addiction Questionnaire (adapted from the Bergen Facebook Addiction Scale).[39] Although there have been some arguments that problematic use of social media should be assessed in a platform-specific manner (given differences in platform design, content, and user motivations),[40,41] the measures listed here primarily capture broader addiction-like features of problematic engagement rather than problems unique to any particular social media platform.

Although problematic use of AI chatbots is a relatively novel field of research, emerging quantitative and qualitative studies have already reported such concerns in youth and adults.[42–45] The self-reported 11 item Generative AI Dependency Scale has been validated in a mixed sample of youth and adults and may be used to assess severity of problematic use of AI chatbots in the context of preoccupation, negative consequences, and withdrawal symptoms.[46] Some items in this measure are more behavior-specific (ie, specific to AI use) than those in screening tools for other addictive behaviors, such as negative consequences (feeling *less confident in one's abilities* without AI) and withdrawal symptoms (feeling *disconnected* when not being able to access AI chatbots).[46] These differences perhaps reflect the uniquely interactive and socially responsive nature of AI chatbots and their capacity to foster anthropomorphism, perceived companionship, and attachment-like or romantic/nonromantic parasocial bonds.[47,48] Although parasocial relationships do occur in pornography and gaming contexts (eg, with video game characters[49] or with pornography actors[50]), AI chatbots may intensify these processes through sycophantic responses and reciprocal, highly personalized, and continuous interaction that is available 24/7 to youth.[16,51]

Addiction-focused screening should not be assumed to capture the full range of clinically relevant AI-chatbot-related risks. As with social media, where problematic/addictive use may coexist with but remain distinct from nonaddiction-related harms (eg, cyberbullying, social comparison, or online sexual exploitation of youth), AI chatbots have also been associated with other various harms (eg, reinforcement of negative thinking and rumination, behaviors influenced by AI misinformation, reduced contact or relationships with people, and romantic/sexualized chatbot engagement among minors).[47,52–54] Thus, clinicians could take a broader approach to screening that not only includes addiction-related questions but also questions about the nature of chatbot interactions, such as (1) What do you talk to the chatbot about? (2) Does the chatbot feel like a friend, partner, or therapist? (3) Have you disclosed things to the chatbot that you have not told anyone else? and (4) What positive and negative experiences have you had from engaging with a chatbot?

Treatment Approaches and Future Directions

Individual and group-based CBT and interventions based on CBT appear to be the most extensively researched intervention type for behavioral addictions in adults, particularly gambling and gaming disorders. The evidence base for CBT in youth with behavioral addictions is steadily developing (eg, a systematic review from 2025 identified 19 interventions based on or delivered in combination with CBT for gaming disorder in youth[17]), with available research suggesting short-term promise in reducing symptoms of gaming disorder,[17,55,56] gambling disorder,[57,58] and problematic use of social media.[59] However, the strength of the current evidence is limited by inconsistent study quality, including lack of randomization, control conditions, and long-term follow-up.[17] Despite these methodological limitations, CBT remains a conceptually strong option for behavioral addictions treatment as it targets the learned and reinforced patterns that maintain dysregulated engagement, including maladaptive cognitions, cue-triggered behavior, limited coping skills, and poor self-efficacy.[60] Several commonly delivered components of CBT[61] also align with treatment needs reported by youth and adults with gaming disorder (eg, enhancement of self-efficacy, goal setting, strategies for urge management, and self-monitoring)[34] as well as opinions on effective change techniques by clinicians with expertise in treating gambling disorder (eg, relapse prevention, goal setting, cognitive restructuring, and problem solving).[62] Additionally, compared with pharmacologic and other psychotherapeutic approaches, CBT offers a skills-based framework that may produce more durable benefits as individuals continue to practice and implement skills, such as cognitive restructuring, emotion regulation, and problem solving, beyond treatment.[63,64] Given some evidence that CBT effects may be weaker in adolescents with behavioral addictions than in adults, researchers and clinicians may pay greater attention to delivering youth-targeted content and further enhancing motivations for change, treatment engagement/adherence, and therapeutic alliance.[55]

Pharmacologic interventions for behavioral addictions have involved opioid receptor antagonists (eg, naltrexone for gambling disorder), selective serotonin reuptake inhibitors (eg, escitalopram for gaming disorder), and other antidepressants (eg, bupropion for individuals with gaming disorder), which have typically been delivered to individuals with co-occurring concerns, such as depression, anxiety, and ADHD in youth.[17,65–67] However, some studies have also examined pharmacologic interventions targeting the behavioral addiction itself among participants without identified co-occurring conditions. Pharmacologic studies in youth are relatively scarce, which may reflect appropriate caution around prescribing during critical developmental periods, particularly given unresolved questions about long-term tolerability and benefits to improving behavioral addiction symptoms.[17] Across the few nonrandomized prepost studies and randomized controlled trials, pharmacologic interventions (including when delivered in combination with psychotherapy or psychoeducation) have shown mixed findings but preliminary promise in short-term reductions in gaming-disorder severity, gaming duration,[17,68–71] and gambling-disorder severity[72] in youth and adults. The current evidence base may be insufficient to directly support clinical recommendations due to the lack of high-quality randomized controlled trials with larger sample sizes and longer term follow-up. However, combined pharmacotherapy and psychotherapy warrants further investigation, given meta-analytic evidence suggesting that this type of polytherapy may produce greater therapeutic responses than either modality alone among youth.[73,74]

If medication is considered in research or clinical contexts, youth-family-provider discussions should include accessible psychoeducation to reduce stigma around behavioral addictions and psychiatric medication,[75,76] trust-building communication with youth,[77] regular monitoring, and shared decision-making that respects the young person's autonomy and preferences.[78] This may be particularly important given youth reports that they want to be included in treatment decisions and feel alienated when clinicians direct communication primarily to parents.[77–79] Although some qualitative studies have examined preferences and experiences of psychological treatment of behavioral addictions,[32,34,80,81] little is known about youth and family attitudes toward medication for these conditions. Conducting this research in the future would be helpful for guiding appropriate youth-family-provider conversations in clinical contexts.

Although studied less frequently, there have been several other promising interventions for youth with behavioral addictions, which span diverse therapeutic approaches and modes of delivery. Such interventions have included mindfulness,[82–84] physical exercise interventions,[85,86] family therapy and family-based eclectic therapy (eg, combining family therapy, solution-focused therapy, and motivational interviewing),[87–89] therapeutic residential camps (typically providing group counseling and outdoor activities),[90,91] attentional bias modification training,[92] response inhibition training,[93] psychoeducation/health education,[94] contingency management,[95] equine-assisted therapy[96] and hypnotic-oriented counseling[97] for gaming disorder, problematic use of social media, and problematic use of smartphones (inclusive of problematic engagement with a variety of activities, including gaming and social media). Many of the listed interventions have the potential to be delivered online in the future. This has been a topic of growing interest in the treatment field, given that individuals with gaming disorder have reported preferences for online support as it reduces barriers to treatment access (eg, time, transport, cost, and stigma), while also offering scalable and potentially cost-effective delivery from a health-systems perspective.[17,34,98,99] Currently, Internet-delivered interventions have been provided in the form of psychoeducation for parents,[100] a brief planning intervention (goal setting, action and coping planning, implementation guidelines, self-monitoring, relapse prevention, and coaching with personalized feedback) for youth and adults with gaming disorder,[17] and a mindfulness-incorporated intervention (goal setting, personalized feedback, mindfulness, and suggestions for behavior change strategies) for youth and adults with problematic use of smartphones, which have all shown promise in reducing symptom severity. As online interventions are easy to access but also easy to discontinue, future clinical and research efforts may prioritize treatment engagement and retention, including through automated or human-delivered weekly check-ins, which have been qualitatively identified as one of the most helpful components of an online intervention for gaming disorder.[32]

Additionally, novel interventions such as noninvasive neuromodulatory approaches have emerged in the behavioral addictions treatment literature, primarily focused on adult populations. Transcranial direct current stimulation and repetitive transcranial magnetic stimulation of the dorsolateral prefrontal cortex have shown preliminary promise in improving self-control, craving regulation, and emotional regulation in individuals with gaming disorder.[101] This warrants further investigation in future large-scale randomized controlled trials targeting youth, as current evidence is based on study samples of 1 to 15 participants with mixed demographics (ie, youth and adults combined).[101] Future neuromodulatory treatment approaches may be further informed by findings from recent neuroimaging studies. For example, recent machine-learning studies using connectome-based predictive modeling reported that increased/decreased functional connectivity between several large-scale networks (ie, sensorimotor, frontoparietal, medial frontal, salience, and default mode networks) may act as neuromarkers of problematic gaming and problematic use of social media severities in youth, and these may represent potential treatment targets or inform individual-level assignment to specific treatments in the future.[102,103] These precision-based individual-level approaches are largely underdeveloped in the behavioral addictions field, but they may be important for advancing early problem detection and personalized interventions.

There are not yet empirically supported interventions for problematic pornography use and problematic AI chatbot use in youth, highlighting a critical gap in the behavioral addictions field as emerging digital behaviors increasingly involve personalized, interactive, and relational forms of engagement. For problematic AI chatbot use, in particular, interventions may need to account for unique engagement characteristics, including emotional reliance, maladaptive reassurance-seeking, which may be reinforced by sycophantic AI responses, perceived companionship or attachment (ie, parasocial relationships), and preferences for chatbot over human engagement.[44,104–107] A valuable first step would be to conduct qualitative studies with youth reporting problematic AI chatbot use to gather lived experience data on problematic engagement characteristics and identify youth-appropriate strategies for reducing or modifying chatbot use, which may inform future interventions.

SUMMARY

Current treatment approaches for behavioral addictions in youth appear to be largely focused on severe problems (eg, individuals diagnosed with Internet gaming disorder based on the DSM-5 criteria) and lack personalization, despite (1) there being individuals with subthreshold yet clinically meaningful problems who are seeking treatment and (2) preferences for tailored, individualized treatment depending on needs and preferences. Although CBT appears to be the most frequently studied and supported approach for behavioral addictions in general, larger randomized controlled trials with longer term follow-up are required to assess effectiveness in youth. Additionally, there is an urgent need to not only expand treatment options but also build a stronger evidence base for each emerging approach, including less-intensive interventions (eg, brief interventions and self-help), more accessible modalities (eg, online interventions), and novel approaches (eg, neuromodulation). Ideally, future health systems for behavioral addictions would allow youth to move flexibly across treatment types, intensities, and modalities according to symptom severity, needs, and preferences.[34]

CLINICS CARE POINTS

- Do not diagnose a behavioral addiction based on duration/frequency of use or high engagement alone. Evidence of significant functional impairment and negative consequences due to the behavior is required.
- When assessing problematic pornography use, ask whether distress is primarily related to functional impairment and impaired control, or whether it reflects conflict with personal, cultural, religious, or family values. The latter (ie, moral incongruence) alone should not be assumed to indicate an addictive behavior.
- When assessing problematic AI chatbot use in youth, pay particular attention to disclosures around perceived companionship, preference for chatbot over human engagement, maladaptive reassurance-seeking, and feelings of being disconnected without chatbot support.
- Offer or refer for CBT when clinically indicated, while adapting treatment to the young person's developmental stage, family context, and co-occurring concerns.
- Currently, pharmacotherapy may be best understood as a potential complement to psychotherapy, given the lack of large-scale randomized controlled trials targeting youth. When medication is considered in clinical/research contexts, involve youth in shared decision-making.
- Match treatment intensity and modality to symptom severity and patient preferences, escalating to specialized or multidisciplinary care when initial strategies (eg, motivational interviewing and CBT) are insufficient.

FUNDING

This study was supported by the Yale Child Study Center Social Media Pilot Research Award.

DISCLOSURE

Dr M.N. Potenza discloses that he has consulted for and advised Neurofinity and Boehringer Ingelheim; been involved in a patent application with Yale University and Novartis; received research support from the Mohegan Sun Casino and the Connecticut Council on Problem Gambling; consulted for or advised legal, nonprofit, health care and gambling entities on issues related to impulse control, Internet use and addictive behaviors; performed grant reviews; edited journals/journal sections; given academic lectures in grand rounds, CME events, and other clinical/scientific venues; and generated books or chapters for publishers of mental health texts. Dr J.J. Park does not report disclosures.

REFERENCES

1. Meredith WJ, Silvers JA. Experience-dependent neurodevelopment of self-regulation in adolescence. Dev Cogn Neurosci 2024;66:101356.
2. Fosco WD, Hawk LW Jr, Colder CR, et al. The development of inhibitory control in adolescence and prospective relations with delinquency. J Adolesc 2019;76:37–47.
3. Geier C, Terwilliger R, Teslovich T, et al. Immaturities in reward processing and its influence on inhibitory control in adolescence. Cerebr Cortex 2010;20(7):1613–29.
4. Kim HS, Son G, Roh E-B, et al. Prevalence of gaming disorder: a meta-analysis. Addict Behav 2022;126:107183.

5. Meng S-Q, Cheng J-L, Li Y-Y, et al. Global prevalence of digital addiction in general population: a systematic review and meta-analysis. Clin Psychol Rev 2022;92:102128.
6. Stevens MW, Dorstyn D, Delfabbro PH, et al. Global prevalence of gaming disorder: a systematic review and meta-analysis. Aust N Z J Psychiatr 2021;55(6):553–68.
7. Cheng C, Lau Y-c, Chan L, et al. Prevalence of social media addiction across 32 nations: meta-analysis with subgroup analysis of classification schemes and cultural values. Addict Behav 2021;117:106845.
8. Giovanelli A, Roundfield KD. Adolescent vulnerability to consumer chatbots—artificial agents and genuine risk. JAMA Netw Open 2025;8(10):e2539028.
9. Calado F, Alexandre J, Griffiths MD. Prevalence of adolescent problem gambling: a systematic review of recent research. J Gambl Stud 2017;33(2):397–424.
10. Efrati Y. Compulsive sexual behavior in adolescents: the roles of personality, attachment orientations, cognitive mechanisms, and psychopathology. Cognit Ther Res 2023;47(3):469–82.
11. Hartmann M, Blaszczynski A. The longitudinal relationships between psychiatric disorders and gambling disorders. Int J Ment Health Addiction 2018;16(1):16–44.
12. Park JJ, Zhao Y, Potenza MN. Gaming disorder and problematic caffeine consumption in adolescents: a narrative review and public health framework. Front Psychol 2025;16:1690304.
13. Park JJ, Han X, Potenza MN, et al. The effect of caffeine use in the relationship between gaming and sleep in adolescents: a mediation analysis. Journal of Behavioral Addictions 2025;14(3):1368–79.
14. Fong TC, Junus A, Wen M, et al. Comorbidity among symptoms of internet gaming disorder, social withdrawal, and depression in 3430 young people in Hong Kong: a network analysis. J Affect Disord 2024;359:319–26.
15. Hassan MR, Mahmud MS, Hasan MK. Social media addiction and its consequences among youth: a developing country perspective. Glob Bus Rev 2024;09721509241276720. https://doi.org/10.1177/09721509241276720.
16. Herbener AB, Damholdt MF. Are lonely youngsters turning to chatbots for companionship? The relationship between chatbot usage and social connectedness in Danish high-school students. Int J Hum Comput Stud 2025;196:103409.
17. Park JJ, Stryjewski A, Chen B, et al. Treatment of gaming disorder in children and adolescents: a systematic review. Journal of the Korean Academy of Child and Adolescent Psychiatry 2025;36(3):106.
18. Pearcy BT, McEvoy PM, Roberts LD. Internet gaming disorder explains unique variance in psychological distress and disability after controlling for comorbid depression, OCD, ADHD, and anxiety. Cyberpsychol, Behav Soc Netw 2017;20(2):126–32.
19. Billieux J, Stein DJ, Castro-Calvo J, et al. Rationale for and usefulness of the inclusion of gaming disorder in the ICD-11. World Psychiatry 2021;20(2):198.
20. King DL, Wölfling K, Potenza MN. Taking gaming disorder treatment to the next level. JAMA Psychiatry 2020;77(8):869–70.
21. World Health Organization. ICD-11: International Classification of diseases (11th revision). 2019.

22. Castro-Calvo J, King DL, Stein DJ, et al. Expert appraisal of criteria for assessing gaming disorder: an international Delphi study. Addiction 2021;116(9): 2463–75.
23. King DL, Billieux J, Behm S, Delfabbro PH. Toward resolving normality-disorder boundary issues in gaming disorder research. J Behav Addict 2025. https://doi.org/10.1556/2006.2024.00081.
24. Grubbs JB, Perry SL. Moral incongruence and pornography use: a critical review and integration. J Sex Res 2019;56(1):29–37.
25. Grubbs JB, Perry SL, Wilt JA, et al. Pornography problems due to moral incongruence: an integrative model with a systematic review and meta-analysis. Arch Sex Behav 2019;48(2):397–415.
26. Bőthe B, Michaud A, Beaulieu V, et al. A global investigation of the Moral Incongruence Model of Pornography Use across genders, religions, and cultures. J Behav Addict 2026. https://doi.org/10.1556/2006.2025.00540.
27. Ko C-H, Yen J-Y, Chen S-H, et al. Evaluation of the diagnostic criteria of internet gaming disorder in the DSM-5 among young adults in Taiwan. J Psychiatr Res 2014;53:103–10.
28. Luo T, Wei D, Guo J, et al. Diagnostic contribution of the DSM-5 criteria for internet gaming disorder. Front Psychiatr 2022;12:777397.
29. American Psychiatric Association. Diagnostic and statistical manual of mental disorders (5th edition). 2013;doi:https://doi.org/10.1176/appi.books.9780890425596.
30. Sleczka P, Braun B, Piontek D, et al. DSM-5 criteria for gambling disorder: underlying structure and applicability to specific groups of gamblers. J Behav Addict 2015;4(4):226–35.
31. Starcevic V, Choi TY, Kim TH, et al. Internet gaming disorder and gaming disorder in the context of seeking and not seeking treatment for video-gaming. J Psychiatr Res 2020;129:31–9.
32. Park JJ, Booth N, Bagot KL, et al. A brief internet-delivered intervention for the reduction of gaming-related harm: a feasibility study. Comput Hum Behav Rep 2020;2:100027.
33. Rodda SN, Merkouris SS, Dowling NA. Current approaches to the identification and management of gambling disorder: a narrative review to inform clinical practice in Australia and New Zealand. Med J Aust 2024;221(9):495–500.
34. Park JJ, Wilkinson-Meyers L, King DL, et al. Person-centred interventions for problem gaming: a stepped care approach. BMC Public Health 2021;21(1):872.
35. Park JJ, King DL, Wilkinson-Meyers L, et al. The practice and feasibility of screening, treatment, and referral for gaming problems in gambling, alcohol and other drugs, and youth services. Int J Ment Health Addiction 2024;22(5): 2633–48.
36. Şahin SS, Ayaz-Alkaya S. The effect of motivational interviewing on internet addiction and digital game addiction in adolescents: a randomized controlled trial. Eur J Pediatr 2026;185(5):336.
37. Han DH, Yoo M, Renshaw PF, et al. A cohort study of patients seeking internet gaming disorder treatment. J Behav Addict 2018;7(4):930–8.
38. Andreassen CS, Pallesen S, Griffiths MD. The relationship between addictive use of social media, narcissism, and self-esteem: findings from a large national survey. Addict Behav 2017;64:287–93.
39. Bagot K, Tomko R, Marshall A, et al. Youth screen use in the ABCD® study. Dev Cogn Neurosci 2022;57:101150.

40. Cataldo I, Billieux J, Esposito G, et al. Assessing problematic use of social media: where do we stand and what can be improved? Curr Opin Behav Sci 2022;45:101145.
41. Brand M, Antons S, Bőthe B, et al. Current advances in behavioral addictions: from fundamental research to clinical practice. Am J Psychiatr 2025;182(2):155–63.
42. Al-Obaydi LH, Pikhart M. Artificial intelligence addiction: exploring the emerging phenomenon of addiction in the AI age. AI Soc 2026;41(2):1577–93.
43. Huang S, Lai X, Ke L, et al. AI technology panic—is AI dependence bad for mental health? A cross-lagged panel model and the mediating roles of motivations for AI use among adolescents. Psychol Res Behav Manag 2024;1087–102.
44. Cheng M, Lee C, Khadpe P, et al. Sycophantic AI decreases prosocial intentions and promotes dependence. Science 2026;391(6792):eaec8352.
45. Zhang X, Li H, Yin M, et al. Investigating AI chatbot dependence: associations with internet and smartphone dependence, mental health outcomes, and the moderating role of usage purposes. Int J Hum Comput Interact 2026;42(7):5592–604.
46. Goh AY, Hartanto A, Majeed NM. Generative artificial intelligence dependency: scale development, validation, and its motivational, behavioral, and psychological correlates. Comput Hum Behav Rep 2025;20:100845.
47. Dohnány S, Kurth-Nelson Z, Spens E, et al. Technological folie à deux: feedback loops between AI chatbots and mental health. Nature Mental Health 2026;1–10.
48. Xie T, Pentina I, Hancock T. Friend, mentor, lover: does chatbot engagement lead to psychological dependence? J Serv Manag 2023;34(4):806–28.
49. Song W, Fox J. Playing for love in a romantic video game: avatar identification, parasocial relationships, and Chinese women's romantic beliefs. Mass Commun Soc 2016;19(2):197–215.
50. Hesse C, Floyd K. Affection substitution: the effect of pornography consumption on close relationships. J Soc Pers Relat 2019;36(11–12):3887–907.
51. Mayor E. Chatbots and mental health: a scoping review of reviews. Curr Psychol 2025;44(15):13619–40.
52. Folk D, Dunn E. How does turning to AI for companionship predict loneliness and vice versa? Psychol Sci 2026;37(4):276–86.
53. Khandpur A. A study on the relational use of artificial intelligence, psychological well-being, and rumination among young adults. International Journal of Interdisciplinary Approaches in Psychology 2025;3(10):77–89.
54. Tandar CE, Bajaj SS, Stanford FC. Social media and artificial intelligence—Understanding medical misinformation through Snapchat's new artificial intelligence chatbot. Mayo Clin Proc: Digit Health 2024;2(2):252–4.
55. Stevens MW, King DL, Dorstyn D, et al. Cognitive–behavioral therapy for internet gaming disorder: a systematic review and meta-analysis. Clin Psychol Psychother 2019;26(2):191–203.
56. Ji Y, Wong DFK. Effectiveness of an integrated motivational cognitive–behavioral group intervention for adolescents with gaming disorder: a randomized controlled trial. Addiction 2023;118(11):2093–104.
57. Larimer ME, Neighbors C, Lostutter TW, et al. Brief motivational feedback and cognitive behavioral interventions for prevention of disordered gambling: a randomized clinical trial. Addiction 2012;107(6):1148–58.
58. Ladouceur R, Boisvert J-M, Dumont J. Cognitive-behavioral treatment for adolescent pathological gamblers. Behav Modif 1994;18(2):230–42.

59. Zhou X, Rau P-LP, Yang C-L, et al. Cognitive behavioral therapy-based short-term abstinence intervention for problematic social media use: improved well-being and underlying mechanisms. Psychiatr Q 2021;92(2):761–79.
60. Bre'Anna L, Smith EH, Ginley MK, et al. Does cognitive-behavioral treatment affect putative mechanisms of change among individuals with problem gambling? A systematic review and exploratory meta-analysis. Addict Behav 2024;158:108110.
61. Radunz M, Stevens MW, Behm S, et al. Common practice elements of cognitive behavioral therapy for gaming disorder: a systematic review and expert panel evaluation. Clin Psychol Rev 2026;126:102740.
62. Keshani IM, Merkouris SS, Guyett A, et al. Clinical consensus statements on change techniques for gambling treatment: a Delphi study with clinicians. Journal of Behavioral Addictions 2025;14(1):430–44.
63. Carroll KM, Rounsaville BJ, Nich C, et al. One-year follow-up of psychotherapy and pharmacotherapy for cocaine dependence: delayed emergence of psychotherapy effects. Arch Gen Psychiatry 1994;51(12):989–97.
64. Carroll KM, Ball SA, Martino S, et al. Enduring effects of a computer-assisted training program for cognitive behavioral therapy: a 6-month follow-up of CBT4CBT. Drug Alcohol Depend 2009;100(1–2):178–81.
65. Lin C, Yeh W-C, Yen J-Y, et al. Can pharmacological interventions have therapeutic effects on internet gaming disorder: a systemic review and meta-analysis. Current Addiction Reports 2025;12(1):32.
66. de Sá RRC, Coelho S, Parmar PK, et al. A systematic review of pharmacological treatments for internet gaming disorder. Psychiatry Investig 2023;20(8):696.
67. Potenza MN, Balodis IM, Derevensky J, et al. Gambling disorder. Nat Rev Dis Primers 2019;5(1):51.
68. Han DH, Hwang JW, Renshaw PF. Bupropion sustained release treatment decreases craving for video games and cue-induced brain activity in patients with internet video game addiction. Exp Clin Psychopharmacol 2010;18(4):297.
69. Han DH, Renshaw PF. Bupropion in the treatment of problematic online game play in patients with major depressive disorder. J Psychopharmacol 2012;26(5):689–96.
70. Kim SM, Han DH, Lee YS, et al. Combined cognitive behavioral therapy and bupropion for the treatment of problematic on-line game play in adolescents with major depressive disorder. Comput Hum Behav 2012;28(5):1954–9.
71. Lim J-A, Lee J-Y, Jung HY, et al. Changes of quality of life and cognitive function in individuals with internet gaming disorder: a 6-month follow-up. Medicine 2016;95(50):e5695.
72. Ghenoiu I, Alexandru I, Manolache R, et al. Therapeutic management of young patients diagnosed with online gambling disorder. Neuroscience Applied 2022;1:100087.
73. Wang X, Zhang Y, Lin J, et al. Treatments of internet gaming disorder and comorbid mental disorders: a systematic review and meta-analysis. Comput Hum Behav 2023;149:107947.
74. Chang C-H, Chang Y-C, Yang L, et al. The comparative efficacy of treatments for children and young adults with internet addiction/internet gaming disorder: an updated meta-analysis. Int J Environ Res Publ Health 2022;19(5):2612.
75. Pescosolido BA, Perry BL, Martin JK, et al. Stigmatizing attitudes and beliefs about treatment and psychiatric medications for children with mental illness. Psychiatr Serv 2007;58(5):613–8.

76. Galanis C, Leske M, Hamamura T, et al. Stigma in substance-based and behavioural addictions: a systematic review. J Behav Addict 2025;14(1):79–99.
77. Dogra N. What do children and young people want from mental health services? Curr Opin Psychiatr 2005;18(4):370–3.
78. O'Brien MS, Crickard EL, Rapp CA, et al. Critical issues for psychiatric medication shared decision making with youth and families. Fam Soc 2011;92(3): 310–6.
79. Kelsey J, Abelson-Mitchell N, Skirton H. Perceptions of young people about decision making in the acute healthcare environment. Nurs Child Young People 2007;19(6):14–8.
80. Bore P, Leo J, Garpenhag L, et al. Adolescents' experiences of psychological treatment for gaming disorder: a qualitative study. Front Psychiatr 2025;16: 1601851.
81. Karhulahti V-M, Behm S, Lukka L. Why do adults seek treatment for gaming (disorder)? A qualitative study. Hum Soc Sci Commun 2023;10(1):299.
82. Lan Y, Ding J-E, Li W, et al. A pilot study of a group mindfulness-based cognitive-behavioral intervention for smartphone addiction among university students. J Behav Addict 2018;7(4):1171–6.
83. Liu F, Zhang Z, Liu S, et al. Effectiveness of brief mindfulness intervention for college students' problematic smartphone use: the mediating role of self-control. PLoS One 2022;17(12):e0279621.
84. Chang H, Meng X, Li Y, et al. The effect of mindfulness on social media addiction among Chinese college students: a serial mediation model. Front Psychiatr 2023;14:1087909.
85. Hong JS, Kim SM, Kang KD, et al. Effect of physical exercise intervention on mood and frontal alpha asymmetry in internet gaming disorder. Mental Health and Physical Activity 2020;18:100318.
86. Liu H, Soh KG, Samsudin S, et al. Effects of exercise and psychological interventions on smartphone addiction among university students: a systematic review. Front Psychol 2022;13:1021285.
87. Pallesen S, Lorvik IM, Bu EH, et al. An exploratory study investigating the effects of a treatment manual for video game addiction. Psychol Rep 2015;117(2): 490–5.
88. Han DH, Kim SM, Lee YS, et al. The effect of family therapy on the changes in the severity of on-line game play and brain activity in adolescents with on-line game addiction. Psychiatry Res 2012;202(2):126–31.
89. Nielsen P, Christensen M, Henderson C, et al. Multidimensional family therapy reduces problematic gaming in adolescents: a randomised controlled trial. J Behav Addict 2021;10(2):234–43.
90. Pornnoppadol C, Ratta-apha W, Chanpen S, et al. A comparative study of psychosocial interventions for internet gaming disorder among adolescents aged 13–17 years. Int J Ment Health Addiction 2020;18:932–48.
91. Sakuma H, Mihara S, Nakayama H, et al. Treatment with the self-discovery camp (SDiC) improves internet gaming disorder. Addict Behav 2017;64:357–62.
92. Nasiry S, Noori M. Online attentional bias modification training for adolescents with internet gaming disorder. J Clin Psychol 2022;10(2):79–90.
93. Zheng Y, He J, Fan L, et al. Reduction of symptom after a combined behavioral intervention for reward sensitivity and rash impulsiveness in internet gaming disorder: a comparative study. J Psychiatr Res 2022;153:159–66.

94. Zamanian H, Sharifzadeh G, Moodi M. The effect of planned behavior theory-based education on computer game dependence in high school male students. J Educ Health Promot 2020;9(1):186.
95. Stinson L, Dallery J. Reducing problematic social media use via a package intervention. J Appl Behav Anal 2023;56(2):323–35.
96. Park H, Jung T. The effects of equine-assisted learning on adolescents with internet gaming disorder. Basel, Switzerland: MDPI; 2024. p. 311.
97. Sugara GS, Fadhilah R. Treatment for social media addiction with hypnotic-oriented counseling. Discover Psychology 2024;4(1):13.
98. Andersson G, Titov N. Advantages and limitations of internet-based interventions for common mental disorders. World Psychiatry 2014;13(1):4–11.
99. Park JJ, King DL, Wilkinson-Meyers L, et al. Content and effectiveness of web-based treatments for online behavioral addictions: systematic review. JMIR Ment Health 2022;9(9):e36662.
100. Marshall B, Warburton WA, Kangas M, et al. Internet gaming disorder (IGD) and smartphone addiction: parent intervention trial. Aust J Psychol 2024;76(1): 2396961.
101. Xu L-x, Geng X-m, Zhang J-l, et al. Neuromodulation treatments of problematic use of the internet. Curr Opin Behav Sci 2022;48:101215.
102. Park JJ, Lacadie CM, Scheinost D. e al., Connectome-based predictive modelling of problematic gaming in youth from the ABCD study. J Behav Addict 2026; 15(1):305–19.
103. Park JJ, Lacadie CM, Zhao Y, Potenza MN. Connectome-based prediction of problematic use of social media in adolescents: findings from the ABCD study. Neuroimage 2026;329:121829.
104. Zhai N, Ma X, Ding X. Unpacking AI chatbot dependency: a dual-path model of cognitive and affective mechanisms. Information 2025;16(12):1025.
105. Hu B, Mao Y, Kim KJ. How social anxiety leads to problematic use of conversational AI: the roles of loneliness, rumination, and mind perception. Comput Hum Behav 2023;145:107760.
106. Barkhuff G. Reassurance robots: OCD in the age of generative AI. 2026:1–5.
107. Zhang K, Xie Y, Chen D, et al. Effects of attractions and social attributes on peoples' usage intention and media dependence towards chatbot: the mediating role of parasocial interaction and emotional support. BMC Psychol 2025; 13(1):986.

United States Postal Service

Statement of Ownership, Management and Circulation

(All Periodicals Publications Except Requester Publications)

1. Publication Title CHILD AND ADOLESCENT PSYCHIATRIC CLINICS OF NORTH AMERICA	2. Publication Number 0 1 1 - 3 6 8	3. Filing Date 08/21/2026
4. Issue Frequency JAN, APR, JUL, OCT	5. Number of Issues Published Annually 4	6. Annual Subscription Price $392.00

7. Complete Mailing Address of Known Office of Publication (Not printer) (Street, city, county, state, and ZIP+4)

Addr 1: Elsevier INC
Addr 2: 230 Park Ave Ste 800
City, State ZIP: New York NY 10169

Contact Person: Mohana Priya Damodharan
Telephone: 91-44-4299-4077

8. Complete Mailing Address of Headquarters or General Business Office of Publisher (Not Printer)

Addr 1: Elsevier INC
Addr 2: 230 Park Ave Ste 800
City, State ZIP: New York NY 10169

9. Full Names and Complete Mailing Addresses of Publisher, Editor and Managing Editor (do not leave blank)

Publisher (Name and complete mailing address)
Name: DOLORES MELONI, ELSEVIER INC.
Addr 1: 1600 JOHN F KENNEDY BLVD. SUITE 1600
Addr 2:
City, State ZIP: PHILADELPHIA PA 19103

Editor (Name and complete mailing address)
Name: JOANNA GASCOINE, ELSEVIER INC.
Addr 1: 1600 JOHN F KENNEDY BLVD. SUITE 1600
Addr 2:
City, State ZIP: PHILADELPHIA PA 19103

Managing Editor (Name and complete mailing address)
Name: PATRICK MANLEY, ELSEVIER INC.
Addr 1: 1600 JOHN F KENNEDY BLVD. SUITE 1600
Addr 2:
City, State ZIP: PHILADELPHIA, PA 19103

10. Owner (Do not leave blank. If the publication is owned by a corporation, give the name and address of the corporation immediately followed by the names and addresses of all stockholders owning or holding 1 Percent or more of the total amount of stock. If not owned by a corporation, give the names and addresses of all the individual owners. If owned by a partnership or other unincorporated firm, give it's name and address as well as those of each individual owner. If the publication is published by a nonprofit organization, give it's name and address.)

Full Name	Complete Mailing Address
WHOLLY OWNED SUBSIDIARY OF REED/ELSEVIER, US HOLDINGS	1600 JOHN F KENNEDY BLVD. SUITE 1600 PHILADELPHIA, PA 19103-2899 PHILADELPHIA, PA 19103-2899

11. Known Bondholders, Mortgagees and Other Security Holders Owning or Holding 1 Percent or more of Total Amount of Bonds, Mortgages, or Other Securities. If none, check box → None

Full Name	Complete Mailing Address
NA	

12. Tax Status (For completion by nonprofit organizations authorized to mail at nonprofit rates) (Check one)
The purpose, function, and nonprofit status of this organization and the exempt status for federal income tax purposes:
[X] Has Not changed During Preceding 12 Months
[ ] Has Changed During Preceding 12 Months (Publisher must submit explanation of change with this statement below)

PS Form 3526, July 2014

13. Publication Title	14. Issue Date for Circulation Data Below	
CHILD AND ADOLESCENT PSYCHIATRIC CLINICS OF NORTH AMERICA	October 2026	

15. Extent and Nature of Circulation	Average No. Copies Each Issue During Preceding 12 Months	No. Copies of Single Issue Published Nearest to filing Date
a. Total Number of Copies (Net press run)	102	111
b. Paid and/or Requested Circulation (1) Mailed Outside-County Paid Subscriptions Stated on PS Form 3541 (Include paid distribution above nominal rate, advertiser's proof copies, and exchange copies)	67	73
(2) Mailed In-County Paid Subscriptions Stated on PS Form 3541 (Include paid distribution above nominal rate, advertiser's proof copies, and exchange copies)	0	0
(3) Paid Distribution Outside the Mails Including Sales Through Dealers and Carriers, Street Vendors, Counter Sales ,and Other Paid Distribution Outside USPS	15	17
(4) Paid Distribution by Other Classes of Mail Through the USPS (e.g. First-Class Mail)	17	18
c. Total Paid Distribution [Sum of 15b. (1), (2), (3), and (4)] ▶	99	108
d. Free or Nominal Rate Distribution (By Mail and Outside the Mail) (1) Free or Nominal Rate Outside-County *Copies Included on PS Form 3541*	2	2
(2) Free or Nominal In-County Copies Included on PS Form 3541	0	0
(3) Free or Nominal Rate Copies Mailed at Other Classes Through the USPS (e.g. First-Class Mail)	0	0
(4) Free or Nominal Rate Distribution Outside the Mail *(Carriers or other means)*	1	1
e. Total Free or Nominal Rate Distribution (Sum of 15d. (1), (2), (3) and (4)) ▶	3	3
f. Total Distribution (Sum of 15c. and 15e.) ▶	102	111
g. Copies not Distributed (See Instructions to Publishers #4 (page #3))	0	0
h. Total (Sum of 15f. and g.) ▶	102	111
i. Percent Paid (15c. Divided by 15f. Times 100) ▶	97.06%	97.30%

* if you are claiming electronic copies, go to line 16 on page 3. If you are not claiming electronic copies, skip to line 17 on page 3.

16. Electronic copy Circulation		
If present, check box		
a. Paid Electronic Copies		
b. Total Paid Print Copies (Line 15c) + Paid Electronic Copies (Line 16a) ▶	99	108
c. Total Print Distribution (Line 15F) + Paid Electronic Copies (Line 16a) ▶	102	111
d. Percentage Paid (Both Print & Electronic Copies (16b divided bt 16c x 100) ▶	97.06%	97.30%

[X] I certify that 50% of all my distribution copies (electronic and Print) are paid above a nominal price

17. Publication of Statement of Ownership
[X] Publication required. Will be printed in the **October 2026** issue of this publication. [ ] Publication not required

18. Signature and Title of Editor, Publisher, Business Manager, or Owner	Title	Date
Mohana Priya Damodharan	Distribution Controller	8/21/2026

I certify that all information furnished on this form is true and complete. I understand that anyone who furnishes false or misleading information on this form or who omits material or information requested on the form may be subject to criminal sanctions (including fines and imprisonment) and/or civil sanctions (including civil penalties)

PS Form 3526, July 2014

9780443432828